Fitness Professional's Guide to
Strength Training Older Adults

Second Edition

Thomas R. Baechle, EdD, CSCS, NSCA-CPT
Creighton University
Omaha, NE

Wayne L. Westcott, PhD, CSCS
Quincy College
Quincy, MA

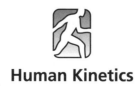

Human Kinetics

Library of Congress Cataloging-in-Publication Data

Baechle, Thomas R., 1943-
  Fitness professional's guide to strength training older adults / Thomas R.
Baechle, Wayne L. Westcott. -- 2nd ed.
    p. cm.
  Rev. ed. of: Strength training for seniors / Wayne L. Westcott, Thomas R.
Baechle. c1999
  Includes bibliographical references and index.
  ISBN-13: 978-0-7360-7581-7 (soft cover)
  ISBN-10: 0-7360-7581-X (soft cover)
  1. Physical fitness for older people. 2. Physical education for older people. 3.
Exercise for older people--
Physiological aspects. 4. Weight training. 5. Muscle strength. I. Westcott,
Wayne L., 1949- II. Westcott, Wayne L.,
1949- Strength training for seniors. III. Title.
  RA781.W42 2010
  613.7'0446--dc22
                              2009054272

ISBN-10: 0-7360-7581-X (print)
ISBN-13: 978-0-7360-7581-7 (print)

This book is a revised edition of *Strength Training for Seniors: An Instructor Guide for Developing Safe and Effective Programs,* published in 1999 by Human Kinetics.

The Web addresses cited in this text were current as of January 4, 2010, unless otherwise noted.

Acquisitions Editors: Michael S. Bahrke, PhD, and Amy N. Tocco; **Developmental Editor:** Judy Park; **Assistant Editors:** Dena P. Mumm and Casey A. Gentis; **Copyeditor:** Bob Replinger; **Indexer:** Bobbi Swanson; **Permission Manager:** Dalene Reeder; **Graphic Designer:** Fred Starbird; **Graphic Artist:** Kathleen Boudreau-Fuoss; **Cover Designer:** Keith Blomberg; **Photographer (cover and interior):** Neil Bernstein; **Photo Asset Manager:** Laura Fitch; **Visual Production Assistant:** Joyce Brumfield; **Photo Production Manager:** Jason Allen; **Art Manager:** Kelly Hendren; **Associate Art Manager:** Alan L. Wilborn; **Illustrator:** Alan L. Wilborn; **Printer:** Sheridan Books

We thank the South Shore YMCA in Quincy, Massachusetts, for assistance in providing the location for the photo shoot for this book.

Printed in the United States of America   10 9 8 7 6 5 4 3 2 1

The paper in this book is certified under a sustainable forestry program.

Human Kinetics
Web site: www.HumanKinetics.com

United States: Human Kinetics
P.O. Box 5076
Champaign, IL 61825-5076
800-747-4457
e-mail: humank@hkusa.com

Canada: Human Kinetics
475 Devonshire Road Unit 100
Windsor, ON N8Y 2L5
800-465-7301 (in Canada only)
e-mail: info@hkcanada.com

Europe: Human Kinetics
107 Bradford Road
Stanningley
Leeds LS28 6AT, United Kingdom
+44 (0) 113 255 5665
e-mail: hk@hkeurope.com

Australia: Human Kinetics
57A Price Avenue
Lower Mitcham, South Australia 5062
08 8372 0999
e-mail: info@hkaustralia.com

New Zealand: Human Kinetics
P.O. Box 80
Torrens Park, South Australia 5062
0800 222 062
e-mail: info@hknewzealand.com

We are honored to dedicate
this book to our wives,
Susan Baechle and Claudia Westcott.

Contents

Chapter 9 Sport-Specific Training.... 247

Chapter 10 Nutrition for Senior Clients 293

Exercise Finder

BALL EXERCISES

BODYWEIGHT EXERCISES

ELASTIC RESISTANCE EXERCISES

Acknowledgments

It is indeed a most reinforcing privilege for us to express our great appreciation to the outstanding individuals who have made it possible and enjoyable to publish this book. First, we acknowledge the invaluable assistance of the most helpful editors at Human Kinetics, especially Michael Bahrke, Judy Park, Dalene Reeder, and Dena Mumm. We are very grateful to our superb photographer, Neil Bernstein, and to our remarkable exercise models, Peggy Leung, Patricia Campbell, James Vranas, and Richard Raymond. We are most thankful for the assistance provided on the nutrition chapter by Debra Wein, MS, RD, and on the special populations chapter by Michelle Streif, as well as for the research support provided by Rita La Rosa Loud. We are especially appreciative for the excellent work produced by our administrative assistants, Susan Stoddard and Susan Thomas. We also gratefully acknowledge the Executive Directors of the South Shore YMCA, Paul Gorman, Ralph Yohe, Mary Moore, Natalie Norton, Mark Free, Kathryn Saunders, and Jen Turner; the President of Quincy College, Martha Sue Harris; the Vice President of Academic Affairs, Patricia Vampatella; and the Chair of Allied Health, Lori Tyszkowski. Finally, we are most thankful for the friendship we share with each other; the support of our wives, Susan Baechle and Claudia Westcott; as well as God's grace in making this writing project an enjoyable and educational endeavor for us.

Introduction

According to the 2007 report on *Physical Activity and Public Health*, copublished by the American College of Sports Medicine (ACSM) and the American Heart Association (AHA), adults and seniors need regular aerobic and strength training exercises to promote and maintain health (Haskell et al. 2007). Unfortunately, most older adults do not perform the minimum amount of physical activity required for health and fitness. Although lack of physical activity is obviously associated with the current obesity epidemic, it is also related to a variety of degenerative conditions including cardiovascular disease, stroke, hypertension, type 2 diabetes, osteoporosis, colon cancer, breast cancer, anxiety, and depression (Kesaniemi et al. 2001).

The good news is that the minimum activity recommendations for older adults from ACSM (2010) are not difficult to achieve. For cardiovascular fitness, the guidelines call for moderate-intensity aerobic activity 5 days a week for a total of at least 150 minutes, or 20 to 25 minutes of vigorous-intensity aerobic activity 3 days each week for a total of 75 minutes, or 20 to 30 minutes of moderate- to vigorous-intensity exercise 3 to 5 days per week. For musculoskeletal fitness the recommendation is 8 to 10 resistance exercises, performed for one set of 10 to 15 repetitions, 2 or 3 days per week. A circuit of 8 to 10 resistance exercises can typically be completed in 15 to 20 minutes.

The time required to exercise on a regular basis, even among time-pressured people, represents a reasonable and doable commitment of time. Although we are strong proponents of aerobic activity, the focus of this book is on designing and directing sensible strength training programs for seniors. Strength training is the foundation on which the strength required in aerobic exercise and everyday tasks can be improved, thus enabling seniors to complete such tasks with less effort. Furthermore, strength training helps to counter the loss of muscle that accompanies the aging process. On average, men and women lose more than 5 pounds (2.3 kg) of muscle tissue each decade between ages 25 and 55, and they experience an even greater rate of muscle loss during their senior years (Forbes 1976; Evans and Rosenberg 1992). Because muscles are the engines of the body, less muscle leads to a lower resting metabolism, which in turn results in fewer calories being burned and more calories being stored as fat. We believe that an important underlying factor in fat gain is muscle loss. With 65 percent of our population classified as overweight (35 percent) or obese (30 percent), participation in strength training should be understood as essential to addressing this problem (Hedley et al. 2004).

Although you may concur that strength training is effective for enhancing muscle development in youth and young adults, you may not be convinced that resistance exercise is a safe activity for seniors. We completed a large-scale study in 2009 with 1,644 men and women

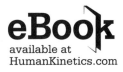

eBook
available at
HumanKinetics.com

who performed one set of 10 resistance exercises, 2 or 3 days a week, for a period of 10 weeks (Westcott 2009). On average, the participants added 3 pounds (1.4 kg) of lean (muscle) weight and lost 4 pounds (1.8 kg) of fat weight and seniors (ages 65 to 80) developed muscle at the same rate as did those in the younger age groups. Be assured that strength training is a highly productive activity for older adults and that the incidence of injury is extremely low. Just as important, seniors find strength training positively reinforcing, and they exhibit excellent exercise compliance. Studies with senior strength trainees have demonstrated 2- to 6-month attendance rates of approximately 90 percent, which indicates a high level of exercise satisfaction (Hedley et al. 2004; Westcott and Guy 1996; Westcott et al. 2008).

Classic studies with postmenopausal women (Nelson et al. 1994), older men (Frontera et al. 1988), and nonagenarians (Fiatarone et al. 1990) have shown significant gains in muscle mass, strength, and functional abilities following several weeks of basic strength training. Additionally, research from Tufts University (Campbell et al. 1994) and the University of Maryland (Pratley et al. 1994) has revealed that 12 to 16 weeks of standard strength training increases resting metabolic rate by more than 7 percent in senior men and women.

If strength training did nothing more than add muscle, elevate metabolic rate, and reduce fat, it would be well worth the effort. Remarkably, in addition to these impressive physical improvements, strength training provides important health benefits. Regular resistance exercise has been shown to reduce the risk of type 2 diabetes by increasing glucose uptake (Hurley 1994); the risk of cardiovascular disease and stroke by decreasing resting blood pressure (Harris and Holy 1987); the risk of colon cancer by increasing gastrointestinal transit speed (Koffler et al. 1992); the risk of low-back pain by strengthening the lumbar spine muscles (Kell and Asmundson 2009; Carpenter and Nelson 1999; Bayramoglu et al. 2001; Risch et al. 1993); the risk of osteoporosis by increasing bone mineral density (Layne and Nelson 1999; Nelson et al. 1994); the risk of falls by improving balance (Campbell et al. 1999; Nelson et al. 1994); and the pain and debilitating effects of arthritis (Hakkinen 2004; Baker et al. 2001), fibromyalgia (Rooks et al. 2002), and clinical depression (Singh et al. 1997). In addition, strength training can restore physical function to the frail elderly (Westcott et al. 2000).

Musculoskeletal weakness is a pervasive problem in the baby boomer generation, and it typically leads to physical frailty among adults in their 70s, 80s, and 90s. One of our studies with wheelchair users in a nursing home clearly demonstrated the benefits of brief strength training sessions for increasing strength, decreasing discomfort, and improving functional abilities in 90-year-old men and women (Westcott et al. 2000). The 19 patients performed just one set of five weight-stack exercises, twice a week, for 14 weeks. The simple and short training sessions produced remarkable results. These elderly participants added 4 pounds (1.8 kg) of muscle, lost 3 pounds (1.4 kg) of fat, increased their upper-body strength by 40 percent, increased their leg strength by 80 percent, and reported significantly less discomfort in their neck, upper-back, and lower-back areas. All but one patient (a double amputee) reduced or discontinued wheelchair use, and one woman made so much physical improvement that she left the nursing facility to rejoin her husband in an independent living apartment.

Although there is no fountain of youth, strength training is clearly the best means for reversing many of the degenerative processes associated with aging (especially muscle loss, metabolic slowdown, and fat gain) and for reducing the risk of several health problems common among older adults. People have gained excellent results with two 20-minute exercise sessions per week, so strength training is a practical physical activity from a time-management perspective.

Today, more than 500 retirement homes have implemented our five-exercise strength training program for their residents. Almost every senior living in a retirement community today has access to a well-equipped strength training room, and most YMCAs, health clubs, fitness facilities, and community centers offer specialized strength training programs for older adults. Many personal trainers specialize in senior strength training using a variety of exercise equipment including portable resistance tools for in-house sessions.

The purpose of this book is to provide instructors of older adults with important information and research-based principles for designing and developing safe and effective strength training programs for this age group. To enable you to put the training principles and exercise protocols into practice, we have included chapters on general guidelines for senior strength training; specific training strategies and training procedures; methods for assessing strength fitness levels; and recommended exercises for machines, free weights, elastic bands, and balls. This text includes basic and advanced sample programs, as well as sport conditioning programs for runners, cyclists, swimmers, skiers, golfers, tennis players, rowers, rock climbers, and hikers. Because of the prevalence of obesity, diabetes, cardiovascular disease, cancer, osteoporosis, low-back pain, arthritis, fibromyalgia, depression, visual and auditory impairments, and strokes among older adults, we have included recommendations for training them and the frail and elderly. In addition, we also address nutritional considerations for older adult exercisers. Perhaps most important, the book includes precise illustrations and biomechanically sound explanations of resistance machine, free-weight, elastic band, and medicine and Swiss-ball exercises, along with key exercises to reduce the risk of injuries typically associated with particular sports or activities.

As older adults realize that muscles are the engines of their bodies, they become more interested in initiating appropriate strength training programs. But many find the field of resistance exercise confusing and intimidating, and they are reluctant to start strength training on their own. Clearly, qualified professional instructors in the area of strength training are needed to work competently and confidently with men and women in their senior years. One of the most useful features of this textbook is the emphasis on physiological adaptations and health benefits associated with strength training, especially for several special populations of older adults. Knowing and sharing this information with older clients is essential to helping them appreciate the true benefits of strength training and make the commitment to training on a regular basis.

By studying the information presented in this book, you will acquire a better understanding of sensible strength training and gain competence and confidence in presenting appropriate strength workouts to older adults. If you use the standard strength training principles, implement the recommended exercise protocols, and follow the sample program designs, you will be able to provide effective leadership for senior strength training participants. The logical and progressive manner in which this information is presented makes it easy to comprehend and apply, allowing you to implement appropriate adaptations for your particular training situation. You should find the figures, tables, and logs especially helpful in setting up specific strength training programs that are relevant to previously sedentary clients.

A successful strength training program can make the difference between older adults who have low strength levels and endure a sedentary existence and those who have high strength levels and enjoy a physically active lifestyle. The tools in this book will enhance your skill as a professional strength training instructor and enable you to become an agent of positive change for the health of older men and women in your community.

1

Why Seniors Should Strength Train

Put yourself in the position of a typical older adult, say a 55-year-old male or female who has been physically inactive and has added 30 pounds (14 kg) of fat. You have been on several diets, but none has produced a permanent reduction in bodyweight. You have tried walking, but your exercise schedule has been inconsistent and your body composition has remained essentially the same. You have read about the benefits of strength training but you're not fully convinced that it would be beneficial to you, and you've heard that it may raise your blood pressure. You're not very athletic, and you've never even tried to lift weights. You're concerned about looking uncoordinated or experiencing an injury, and you're wondering whether the benefits of strength training are really worth the time and effort. Unless someone clearly explains why you should undertake a strength training program and carefully shows you how to perform the exercises, chances are that you will not attempt this unfamiliar physical activity. A fitness professional who has expertise in strength training older adults can play a vital role in helping you and the growing number of older adults get on track with respect to improving musculoskeletal fitness. In fact, research shows that strength training has many health and fitness applications beyond building stronger muscles.

The purpose of this chapter is to present the beneficial effects of strength training—including replacing muscle, reducing fat, increasing metabolic rate, decreasing low-back discomfort, relieving arthritic pain, minimizing osteoporosis, enhancing glucose utilization, speeding up gastrointestinal transit, lowering resting blood pressure, improving blood lipid levels, and improving postcoronary performance, as well as boosting self-confidence and beating depression. When discussed with older clients, this information can help you, the fitness professional, convince them that strength training is an important physical activity that they can do and that can do them a lot of good (American Heart Association and American College of Sports Medicine 2007).

BODY COMPOSITION

Most people realize that strength training is the best way to develop larger and stronger muscles. They know that bodybuilders perform strength training to build exceptionally large muscles, and that weightlifters do it so that they can lift exceptionally heavy weights. Because most older adults have no desire to compete in bodybuilding or weightlifting events, they tend to avoid strength training altogether. This circumstance is unfortunate because everyone, especially people over age 50, can benefit from larger and stronger muscles. Contrary to what some may think, few people have the genetic potential to develop exceptionally large muscles, and those who do must work deliberately for many years to achieve the profound muscularity that they exhibit. Fears of becoming huge overnight or too strong are without scientific basis.

Too Little Muscle, Too Much Fat

For almost all men and women, the reality is typically the opposite. Rather than being concerned about too much muscle, older adults should be concerned about too little muscle. Adults who do not regularly perform strength training exercises lose about 0.5 pound (0.23 kg) of muscle per year during their 30s and 40s (Evans and Rosenberg 1992). Unfortunately, evidence indicates that the rate of muscle loss may double (to 1 pound, or 0.45 kg, per year) in people over 50 years of age (Nelson et al. 1994). Even more disturbing, the number of type II (fast-twitch) muscle fibers in sedentary males decreases more than 50 percent by age 80 (Larsson 1983). These are the fibers that are most involved in movements requiring high levels of strength (e.g., ascending and descending stairs) among older adults. Because muscles are the engines of the body, the loss in muscle tissue is comparable to going from an eight-cylinder engine car to one with four cylinders, while the weight of the automobile (the person's bodyweight) remains the same or even increases.

Having less muscle and more fat compromises physical fitness and contributes to health problems, including a variety of degenerative diseases such as diabetes, osteoporosis, heart disease, and colon cancer. Although most seniors know that they have more fat than they should and are not as strong as they once were, many do not realize that they have lost muscle as they have become older. Even fewer older adults understand that muscle loss contributes to a decrease in their metabolic rate, which plays a major role in their fat gain.

Muscle Loss

Muscle loss causes two of life's major problems and is associated with a variety of health-related consequences:

1. Reduced functional capacity, which leads to less physical activity and further muscle loss

2. Reduced calorie utilization, which leads to slower metabolism and fat accumulation

---

The typical approach taken by many who desire to lose fat is to undertake a low-calorie diet plan. Although almost half of the adult population is dieting (Tufts 1992), fewer than 5 percent will be successful (Brehm and Keller 1990). According to an exhaustive review of the research by Mann and colleagues (2007), essentially all those who shed weight through dieting will regain all the weight lost within a relatively short postdiet period. The inability to keep the weight lost off is as much a matter of physiology as it is willpower. On most diets, approximately 25 percent of the weight lost is muscle tissue (Ballor and

Poehlman 1994), which in turn results in a reduction in resting metabolic rate that may exceed 125 calories per day (Alexander 2002). Consequently, among dieters, the eventual return to normal eating provides too many calories for the slower metabolism and lower postdiet energy requirements. Older adults must understand that too much fat is only part of the body composition problem, and that dieting is not an effective solution (Westcott 2005).

Adding Muscle to Lose Fat

The less obvious but more important issue to discuss with your clients is that they have too little muscle. Adding muscle has the two-fold effect of increasing both physical capacity (a larger engine) and resting metabolism (higher daily energy requirement). Research clearly demonstrates that regular strength training can replace muscle lost by older adults (Grimby et al. 1992; McCartney et al. 1996) and increase resting metabolic rate (Pratley et al. 1994; Hunter et al. 2000; Ades et al. 2005) in older adults.

One of the earlier studies in this area was conducted at Tufts University with previously sedentary men and women between 56 and 80 years of age (Campbell et al. 1994). The 12 subjects performed three 30-minute strength training sessions each week for 3 months and did not engage in other forms of exercise during the study. Their strength training program consisted of three sets of four exercises that collectively addressed all the major muscle groups. At the conclusion of the study participants demonstrated, on average, an increase of 3 pounds (1.4 kg) of lean (muscle) weight and a loss of 4 pounds (1.8 kg) in fat weight, even though they were eating about 250 more calories per day than they were at the beginning of the study. How did this happen? The muscle development from strength training apparently increased resting metabolic rates by almost 7 percent, while the training increased daily energy utilization by approximately 15 percent. Similar results in resting metabolic rate were reported by Pratley and colleagues (1994) and by Paffenbarger and Olsen (1996).

Unlike dieting, which decreases the number of calories eaten per day (and results in muscle loss among inactive people), strength training increases the number of calories used each day. Besides raising the resting metabolic rate, stronger muscles enable older adults to perform essentially all physical activities with less effort.

In another early study, Butts and Price (1994) examined the effects of a relatively high-effort strength training program on body composition in adult and senior-aged women. The participants completed one set in each of 12 exercises 3 days per week for 12 weeks. After the 3-month training period, women increased their lean (muscle) weight by 2.9 pounds (1.3 kg) and decreased their fat weight by 3.0 pounds (1.4), for a 5.9-pound (2.7 kg) improvement in body composition.

In a similar study with mostly male subjects (Draovitch and Westcott 1999), 77 older adults performed relatively high-effort strength training sessions (one set in each of 12 exercises), 3 days per week for 8 weeks. After 2 months of training, participants increased lean (muscle) weight by 3.9 pounds (1.8 kg) and decreased fat weight by 4.1 pounds (1.9 kg), for an 8.0-pound (3.6 kg) improvement in body composition.

TABLE 1.1

Lean Muscle Weight Changes After Exercise

Age	Lean weight change
21–44 years	+2.5 lb (1.1 kg)
45–54 years	+3.1 lbs (1.4 kg)
55–64 years	+2.9 lbs (1.3 kg)
65–80 years	+3.2 lbs (1.4 kg)

Changes in lean muscle weight for men and women between 21 and 80 years of age after 10 weeks of strength training (1,644 subjects). No significant differences occurred among the age groups.

From Westcott 2009. ACSM strength training guidelines. *ACSM's Health & Fitness Journal* 13(4): 14-22.

Seniors sometimes question whether they are too old to make meaningful changes in their body composition. But a study by Westcott (2009) involving 1,644 men and women reported significant positive changes in body composition. The older adults in this study performed about 25 minutes of relatively high-effort strength training (one set in each of 12 exercises) and about 20 minutes of moderate-effort aerobic activity (treadmill walking or stationary cycling) 2 or 3 days per week for 10 weeks. As shown in table 1.1, lean weight in all age categories (21 through 80 years) showed statistically similar gains. These results are similar to those found in an earlier 8-week study conducted by Westcott and Guy (1996) involving 1,132 seniors. Both studies also revealed that men added about twice as much lean (muscle) weight and lost about twice as much fat weight as the women did. The faster rate of body composition change in males is most likely due to several genetic factors, including greater body weight, more muscle mass, and higher levels of anabolic hormones such as testosterone.

Other researchers who studied the effects of strength training on body composition in older men (Frontera et al. 1988), women (Nelson et al. 1994), and frail elderly people (Fiatarone et al. 1990) also reported lean weight gains and fat losses.

In case you believe that an age limit governs body composition adaptations, consider the results of a 14-week study involving frail nursing home patients who averaged almost 90 years of age (Westcott et al. 2000). Resistance training just 10 minutes a day (one set of five exercises) on 2 days per week produced an average gain of 3.8 pounds (1.7 kg) in lean (muscle) weight and a loss of 2.9 pounds (1.3 kg) in fat. Seniors in this

General Frailty

Numerous strength training studies such as those pioneered at Tufts University involving older adults (Campbell et al. 1994; Fiatarone et al. 1990; Frontera et al. 1988; Nelson et al. 1994) reported significant musculoskeletal improvements and no exercise-related injuries. Load assignments as heavy as 80 percent of 1RM were well tolerated by healthy and frail clients up to 100 years of age (Fiatarone and Singh 2002; Fiatarone et al. 1994). Strength training offers one of the most beneficial forms of exercise to frail clients, providing them higher levels of muscle strength and endurance to help them maintain their independence and reduce the frequency of falls (Grimby et al. 1992).

study also increased their leg strength by more than 80 percent and their upper-body strength by almost 40 percent. Be assured that seniors are never too old to improve their body composition and increase their muscular strength.

METABOLIC RATE

Muscle tissue is active, so it uses large amounts of energy during exercise and requires a significant energy supply at rest. The latter energy requirement is due to the tissue remodeling processes that take place 24 hours a day. Even during sleep, the muscle remodeling process may account for 25 percent of the calories used by the body. You will recall that the senior subjects in the Tufts University study (Campbell et al. 1994) added 3 pounds (1.4 kg) of muscle and raised their resting metabolic rate by almost 7 percent after 12 weeks of strength training. Similarly, older men in a 16-week strength training study at the University of Maryland (Pratley et al. 1994) increased their lean weight by 3.5 pounds (1.6 kg) and their resting metabolism by almost 8 percent. A 24-week research program at the University of Alabama by Hunter and colleagues (2000) also revealed metabolic rate benefits from regular strength training. In their study older adults added 4.5 pounds (2.0 kg) of lean weight and increased their resting metabolism by almost 7 percent. Assuming an average resting metabolism of 1,500 calories a day, this additional muscle accounts for more than 100 additional calories used at rest on a daily basis.

The increase in resting metabolism, however, is only part of the increased energy expenditure attributable to strength training. The strength training session itself is also responsible for burning a considerable number of calories (Ades et al. 2005). For example, a 25-minute circuit strength training program may use up 200 calories (about 8 calories per minute) according to research by Hempel and Wells (1985) and by Haltom et al. (1999). The body also burns additional calories during the transition from reliance on the anaerobic energy system (dominant energy source during strength training) back to the aerobic energy system used at rest. This process is referred to as the postexercise energy expenditure, and its magnitude is directly related to the intensity and duration of the strength training session. Research by Gillette et al. (1994) showed significantly higher energy utilization for 90 minutes following strength exercise as compared with endurance exercise. Melby and associates (1993) found a 12 percent increase in metabolic rate 2 hours after a high-intensity, high-volume strength workout. A study on circuit

Key Strength Training Effects

In summary, strength training appears to have a threefold effect on metabolic function and energy utilization. First, strength training produces a large increase in energy use during the exercise session. Second, strength training results in a moderate increase in metabolism during the postexercise recovery period. Third, strength-trained muscle requires more energy all day long, which leads to a significant (7 to 8 percent) increase in resting metabolic rate. Clearly, developing larger and stronger muscles through sensible strength training is an effective means of enhancing metabolism.

strength training by Haltom and colleagues (1999) revealed that participants used 15 to 25 percent as many calories as they burned in their exercise session during the hour following the workout. In other words, a circuit strength training session that burns 200 calories may actually burn 250 calories when the postexercise energy expenditure is included. Although it may not be advisable for seniors new to strength training to undertake a circuit weight training program, even a moderate-intensity strength training program should produce some postexercise elevation over resting metabolic rates (Campbell et al. 1994). Circuit weight training is a variation of interval training in which timed work and rest periods are used while alternating weight training exercises (e.g., push–pull, upper body–lower body). The rest periods used are typically 30 seconds or shorter (Baechle and Earle 2006). The higher percentage of exercise time and lower percentage of recovery time elicits relatively high energy expenditure and cardiovascular activity (Messier and Dill 1985).

DIABETES

The inability of body cells to utilize glucose effectively is a metabolic disorder that may lead to diabetes mellitus. Exercise promotes glucose utilization, and most diabetics find regular physical activity useful for maintaining consistent glucose levels. Although aerobic exercise has traditionally been recommended for enhancing glucose utilization (Council on Exercise of the American Diabetes Association 1990), research suggests that strength training may be equally effective (Durak, Jovanovis-Peterson, and Peterson 1990; Miller et al. 1984).

Diabetes and Strength Training

People with diabetes may benefit from strength training in many ways. First, strength training may reverse muscle myopathy, a problem associated with poor glucose utilization and a predisposing factor for adult-onset diabetes (Durak 1989). Second, strength training may preserve lean body mass in people who follow low-calorie diets to reduce body fat (Ballor et al. 1988). Third, trained muscles have higher glucose uptake and lower insulin resistance (Ibanez et al. 2005) than untrained muscles do (Lohmann and Liebold 1978).

Studies involving older (>55 years) people with diabetes in resistance training programs such as one by Castaneda et al. (2002), in which subjects performed three sets of eight repetitions twice a week at 60 to 80 percent of 1RM during weeks 1 through 8 and 70 to 80 percent of 1RM during weeks 10 through 14, reported significantly improved glycemic control, greater fat-free mass, reduced abdominal adiposity, reduced need for diabetes medications, lower systolic blood pressure, and increased strength. (One-repetition maximum, or 1RM, represents the heaviest resistance or load that a person can lift one time.) In earlier studies by Hurley (1994) glucose utilization increased in older men 23 percent after 4 months of strength training. Eriksson et al. (1997) found that an 11-station circuit weight training program (one set of each exercise, twice a week, for 3 months) significantly improved glycemic control in previously sedentary seniors with type 2 diabetes. Although resistance training has been shown to bring about significant improvements in glycemic control, studies that have focused on the effects of incorporating both forms of exercise (Sigal et al. 2007; Balducci et al., 2004; Tokmakidis et al. 2004) have shown even better results.

Because poor glucose metabolism is a predisposing factor in type 2 diabetes, the positive effect of strength training on glucose uptake may help prevent this serious disease, which is increasingly prevalent in older adults (Craig et al. 1989).

GASTROINTESTINAL TRANSIT

Gastrointestinal transit refers to the time required for food to move through the digestive system. Slow gastrointestinal transit speed appears to be associated with increased risk for colon cancer (Hurley 1994). As far back as 1986 (Cordain, Latin, and Behnke), aerobic activity such as running was shown to speed up gastrointestinal transit. Since then, researchers at the University of Maryland found that strength training improved gastrointestinal transit time 56 percent in middle-aged and older men after 3 months of strength training. The researchers concluded that strength training might be an effective way to address age-related gastrointestinal motility disorders, as well as reduce the risk of colon cancer (Koffler et al. 1992).

CARDIOVASCULAR DISEASE

All types of exercise increase oxygen delivery demands on the cardiovascular system, resulting in both higher heart rates and higher systolic blood pressures, which increase in a parallel manner. Traditionally, strength training has been misrepresented as an activity that elevates blood pressure to extreme levels, both during performance and after a period of training. Although prolonged static contractions sometimes used in isometric exercise can raise blood pressure to undesirable levels, this circumstance is unlikely to occur in properly supervised strength training activities.

Blood Pressure

Consider that pedaling a stationary cycle at a normal effort level (75 percent of maximum heart rate) increases systolic blood pressure approximately 35 percent above resting pressure (Westcott 1986). That is, if your resting systolic blood pressure is 120 mmHg, it would average about 162 mmHg throughout a stationary cycling session. By way of comparison, a set of 10 repetitions in the dumbbell curl, taken to temporary muscle failure, raises systolic blood pressure about 35 percent above resting (Westcott and Howes 1983), and a set of 10 repetitions to temporary muscle failure in the leg press raises systolic blood pressure about 50 percent above resting (Westcott 2004b). The increase in systolic blood pressure (and heart rate) during a set of resistance exercise is linear, progressive, and consistent on a repetition-by-repetition basis. Given a resting systolic blood pressure of 120 mmHg, the 50 percent increase observed in high-effort leg presses would result in a peak reading of 180 mmHg, which is well below the 250 mmHg ceiling level for exercise-related systolic blood pressure recommended by the American College of Sports Medicine (2010). The blood pressure response to strength training, even among older adults in cardiac rehabilitation programs, has been found to be clinically acceptable when participants trained at moderate (40–60 percent of 1RM) intensity (Haslam et al. 1988). The study by DeGroot et al. (1998) reported that the blood pressure response to the same 1RM intensity was lower than the response to treadmill training at 85 percent of $\dot{V}O_2$max. Additionally, in our study with leg presses we found a 10 mmHg decrease in diastolic pressure (below resting level) immediately following the training set, because the increased vascular network reduced resistance to blood flow (Westcott 2004b).

Although resistance training temporarily elevates blood pressure during exercise sets, it does not result in higher resting blood pressure levels following a properly designed program of strength training (Hurley 1994). In fact, circuit weight training studies by Harris and Holly (1987) and Hurley et al. (1988), which were 9 and 16 weeks in length respectively, also showed significant reductions in diastolic blood pressure. In a study by Westcott et al. (2009) involving 1,725 adults and older adults who participated in 20 minutes of strength training and 20 minutes of aerobic training, systolic blood pressure was found to decrease an average of 4 mmHg and diastolic blood pressure to decrease 2 mmHg after 10 weeks of training. Although the aerobic activity undoubtedly contributed to better blood pressure readings, at least one comparative study has shown that strength training and endurance exercise are equally effective for reducing resting blood pressure (Smutok et al. 1993).

Thus, contrary to popular misconceptions, sensible strength training does not appear to have any detrimental effects on blood pressure. Numerous studies have demonstrated reductions in resting blood pressure readings, especially in response to circuit weight training programs (Katz and Wilson 1992; Kelley 1997).

Blood Lipids

Blood lipid profiles appear to be important predictors of cardiovascular disease. Unfortunately, many older adults have levels of total cholesterol, LDL (bad) cholesterol, and triglycerides that are higher than desirable, and levels of HDL (good) cholesterol that are lower than ideal. Although genetics is a major factor in this area, research indicates that diet and exercise can have a positive influence on blood lipid profiles.

Perhaps the best-known study on this topic was conducted over 20 years ago (Hurley et al. in 1988). The subjects (40- to 55-year-old men) demonstrated significant decreases in LDL cholesterol and increases in HDL cholesterol following a 16-week circuit weight training program. But subsequent research (Kokkinos et al. 1988, 1991; Smutok et al. 1993) was not able to demonstrate similar results. A recent review of 84 studies (Tambalis et al. 2008) published between 1990 and 2006 on the effects of aerobic training, resistance training, and combined training disclosed that reductions in LDL were commonly reported in response to resistance training, whereas combined training brought about improvements in LDL and HDL cholesterol levels. A meta-analysis by Kelley and Kelley (2009) found that strength training reduced LDL cholesterol and total cholesterol as well as the ratio of total cholesterol to HDL cholesterol.

Because the studies on the effectiveness of strength training for improving blood lipid profiles are not conclusive, more research is warranted. We at least can be confident in saying that regular strength exercise does not adversely affect blood lipid profiles and may produce desirable changes in LDL and HDL cholesterol levels (Johnson et al. 1982; Stone et al. 1982; Blessing et al. 1987; Ulrich et al.1987; Boyden et al. 1993; Goldberg et al. 1984; Tucker and Sylvester 1996).

Postcoronary Performance

Coronary artery disease, the leading medical problem in the United States, is particularly prevalent among older adults. Fortunately, treatment of coronary artery disease has progressed to the point where many heart attack survivors and post-bypass patients lead relatively normal lives. Although usually encouraged to follow an aerobic training regimen, patients with cardiovascular problems have traditionally been advised against resistance exercise. This recommendation is unfortunate because recovering people often experience muscle atrophy when they are inactive during their rehabilitation period. They, like all of us, depend on muscular strength and endurance to perform physical tasks and daily activities. In the absence of good muscular fitness, everyday tasks require more effort.

Several studies have shown that strength training can be a safe and productive activity for most postcoronary patients (Butler et al. 1987; Stewart et al. 1988; Faigenbaum et al. 1990; Ghilarducci, Holly, and Amsterdam 1989; Haennel, Quinney, and Kappagoda 1991; Vander et al. 1986). Harris and Holly (1987) found that strength training could be a safe activity among patients with controlled hypertension. Pierson et al. (2001) found that a 6-month program of either resistance training or aerobic training produced improvements in peak oxygen consumption at maximal levels of exercise. Furthermore, when patients included both types of exercise in their workouts, muscular strength increased substantially, body composition improved, and cardiovascular demand at a fixed submaximal aerobic exercise load decreased.

Although postcoronary clients will benefit from a stronger musculoskeletal system that will reduce stress on the cardiovascular system, thereby reducing cardiac risk, caution must always be exercised when training them and others with special conditions and needs. The American College of Sports Medicine (2010) has suggested that asymptomatic cardiac patients begin low-level resistance training as early as 7 to 8 weeks after their event, and the American Association of Cardiovascular and Pulmonary Rehabilitation (1995) has developed a comprehensive set of strength training recommendations for postcoronary individuals. Prior medical approval is, of course, an essential prerequisite to placing a postcoronary client on a strength training program.

OSTEOPOROSIS

Osteoporosis is a degenerative disease of the skeletal system characterized by gradual loss of bone proteins and minerals that leads to fragile bones, which are at increased risk of fracture. Because bone condition essentially parallels muscle condition, weak muscles are associated with weak bones and strong muscles with strong bones. According to the National Osteoporosis Foundation (NOF 2008), 10 million Americans probably have osteoporosis, and another 34 million have low bone mass or osteopenia, which places them at increased risk for the disease. Osteoporosis has no obvious symptoms, and unfortunately it is usually determined after an injury. Therefore, as a trainer, you should ask older clients, especially women, if they have had a bone scan, and if they have, you should request a copy of the report.

Because osteoporosis is highly correlated with muscle weakness, it is a condition that can benefit greatly from strength training (Bell 1988; Colletti et al. 1989; Marks 1993; Layne and Nelson 1999; Ryan et al. 1994; Snow-Harter et al. 1992). As muscles become stronger in response to training, bones become stronger (Hughes et al. 1995). Research that has investigated the relationship has shown that strength training can help maintain or increase bone mineral density in men and women over 50 years of age (Kerr et al. 2001; Rhodes et al. 2000; Nelson et al. 1994; Menkes et al. 1993). Dr. Robert A. Gurtler, fellow of both the American Academy of Orthopaedic Surgeons and the American Orthopedic Society of Sports Medicine, says, "Both having the right genetics and practicing good eating habits are essential for the prevention of osteoporosis. But an equally important factor is whether you are performing weight-bearing exercise on a regular basis" (personal communication, May 1998).

Logically, the same activities that build myoproteins in muscles also enhance the protein and mineral content in bones. Although genetics, hormones, nutrition, and other factors affect bone remodeling (an ongoing process by which bone absorption and formation occur at the same rate) and influence the course of osteoporosis, strength training is an excellent way to develop and maintain strong and functional musculoskeletal systems that resist deterioration and osteoporosis.

Research with older men (Menkes et al. 1993) and postmenopausal women (Nelson et al. 1994) indicates that bone loss can be changed to bone gain through regular and progressive strength training.

For instance, the study by Menkes et al. (1993) showed significant increases in bone mineral density at the spine (2 percent) and neck of the femur (3.8 percent). This finding is important, especially because it concerns the femoral neck, which is a common area of fractures in older people.

Supporting Menkes' results was a study by Nelson and her colleagues at Tufts University (1994) that involved 39 postmenopausal women (ages 50 to 70 years) who engaged in a full year of strength training workouts. Their program consisted of five exercises (hip extension, knee extension, lat pull-down, back extension, abdominal flexion), which were performed for three sets of eight repetitions, 2 days per week. In the women who strength trained, 1 percent increases in bone mineral density in the lumbar spine and femoral neck were reported, whereas those who did not train experienced a 2 percent decline. The strength-trained group also experienced a 3-pound (1.4 kg) increase in muscle, whereas the control group lost 1 pound (0.45 kg) of muscle.

Another 12-month study of menopausal women clearly demonstrated the importance of strength training for increasing bone mineral density (Notelovitz et al. 1991). Subjects who combined strength training and estrogen therapy increased total bone mineral density by 2.1 percent, whereas those who received only estrogen therapy experienced no change in bone mineral density. Taunton (1997) replicated the results of Notelovitz's (1991) work, showing that strength training significantly increased bone mineral density of the lumbar spine (and a trend toward improved hip bone mineral density) in 65- to 75-year-old women. Rhodes and colleagues (2000), in a strength training study involving DEXA (dual-energy X-ray absorptiometry) measurements of bone mineral density changes in older adults, also reported significant increases. Charette et al. (1991) suggested that bone remodeling requires 4 to 6 months, but it is possible that strength training programs of shorter duration will elicit positive changes in bone mineral density.

Collectively, these studies provide convincing evidence that strength training can produce positive changes in bone mineral density that help provide some degree of protection from osteoporosis.

Reduction in Falls

"While thinning bones render the skeleton prone to fractures, it is the gradual erosion of muscle and the ensuing frailty which leads to falls" (Dudley 2001). The erosion of muscle and the concomitant loss of strength compromise balance and stability and all too often lead to falls among older adults. Such falls result in further disuse and muscle atrophy. A further decline in functional ability is likely to occur, leading to a permanent loss in independence (Borst 2004). Well-designed strength training programs undertaken by seniors have been found to improve dynamic balance (Campbell et al. 1997) and reduce falls (Sequin et al. 2003) while also improving walking endurance (Ades et al. 1996) and walking speed (Fiatarone et al. 1994). In fact, in the study by Borst (2004) that investigated the effects of resistance training on sarcopenia and muscle weakness, the researchers stated, "Resistance training remains the most effective intervention for increasing muscle mass and strength in older people." Developing and maintaining leg strength and balance should be one of the primary goals in strength training programs designed for older adults because of their importance in reducing falls, maintaining independence, and helping them enjoy a higher quality of life.

LOW-BACK PAIN

The chances are good that the average older adult will experience one or more bouts of low-back pain. Medical professionals estimate that four out of five American adults encounter occasional or chronic low-back discomfort. This pervasive problem is responsible for more employee absenteeism and medical expense than any other malady except cold and flu illnesses. A surprise to many is that a highly effective intervention for low-back pain is a low-back strengthening program (Jones et al. 1988; Bayramoglu et al. 2001)—a simple remedy that works for many who suffer from low-back pain.

Such a program is effective because there is a strong, positive relationship between weak low-back muscles and low-back discomfort. Several years of low-back pain studies conducted at the University of Florida demonstrated that systematic strengthening of the low-back muscles significantly reduced or eliminated discomfort in up to 80 percent of their patients (Risch et al. 1993).

The University of Florida strength training program was as simple as it was effective. All the program participants performed one set of low-back extensions on a machine using a resistance that permitted between 8 and 15 repetitions. On average, they trained 3 days per week for a period of 10 weeks. Carpenter and Nelson (1999) found that performance by older adults of one set of lumbar extension exercises on only 1 day a week (8–15 repetitions) to muscular fatigue was as effective at strengthening the low back and reducing pain as multiple-set training was. Limke and Rainville (2008) also reported that one-set training was as effective as multiple-set training for reducing low-back pain and increasing strength. These studies and our work with laborers at a large automotive plant who experienced low-back pain indicate that developing a stronger midsection (rectus abdominis, internal obliques, external obliques) may also complement stronger low-back muscles and further reduce the risk of injury or reinjury (Westcott 2004a).

Although low-back pain is a complex medical issue, an appropriate program of low-back and abdominal strengthening exercises appears to provide better musculoskeletal function, support for vertebral column components, and shock absorption that reduces stress and excessive wear and tear on sensitive low-back structures, which in turn reduces the risk of low-back injury and structural degeneration.

ARTHRITIS

According to the Arthritis Foundation (2009) arthritis is a term that describes more than 100 conditions that cause pain, swelling, and movement restrictions in joints and connective tissue throughout the body. The number of American adults afflicted is greater than 46 million (National Center for Health Statistics 2009), and the two most prevalent forms of arthritis are rheumatoid and osteoarthritis. Rheumatoid arthritis is an inflammatory disease involving the synovial membrane, whereas osteoarthritis is characterized by a wearing away of articular cartilage. Rheumatoid arthritis can affect joints as well as blood vessels, skin, cardiac muscle, and the lungs. In contrast, osteoarthritis is a degenerative disease that results in the thinning of articular cartilage of the knees, hips, feet, spine, and hands. Physicians traditionally have cautioned those with arthritis to avoid strenuous exercise in general and strength training in particular. But that practice is changing thanks to research such as that conducted at Tufts University (Baker et al. 2001), where researchers found that adults (55 and older) with osteoarthritis who strength trained achieved significant reductions in pain and improved in muscular strength, functional performance, physical ability, and quality of life.

Although the exact mechanisms by which strength exercise provides relief are not understood, it has become almost common knowledge that strength training can ease the pain of osteoarthritis and rheumatoid arthritis while strengthening the musculoskeletal system and enhancing the functional capacity of joints (Marks 1993; Quirk et al. 1985).

FIBROMYALGIA

Fibromyalgia, along with osteoarthritis, rheumatoid arthritis, systemic lupus, erythematosus, gout, and bursitis, is a rheumatic disease (ACSM 2010). Fibromyalgia affects approximately 5 million Americans, predominantly women (National Institute of Arthritis and Musculoskeletal and Skin Diseases 2005). It is a chronic disorder characterized by widespread pain and pain-specific tender points (Wolfe et al. 1990), and it may be accompanied by sensitivity to touch and noises, irritable bowel syndrome, trouble sleeping, numbness in extremities, depression, mood changes, and memory loss. Two studies have provided excitement about the benefits of strength training for people with fibromyalgia, such as the study by Hakkinen et al. (2001) involving premenopausal women and a study by Rooks and colleagues (2002) that involved women in a 20-week program of strength training and aerobic training.

DEPRESSION AND SELF-CONFIDENCE

In a study (Singh, Clements, and Fiatarone 1997) conducted at Harvard Medical School researchers suggested that older adults who suffer from depression may benefit from strength training. The 32 subjects (age range of 60 to 84 years) met the diagnostic criteria for mild to moderate depression and were assigned to either a strength training program or a lecture and discussion series on health-related topics. After 10 weeks, 82 percent of the strength exercisers no longer met the depression criteria, compared with 40 percent of those who attended class lectures and discussions. A subsequent study by Singh, Clements, and Singh (2001) demonstrated that a 20-week (10 supervised, 10 unsupervised) resistance training program significantly reduced depression levels after 20 weeks of training and a 26-month follow-up. Westcott (1995), using a self-administered questionnaire to 49 middle-aged and older adults, attempted to ascertain whether an 8-week program of strength and endurance exercises would affect the self-confidence of participants. Although statistical analyses were not performed, a tabulation of ratings suggested that the exercise program had a positive effect on the participants' self-confidence. Although more research is needed in these areas, it appears that strength training has the potential to help counteract depression and enhance self-confidence in older adults.

VISUAL AND AUDITORY IMPAIRMENTS

Fitness professionals commonly have older clients with visual or hearing impairments, so recommendations about how to train such clients is included in chapter 8. Although some have expressed concern about the effects of resistance training on intraocular pressure, recent research (Conte et al. 2009; Chromiak et al. 2003) has shown significant decreases in postexercise pressure. Because people with sight and hearing problems often have balance problems as well, they may benefit from a fall-reduction program that includes leg strengthening and balance exercises.

STROKES

The National Stroke Association (2008) reported that 6 million people in the United States have survived strokes. Although not all research has supported the use of resistance training by those who have strokes (Moreland et al. 2003), research by Weiss et al. (2000) provides evidence that such training 1 year after a stroke can improve the lower-limb strength of the affected side and bring about improvements in chair stand time, balance, and motor performance. Each client who has experienced a stroke brings a unique set of limitations and capacities. Spasticity presents one of the major challenges, because it may cause a loss of balance and uncontrolled movements in the involved limbs.

Summary
of Strength Training Principles for Older Adults

Research indicates that older adults may experience many health-related benefits from a sensible program of strength exercise that is performed at a relatively high effort level. Some of the possible benefits include the following:

- Better body composition, with up to 4 pounds (1.8 kg) more lean weight and 4 pounds less fat weight after 2 months of regular strength training

- Increased metabolic rate of up to 7 percent higher resting metabolism and up to 15 percent greater daily calorie requirements after 3 months of regular strength exercise

- Decreased low-back discomfort, as evidenced by approximately 80 percent of patients reporting less or no pain after about 3 months of specific low-back strengthening exercise

- Reduced arthritic pain, as indicated by subjective ratings of symptoms in strength-trained adults who have arthritis

- Increased bone mineral density that may minimize age-related bone loss and offer protection against osteoporosis

- Enhanced glucose utilization that may reduce the risk of type 2 diabetes

- Faster gastrointestinal transit that may reduce the risk of colon cancer and other motility disorders of the gastrointestinal system

- Reduced resting blood pressure, including lower diastolic readings and lower systolic readings

- Improved blood lipid profiles, including lower levels of LDL cholesterol and higher levels of HDL cholesterol

- Improved postcoronary performance resulting from higher muscular functional capacity and lower cardiovascular stress from routine and unplanned physical activity

- Enhanced self-confidence, as reported by previously sedentary men and women following 2 months of regular strength training

- Relieved depression in older adults clinically diagnosed with mild to moderate depression

Training Principles and Teaching Strategies

Muscle strength can be developed by almost any training program that progressively increases the resistance or load during exercises. Unfortunately, some of the popular strength training programs carry a high risk of injury, and others provide a low rate of improvement. A well-designed strength training program for older adults should maximize the training outcomes while minimizing the likelihood of injury. Exercises included should be simple to perform and organized in a time-efficient manner. Those who train seniors should understand that older adults are often capable of training at relatively high effort levels (Frontera et al. 1988; Fiatarone et al. 1990; Nelson et al. 1994). At the same time, care should be taken not to push them so hard that their muscles are sore on the days between workouts (Miles et al. 1997).

According to the ACSM (2010), a basic program of strength training should include at least one set of 8 to 12 repetitions in 8 to 10 exercises involving the major muscle groups, performed at a controlled movement speed, on 2 or 3 nonconsecutive days a week.

Although ACSM's strength training guidelines apply to all adults, specific recommendations apply to older people. The first priority is for fitness professionals who understand the special needs and abilities of older people and can provide carefully instructed and supervised training sessions. Second, ACSM advocates that strength training programs for older participants should have a higher repetition range with relatively less resistance (10 to 15 reps rather than 8 to 12 reps), especially during the initial 8 weeks of the exercise program. Third, older exercisers should be encouraged to strength train at controlled speeds (without momentum) through a full range of pain-free movement while breathing continuously (no held breaths). Finally, ACSM suggests that older people begin with machine exercises for greater body stabilization, range control, and movement precision.

This chapter presents research-based guidelines for designing safe and effective strength training programs for older adults, including those age 75 years or older, and covers the following essential strength training principles:

1. Training frequency
2. Number of sets
3. Training load or resistance

4. Number of repetitions

5. Exercise selection

6. Training progression

Besides understanding the essential strength training principles, you, as a fitness professional, need to know effective teaching strategies for educating and motivating your clients. Therefore, the last section of this chapter presents an instructional model and the following 10 components of interactive teaching for improved communications and enhanced exercise outcomes:

1. Understandable performance objectives

2. Concise instruction with precise demonstration

3. Attentive supervision

4. Appropriate assistance

5. One task at a time

6. Gradual progression

7. Positive reinforcement

8. Specific feedback

9. Careful questioning

10. Pre- and postexercise dialogue

The correct combination of training principles and teaching strategies will greatly enhance the exercise experience of older adults and facilitate their success as competent and confident senior strength trainers.

PRINCIPLE 1: TRAINING FREQUENCY

Properly planned strength training workouts that progressively stress the prime mover muscles will produce some degree of tissue microtrauma. Following each exercise session, the stressed tissues undergo repair and building processes (muscle remodeling) that result in slightly larger and stronger muscles over time. These beneficial physiological adaptations typically require 48 to 72 hours to occur, and it is during this time that the next strength workout should be undertaken for best training results. Thus, strength development is enhanced by training the same muscles again 2 or 3 days after the last workout. Training less frequently passes over the optimal period for stimulating progressively greater levels of strength. Conversely, training too frequently prevents muscles from recovering adequately and ultimately from developing to their full

> ### *Tissue Microtrauma*
>
> Microscopic tears in muscle and connective tissue that require about 48 to 72 hours recovery time for remodeling and building processes to be completed.

potential. The actual amount of recovery time needed to achieve maximum muscle-building benefit will vary because of individual differences. Therefore, you must monitor your clients' improvement carefully to determine the most productive training frequency for them.

Because the only way to determine a client's most productive training frequency is through trial and error, maintaining a detailed record of each client's training sessions is important. When the muscle recovery and building period between workouts is appropriate, a consistent and progressive increase in loads used and repetitions performed should be possible.

Although most strength training textbooks recommend three strength training sessions per week (Baechle and Earle 2005; Baechle and Earle 2008; Fleck and Kraemer 1997; Westcott 1995a), some research indicates that two strength workouts per week may be as effective (Braith et al. 1989; DeMichele et al. 1997). Specifically, twice-a-week strength training appears to be highly productive for developing strength in men and women over the age of 50 (Stadler, Stubbs, and Vukovich 1997; Westcott and Guy 1996; Westcott et al. 2009).

In 1989 Braith et al. found that two exercise sessions per week produced only 75 percent as much strength gain as three training sessions per week. But a 1997 study from the same university (DeMichele et al. 1997) showed the same strength development from two or three weight training workouts per week. The 2- and 3-day trainees showed similar strength gains (figure 2.1), but the subjects who trained only once a week did not achieve significant strength gains.

In a study by Westcott et al. (2009), 1,725 adult and senior subjects showed no differences in muscle development between the 2-day-a-week and 3-day-a-week exercise groups after 10 weeks of strength training. All the participants trained according to the ACSM guidelines, in small classes under close supervision. Both the Tuesday–Thursday trainees and the Monday–Wednesday–Friday trainees added 3.1 pounds (1.4 kg) of lean (muscle) weight over the training period. The results of these studies indicate that for older adults, strength training on 2 nonconsecutive days per week may be as effective as more frequent exercise sessions.

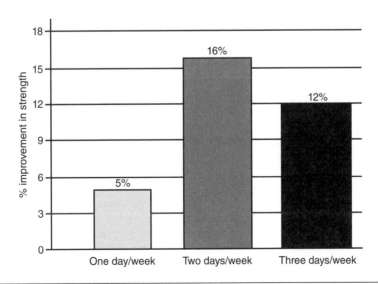

Figure 2.1 Strength gains after 12 weeks of training 1, 2, or 3 days per week.

Data from DeMichele et al. 1997.

Apparently, during the first few months of strength training, two exercise sessions per week provide the essential stimulus for muscle development, and little or no additional muscle-building benefit results from a third weekly workout.

A well-designed study by McLester and colleagues (2003) revealed that advanced strength exercisers, both young and old, required more than 2 days of recovery time to maximize their training response. Following a relatively hard strength training session on Monday, muscle strength was well below baseline (initial) level on Tuesday, slightly below baseline level on Wednesday, significantly above baseline level on Thursday, and the same amount over baseline on Friday. That is, these subjects were not fully recovered in 48 hours, but had optimized their muscular response to the training stimulus after 72 hours.

Training consistency is as important as frequency. Clients who miss scheduled training sessions undermine the ability of the body to achieve progressive adaptation to the strength-building stimulus—because it is absent. Training the same muscles too frequently, say, 2 days in succession, is also counterproductive because time is insufficient for muscle recovery and remodeling. Using some of the strategies discussed later in this chapter, you can find ways to motivate older adults so that they do not miss scheduled workouts.

PRINCIPLE 2: NUMBER OF SETS

According to the 2006 training guidelines of the American College of Sports Medicine, one or more sets of resistance exercise are recommended for developing muscle strength. Although some trainers prefer their clients to follow multiple-set training programs, one set is the minimum requirement for stimulating strength gains. Because single-set strength training provides a user-friendly and time-efficient approach to muscle fitness, it is a suggested starting point for most older adults new to strength training.

Although competitive weightlifters and bodybuilders perform several sets of each exercise, high-volume strength training (large numbers of sets and repetitions) may not be necessary for improving muscle fitness in the average adult. In fact, several studies, such as those described next, have demonstrated similar results from single-set and multiple-set strength training, at least for the first 4 months of exercise.

◆ GUIDELINES ◆

The general guideline for training frequency with clients who are new to training is for them to train two or three times per week on non-consecutive days. For advanced exercisers, 72 hours between successive high-effort training sessions is recommended. For example, schedule workouts on Mondays, Wednesdays, and Fridays or Tuesdays, Thursdays, and Saturdays if your beginning clients are going to train 3 days a week, and Mondays and Thursdays or Tuesdays and Fridays for your advanced clients who are following a 2-day-per-week program.

A 14-week study by Starkey et al. (1996) compared lower-body strength gains for 38 untrained adults who completed one or three sets of exercise. Both exercise groups attained similar increases in lower-body strength, as indicated by their changes in performance in knee extension and knee flexion exercises. Kraemer, Purvis, and Westcott (1996) reported on a 9-month study with college athletes who performed either single-set or multiple-set strength training. Both groups experienced similar strength improvement over the first 4 months of training, after which the multiple-set exercise program produced better results. In a more recent study by Kelly et al. (2007), also involving college-age students, superior strength gains were reported in knee extension exercises after 2 months using the multiple- (three-) set approach.

Studies involving older adults are especially relevant to understanding how to design programs for those over 50 years of age. For instance, Westcott, Greenberger, and Milius (1989) examined muscle endurance changes in 77 middle-aged men and women who completed one, two, or three sets of exercise over a 10-week training period. All three exercise groups experienced similar increases in upper-body muscle endurance, as indicated by their performance improvement in chin-ups and bar dips. With respect to muscle and body composition changes, both of the earlier mentioned studies involving 21- to 80-year-olds by Westcott and Guy (1996) and Westcott et al. (2009) resulted in increases of 2.4 and 3.1 pounds (1.1 and 1.4 kg), respectively, in lean muscle mass in response to single-set training. Recently, Westcott and associates (2008) conducted a 6-month study with senior women, all of whom performed single-set strength training (one set of 12 exercises). During the first 12 weeks they added 2.2 pounds (1.0 kg) of lean weight, and during the second 12 weeks they gained 2.5 pounds (1.1 kg) of lean weight. These findings indicate that older individuals can experience significant muscle development for at least 6 months using a single-set exercise protocol.

A 12-week study with senior subjects between 56 and 80 years of age (Campbell et al. 1994) incorporated multiple-set strength training (three sets of four

◆ GUIDELINES ◆

The general guideline to use when training clients new to strength training is to have them perform one set of each exercise. As training continues and their muscle fitness improves, you may want to have your clients perform additional sets. Advanced trainees who have a desire to develop higher levels of strength fitness and have the time should be encouraged to perform two or three sets of each exercise.

To get the best training effect when performing two or more sets of the same exercise, we suggest that you instruct your clients to rest approximately 2 minutes between sets. This break provides the time needed to replenish about 95 percent of the energy stores (creatine-phosphate) used during the previous exercise set. Taking shorter rest periods may reduce the number of repetitions completed on subsequent sets of an exercise (Miranda et al. 2007).

exercises). These older men and women averaged a 3-pound (1.4 kg) gain in lean weight (accompanied by a 7 percent increase in resting metabolic rate).

The results of these studies indicate that both single-set and multiple-set strength training protocols are effective for building muscle in beginning adult and older adult exercisers during the first 2 to 6 months of exercise. After the introductory strength training program begins to plateau, you will want to change your clients' exercise protocol in some way to facilitate further progress. If they have been performing one set of each exercise, consider switching them to a multiple-set training program (two or three sets per exercise depending on time availability). On the other hand, if they have been completing multiple sets of each exercise, additional benefits may be derived from reducing the training volume for a couple of weeks or by incorporating some of the high-intensity strength training programs presented in chapter 5.

PRINCIPLE 3: TRAINING RESISTANCE OR LOADS

The basic premise for developing strength training is that the amount of resistance or load used should challenge muscles to work harder than they are accustomed to working. This premise or process has traditionally been called the overload principle, and it indicates that training with progressively heavier resistance or loads will stimulate further strength development. For example, increasing a training load of 50 pounds (23 kg) in an exercise in one workout to 52.5 pounds (24 kg) in the next will create an overload on the muscles involved from the previous workout.

Trainers commonly assign training loads using a percentage of the client's one-repetition maximum, which represents the heaviest resistance or load that the person can lift one time. An abbreviation for the term *maximum load* is 1RM (repetition maximum). Loads and the number of repetitions that can be performed with a percentage of 1RM are inversely related: Lower resistance or loads permit more repetitions, and higher resistance or loads result in fewer repetitions. For example, a client may complete 16 repetitions with 60 percent of 1RM but only 4 repetitions with 90 percent of 1RM. Thus, as load assignments become heavier, the number of repetitions possible decreases. Most authorities advise that training loads between 60 and 90 percent of 1RM (Baechle and Earle 2006) are sufficient to create an overload. It is generally accepted that using 60 percent of maximum resistance has both a lower strength-building stimulus and a lower risk of injury, whereas training at 90 percent of maximum resistance provides a higher strength-building stimulus but a higher risk of injury. Several studies, however, have shown similar strength gains in adults and seniors working within the range of 60 to 90 percent of 1RM (Taaffe et al. 1996; Kerr et al. 1996; Chestnut and Docherty 1999; Bemben et al. 2000; Westcott 2002; Behm et al. 2002; Vincent and Braith 2002; Harris et al. 2004). Likewise, we are unaware of any studies that indicate that training with heavier loads carries a higher injury risk than training with lighter loads, as long as all repetitions are performed properly. For advanced participants, empirical evidence indicates that performing more repetitions with lower loads (e.g., 12 to 16 reps) places greater emphasis on muscle endurance and that doing fewer repetitions with higher loads (e.g., 4 to 8 reps) places greater emphasis on muscle strength. Nonetheless, it appears that older adults can safely and successfully attain relatively high levels of muscular conditioning by training with exercise loads between 60 and 90 percent of maximum.

Our recommendation for beginning older adult exercisers is to train with higher repetitions and lower loads (e.g., 12 to 16 reps), because this protocol provides more motor-learning opportunity and places less stress on unconditioned joint structures (tendons, ligaments, and fascia). As they increase their strength and musculoskeletal fitness, older adults may progressively train with higher loads and fewer repetitions (e.g., 8 to 12 reps). Seasoned senior strength trainers who are most interested in maximizing their muscle strength may then progress to relatively heavy loads (e.g., 4 to 8 reps) in selected multimuscle exercises (e.g., bench press, squat). Warm-up sets with lighter loads and more repetitions are highly recommended before performing relatively heavy exercise sets.

The American College of Sports Medicine (2010) exercise guidelines recommend that older adults begin strength training with loads or resistance that permits 10 to 15 repetitions, which corresponds to approximately 65 to 75 percent of 1RM. We concur with this recommendation, especially for frail older individuals. Most of the studies on senior strength training, however, have used between 8 and 12 repetitions, which corresponds to approximately 70 and 80 percent of 1RM. These include the studies conducted at Tufts University (Frontera et al. 1988; Fiatarone et al. 1990; Nelson et al. 1994), the University of Maryland (Koffler et al. 1992; Menkes et al. 1993; Pratley et al. 1994), and the South Shore YMCA (Westcott and Guy 1996; Westcott et al. 2009; Westcott et al. 2008).

Overall, research studies with subjects in their 60s, 70s, 80s, and 90s have shown excellent results with training loads between 70 and 80 percent of 1RM.

When using a multiple-set approach with clients, two popular options for assigning loads are available. One method involves instructing clients to perform all repetitions with the same load in each set of a given exercise. For example, a client could be instructed to complete three sets of 10 leg presses using 100 pounds (45 kg) for each set. Another approach to multiple-set training is to instruct clients to do the same number of repetitions with progressively heavier loads in each set

◆ GUIDELINES ◆

The general guideline for the amount of resistance or load that should be assigned is between 60 and 90 percent of 1RM. Assigning loads between 50 and 60 percent of 1RM may be preferable when training frail, older individuals during the initial weeks of a strength training program. For typically healthy adults, however, years of empirical evidence and several research studies clearly support assigning training loads between 70 and 80 percent of 1RM for older adults, which corresponds with 8 to 12 repetitions for most exercises. Periodically training with different percentages of 1RM will provide a change of pace that may have both physiological and psychological benefits. That approach, therefore, is strongly recommended.

of a given exercise. For example, the first set of 10 leg presses could be performed with 60 pounds (27 kg), the second set with 80 pounds (36 kg), and the third set with 100 pounds (45 kg). Some evidence (Faigenbaum et al. 1993, 1996) suggests that, for beginning participants, three exercise sets with progressively heavier loads may have a greater effect than three sets with the same resistance.

PRINCIPLE 4: NUMBER OF REPETITIONS

As noted in the previous section, an inverse relationship exists between the resistance used and the number of repetitions that can be completed. Most adults can complete about 4 repetitions with 90 percent of their 1RM, 8 repetitions with 80 percent of their 1RM, 12 repetitions with 70 percent of their 1RM, and 16 repetitions with 60 percent of their 1RM. In one study (Westcott 2002), 141 men and women completed as many repetitions as possible in a standard chest exercise using 75 percent of their 1RM. As shown in figure 2.2, the subjects performed an average of 10 repetitions at 75 percent of their 1RM. A small percentage of the participants performed fewer than 8 repetitions. These were power athletes who typically have a high percentage of type II (low-endurance) muscle fibers. Likewise, a small percentage of the participants completed more than 12 repetitions. These were aerobic athletes who typically have a high percentage of type I (high-endurance) muscle fibers. In a more recent study involving trained and untrained men (Shimano et al. 2006), it was determined that the training status of individuals has a minimal impact on the number of repetitions performed at a relative exercise intensity. While there are many repetition range options, we believe that most adults and seniors will experience excellent results training with between 8 and 12 repetitions.

For practical purposes it is not necessary to test to determine an individual's 1RM to find the correct training load. In most cases, if your client can complete

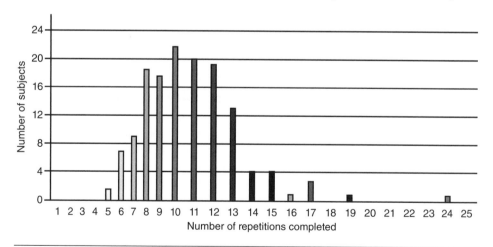

Figure 2.2 Distribution of repetitions completed with 75 percent of maximum weight load (*n* = 141).

Reprinted, by permission, from W.L. Westcott, 2007, *Strength training past 50,* 2nd ed. (Champaign, IL: Human Kinetics), 147.

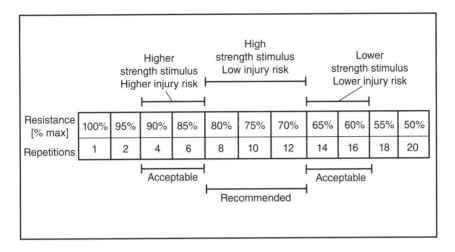

Figure 2.3 Resistance and repetitions relationships for the recommended training protocols.

8 to 12 repetitions with proper form, the load is equal to approximately 70 to 80 percent of 1RM and is therefore an appropriate training resistance.

Just as productive load assignments fall within a range, effective training has a corresponding repetition range. Figure 2.3 illustrates a continuum of resistance and repetitions relationships for the recommended strength training protocols.

Higher repetitions (more than 12 reps) with lower loads may be advisable during the initial training period, especially for frail older people and older adults who are just learning proper exercise technique. Fewer repetitions (fewer than 8 reps) may be advisable as clients become stronger and want to train with a higher percentage of their maximum resistance.

◆ GUIDELINES ◆

The general guideline for older adults is to perform 8 to 12 repetitions per set, performed with proper technique and to the point of muscle fatigue. This effort is typically accomplished with loads between 70 and 80 percent of 1RM.

PRINCIPLE 5: EXERCISE SELECTION

Although a sound strength training program should address all the major muscle groups (ACSM 2006), some follow a preferred-exercise approach. That is, they select certain exercises that are more popular, more convenient, or more satisfying to perform. For example, many strength training enthusiasts emphasize the bench press, which is an excellent exercise for the pectoralis major, anterior deltoid, and triceps muscles. But if equal attention is not given to the opposing muscles (latissimus dorsi, teres major, posterior deltoid, and biceps), muscle imbalance is likely to develop around the shoulder joint because of a relatively strong chest musculature and a relatively weak upper-back musculature. Such imbalances may lead to poor posture and musculoskeletal injuries.

Major Muscle Groups

To encourage balanced muscle development, the program that you design for your clients should include exercises for opposing muscle groups. For example, the leg extension for the quadriceps muscles could be paired with the leg curl for the hamstrings muscles in a machine exercise workout, and the biceps curl for the front of the arm could be followed by the triceps extension for the back of the arm in a free-weight workout.

> ### Muscle Imbalance
>
> The condition in which one muscle is disproportionately stronger than its opposing muscle.

Also important is to include at least one exercise for the quadriceps, hamstrings, pectoralis major, latissimus dorsi, deltoids, biceps, triceps, low back, abdominal muscles, and upper trapezius.

Arrangement of Exercises

The following are examples of machine and free-weight exercise selections and a suggested order for their inclusion in the workout (see table 2.1). The order follows the principle of exercising the larger muscles first. A machine program might begin with the leg extension for the quadriceps muscles followed by the leg curl for the hamstrings muscles, whereas a free-weight program might begin with dumbbell squats that work the front and back leg muscles concurrently.

> ### Opposing Muscles
>
> Muscles that produce the opposite joint movements of the prime mover muscles. For example, the biceps and triceps muscles of the arm act as opposing muscles; the biceps serve as prime movers for elbow flexion, and the triceps serve as prime movers for elbow extension.

The next group of exercises work the torso muscles, including the pectoralis major, latissimus dorsi, and deltoid groups. Sample machine and free-weight exercises, respectively, that could be selected are chest crossovers or dumbbell flys for the pectoralis major, pullovers or dumbbell one-arm rows for the latissimus dorsi, and lateral raises or dumbbell lateral raises for the deltoids.

The next training sequence exercises the biceps and triceps muscles, which may be worked effectively with machine or dumbbell arm curls and machine or dumbbell arm extensions. Performing these exercises toward the end of the workout avoids fatiguing the arm muscles, which would reduce the number of repetitions performed in the upper body exercises.

TABLE 2.1

Recommended Performance Sequence of Machine and Free-Weight Exercises

Muscle group	Machine exercise	Free-weight exercise
Quadriceps	Leg extension (p. 40)	Dumbbell squat (p. 52)
Hamstrings	Leg curl (p. 42)	Dumbbell squat (p. 52)
Hip adductors	Hip adduction (p. 46)	
Hip abductors	Hip abduction (p. 48)	
Gastrocnemius	Heel raise (p. 50)	Dumbbell heel raise (p. 60)
Pectoralis major	Chest crossover (p. 86)	Dumbbell bench press (p. 110)
Latissimus dorsi	Pullover (p. 96)	Dumbbell one-arm row (p. 114)
Deltoids	Lateral raise (p. 92)	Dumbbell lateral raise (p. 116)
Biceps	Biceps curl (p. 132)	Dumbbell standing curl (p. 142)
Triceps	Triceps extension (p. 134)	Dumbbell overhead triceps extension (p. 150)
Low back	Low-back extension (p. 70)	Trunk extension (p. 80)
Abdominals	Abdominal flexion (p. 72)	Exercise ball trunk curl (p. 84)
Obliques	Rotary torso (p. 74)	Twisting trunk curl (p. 82)
Neck extensors	Neck extension (p. 158)	Dumbbell shrug (p. 162)
Neck flexors	Neck flexion (p. 160)	
Forearms	Wrist roller (p. 272)	Dumbbell incline curl (p. 144)

The muscle groups worked last in the workout should be the midsection and neck. Because these muscles serve as stabilizers in most exercises, the best approach is to avoid fatiguing them until the end of the workout. Recommended midsection exercises include the low-back machine and abdominal machine, as well as trunk extensions and trunk curls with bodyweight resistance. The neck muscles may be exercised safely and effectively on the neck machine or with dumbbell shoulder shrugs. Our research with frail nursing home patients revealed excellent

◆ GUIDELINES ◆

Include at least one exercise for the quadriceps, hamstrings, pectoralis major, latissimus dorsi, deltoids, biceps, triceps, low back, abdominal, and upper trapezius muscles or include multimuscle exercises that cumulatively address all these muscle groups. Besides performing these exercises, older adults may benefit from exercises that strengthen the adductor and abductor muscles of the hip, the oblique muscles that surround the midsection, the calf muscles, and the forearm muscles. Also, exercises should be arranged in the workout so that larger muscle groups are exercised first.

results with neck strengthening exercises, enabling clients to hold their heads erect for enhanced breathing, swallowing, speaking, and seeing (Westcott 2009).

Besides using the basic exercises, older adults may benefit by strengthening the adductor and abductor muscles of the hip, the oblique muscles that surround the midsection, the calf muscles, and the forearm muscles. Consider including exercises for these muscle groups in the overall training program on a regular basis if possible.

For frail older people and poorly conditioned seniors, a few multimuscle exercises may be more appropriate than a program of several single-muscle exercises. For example, performing a set of leg presses (quadriceps and hamstrings), chest presses (pectoralis major, anterior deltoids, triceps), seated rows (latissimus dorsi, posterior deltoids, biceps), abdominal curls (rectus abdominis), and low-back extensions (erector spinae) works essentially all the major muscle groups in a brief (10-minute) training session.

Single-Muscle Exercises

Exercises that address one major muscle group in a rotary movement, such as leg extensions for the quadriceps muscles. Rotary exercises feature one joint action with a circular movement around the joint axis.

Multiple-Muscle Exercises

Exercises that use two or more major muscle groups simultaneously to perform a linear movement, such as leg presses for the quadriceps and hamstrings muscles. Linear exercises involve two joint actions that produce a straight pushing or pulling movement.

Although performing a specific exercise for each of the muscle groups previously mentioned may be advisable, time and equipment limitations may make this difficult to accomplish. If this is the case, a smaller number of multiple-muscle exercises may provide a similar conditioning effect. Whether clients perform many or few exercises, they should train the major muscle groups in a comprehensive manner that increases overall strength and function.

PRINCIPLE 6: TRAINING PROGRESSION

As training continues and muscles become stronger, people can complete more repetitions with a given load. Increasing the number of repetitions is a logical approach to training progression and is a productive procedure up to a point. For best results, however, individuals should complete each exercise set within the time frame of the anaerobic energy system—typically a range of 8 to 12 repetitions, which corresponds to about 50 to 70 seconds (6-second repetitions) of continuous training effort. Based on this standard training protocol of 8 to 12 repetitions, you should slightly increase loads whenever clients can complete 12 repetitions with proper form during two consecutive workouts. Although no studies address specific load increments, our observations suggest that resistance increases of 5 percent or less provide a safe and productive training progression. As mentioned previously, periodically instructing clients to use a different percentage of 1RM will provide a change of pace that may have both physiological and psychological benefits and is therefore strongly recommended.

Encourage clients to increase the number of repetitions first and then instruct them to increase the amount of the load or resistance in an exercise. This protocol is known as a double progressive program—a conservative training approach that reduces risks of overtraining injuries and may be applied to a variety of exercise programs.

> ### Double Progressive Program
>
> Systematically increasing the training demand by first adding more repetitions and then adding more resistance.

Summary
of Strength Training Principles for Older Adults

- **Training frequency:** The general guideline for training frequency with clients who are new to training is for them to train two or three times per week on nonconsecutive days. For advanced exercisers, 72 hours between successive high-effort training sessions is recommended. For example, schedule workouts on Mondays, Wednesdays, and Fridays or Tuesdays, Thursdays, and Saturdays if clients are going to train 3 days a week, and Mondays and Thursdays or Tuesdays and Fridays if they are following a 2-day-per-week program.

- **Number of sets:** The general guideline to use when training clients new to strength training is to have them perform one set of each exercise. As training continues and their muscle fitness improves, you may want to have your clients perform additional sets. Advanced trainees who have a desire to develop higher levels of strength fitness and have the time should be encouraged to perform two or three sets of each exercise.

  To get the best training effect when performing two or more sets of the same exercise, we suggest that you instruct your clients to rest approximately 2 minutes between sets. This break provides the time needed to replenish about 95 percent of the energy stores (creatine-phosphate) used during the previous exercise set. Taking shorter rest periods may reduce the number of repetitions completed on subsequent sets of an exercise (Miranda et al. 2007).

- **Training resistance or loads:** The general guideline for the amount of resistance or load that should be assigned is between 60 and 90 percent of 1RM. Assigning loads between 50 and 60 percent of 1RM, however, may be preferable when training frail, older people during the initial weeks of a strength training program. But for typically healthy older adults, years of empirical evidence and several research studies clearly

(continued)

Summary *(continued)*

support assigning training loads between 70 and 80 percent of 1RM. Periodically training with different percentages of 1RM will provide a change of pace that may have both physiological and psychological benefits.

- *Number of repetitions:* The general guideline for older adults is to perform 8 to 12 repetitions per set, performed with proper technique and to the point of muscle fatigue. This effort is typically accomplished with loads between 70 and 80 percent of 1RM.

- *Exercise selection:* Include at least one exercise for the quadriceps, hamstrings, pectoralis major, latissimus dorsi, deltoids, biceps, triceps, erector spinae, rectus abdominis, and upper trapezius, or use multi-muscle exercises that cumulatively address all these muscle groups. Besides performing these exercises, older adults may benefit from exercises that strengthen the adductor and abductor muscles of the hip, the oblique muscles that surround the midsection, the calf muscles, and the forearm muscles. Also, exercises should be arranged in the workout so that larger muscle groups are exercised first.

- *Training progression:* For practical purposes, load increases of 1.0 to 2.5 pounds (0.5 to 1.0 kg) are recommended, depending on the client's strength level. Most dumbbell sets should be increased by 1 pound (0.5 kg) up to 15 pounds (7 kg) and then increased in 5-pound (2.3 kg) increments. The use of 1-pound (0.5 kg) magnetic add-on weights with larger dumbbells is an option. Another option for clients who are using weight-stack machines that do not have a 1-pound (0.5 kg) increment is to use lighter add-on weights to keep the resistance progressions less than 5 percent.

TEACHING STRATEGIES

Teaching strength training principles, concepts, and techniques to older adults requires a thorough knowledge of program design variables and correct exercise movements, as well as strong sensitivity to the uniqueness of this group of clients. Successful instruction of the various exercises also involves a well-planned and sequential presentation of exercise techniques, as well as an understanding of strength training procedures that will make your teaching approaches safe and effective. Just as important as being able to educate older adults is determining how to motivate them to begin and continue a personal program of strength training that you have designed for them.

Motivating older adults to train correctly and consistently can be a challenging task. Although some older adults may be enthusiastic about starting an exercise program, most require some extrinsic motivation to maintain their interest and adherence, especially during the first few weeks of training. Furthermore, the newness of the activity, the fear of injury, the potential embarrassment of appearing weak or uncoordinated, the concern about giving a good effort without getting noticeable results, as well as various misconceptions and distractions, are all factors that make it more difficult for older adults, compared with those who are younger, to master strength training skills.

Successful instructors do not merely teach how to perform exercises—they actually shape seniors' attitudes towards strength training. For best results, both the process and the product of sensible strength training must be positive experiences. The following teaching strategies have proved effective for motivating adults to participate in strength training activities with higher levels of confidence and competence, all of which serve to reinforce their exercise efforts.

Four Key Focus Phrases

You should say four key phrases to each participant during every exercise session: *Hello, Goodbye, Thank you*, and the person's name. Of course, *Hello* and *Goodbye* need be used only once, when the client arrives and departs. *Thank you* may be used as often as appropriate, and you should frequently speak the person's name. These four focus phrases make new exercisers feel noticed, valued, and appreciated as participants in the strength training program.

> ### Four Key Focus Phrases
>
> Use with each participant during every class:
>
> - Hello!
> - Goodbye!
> - Thank you!
> - Person's name (Jim, Mrs. Brown, Dr. Finley)

10 Components of Interactive Teaching

Although the four key focus phrases represent common courtesy, several suggested dialogues should be standard language when training older adults, especially during the learning stages of strength training. We refer to these as the 10 teaching components. These instructional interactions have proved helpful in large-scale senior strength training programs (Westcott 1995b) and should facilitate positive and productive exercise experiences for new participants.

1. *Understandable performance objectives.* The first and perhaps most important instructional step is clearly communicating to your client the primary performance objective for a particular class session. That is, you tell the exerciser specifically what you want him or her to accomplish during the workout. This step provides training direction and enables the client to focus on the major task rather than less substantive details.

2. *Concise instruction with precise demonstration.* After you have presented the performance objective, provide simple instructions about how to accomplish it by telling the client exactly what he or she should do. Because showing is typically more effective than telling, the next instructional step is modeling the desired exercise actions. The demonstration phase should be deliberate rather than rushed, and you should repeat it as many times as necessary. Introduce

additional exercises only after your clients' exercise form and breathing patterns are flawless. Always point out key aspects of proper technique during the demonstration.

3. *Attentive supervision.* Never assume that people understand exactly how to do what you have just demonstrated or that they can do so without coaching. Staying beside your client during his or her first attempts to replicate the correct exercise movement patterns is an effective approach. Many older people lack confidence in their physical ability, and others may have limited neuromuscular coordination. In either case, by being watchful you can boost your clients' confidence and reduce their fear of making a mistake. Attentive supervision is a powerful motivator for most new exercisers.

4. *Appropriate assistance.* To assure safe and successful workout performance among older adults, you may need to provide some form of manual assistance. This may include assisting clients onto a machine and making needed adjustments, helping them fasten a seat belt, handing them free weights, guiding them through an exercise movement, reminding them when to exhale and inhale, stabilizing their posture, or making minor adjustments to body-part positions during the execution of exercises. Although younger exercisers may not be receptive to manual assistance, most older adults appreciate a helping hand as they attempt to master new exercises.

> ## Recommended Reading
>
> Baechle, T., and R. Earle. (2006). *Weight Training: Steps to Success* (3rd edition). Champaign, IL: Human Kinetics.
>
> Baechle, T., and R. Earle. (2005). *Fitness Weight Training* (2nd edition). Champaign, IL: Human Kinetics.
>
> Wilmore, J., D. Costill, and W.L. Kenney. (2008). *Physiology of Sport and Exercise* (4th edition). Champaign, IL: Human Kinetics.

5. *One task at a time.* Presenting several exercises simultaneously or requesting that older adults complete sequential performance tasks may be confusing or even overwhelming. Make only one instructional request at a time. Providing a single directive increases the probability that your client will successfully complete each task and feel more physically competent and mentally confident.

6. *Gradual progression.* Although training progression is important in strength training, the progression should occur relatively slowly with seniors. You should never introduce a follow-up task until the first task has been performed properly, and you should always present simple actions before more complex ones. For older people, the approach to strength training should resemble a series of hurdles; the first hurdle should be very low and each successive hurdle should be just a little bit higher.

7. *Positive reinforcement.* Most older exercisers experience some degree of uncertainty over the effectiveness of their efforts. Positive reinforcement in the form of encouraging comments, personal compliments, and pats on the shoulder are simple ways to support a person's training progress. Make such comments immediately, or as soon as possible, following the correct execution of an exer-

cise or the accomplishment of a primary goal for the workout. Although you should frequently give positive reinforcement, such performance affirmations must be merited and sincerely offered if they are to be meaningful.

8. *Specific feedback.* Positive reinforcement is also more effective when coupled with specific feedback that provides useful information about the exercise performance. Giving a reason for a positive comment makes it more valuable as an educational and motivational tool. Saying "Good job, Jim," may be emotionally reinforcing, but saying "Good job, Jim—you performed all 10 leg curls through a full range of movement" is more informative and more powerful. First, it shows Jim that you were actually observing his exercise form; second, it increases the likelihood that Jim will again use full movement range the next time he performs leg curls.

9. *Careful questioning.* Older adults are usually communicative, but they may not volunteer information that could be useful in fine-tuning their training program. By asking relevant questions you can learn how your clients are responding to the exercise experience. Whenever possible, phrase questions in a manner that promotes thoughtful answers rather than yes or no responses. For example, instead of asking Mrs. Jones if she felt muscle fatigue on a set of leg extensions, you could ask her where she felt fatigue (quadriceps muscles, knee joint, and so on) and how much fatigue she experienced (low, moderate, high).

10. *Pre- and postexercise dialogue.* Dialogue should proceed and follow each exercise session. You should take a couple of minutes before and after each workout to learn some of the participant's perspectives. Pre- and post-training conversations provide opportunities for encouragement and reinforcement, as well as time to become better acquainted with the client.

Summary
of Teaching Strategies

A successful educational and motivational strategy for older adult exercisers should include

- understandable performance objectives,
- concise instruction with precise demonstration,
- attentive supervision,
- appropriate assistance,
- a request to perform one task at a time,
- gradual progression in complexity,
- positive reinforcement following correct performances,
- specific feedback,
- careful questioning, and
- pre- and postexercise dialogue (which should always involve the key phrases, such as Hello, Goodbye, Thank you, and the client's name).

Table 2.2 presents detailed information about teaching strategies, related sample instructional statements, and specific task descriptions. These simple dialogues are only examples of how to implement the 10 suggested client interactions.

TABLE 2.2

Sample Instructional Statements
for Implementing Desired Teaching Strategies

	General teaching strategy	Sample instructional statement	Specific task description
1.	Understandable performance objective	This is what I would like you to accomplish today.	Your primary task is to exhale during the lifting phase of every repetition.
2.	Concise instruction with precise demonstration	This is how I would like you to breathe when you lift the weight stack.	Watch me breathe out through my mouth during every lifting action.
3.	Attentive supervision	I will watch you as you perform the leg extension exercise.	Let me hear you exhale every time you lift the weight stack.
4.	Appropriate assistance	I will exhale loud enough for you to hear me during each of your lifting repetitions.	Try to exhale when you hear me breathing out.
5.	One task at a time	Remember, all I want you to do is exhale when you lift the weight.	Just try to breathe out when you hear me breathe out.
6.	Gradual progression	Don't worry about when to inhale. That will be our next task.	If you breathe out when you lift the dumbbell, you should automatically breathe in when you lower the dumbbell.
7.	Positive reinforcement	You are doing very well today.	I'm really pleased with your progress.
8.	Specific feedback	Your breathing technique is right on target.	You are exhaling evenly throughout every lifting movement.
9.	Careful questioning	Do you understand the proper breathing for this exercise?	How does the breathing pattern feel to you?
10.	Pre- and postexercise dialogue	Let's talk for a couple minutes about today's exercise experience.	I think you had a great workout, and it looks as if you've mastered the breathing technique. Please tell me how you feel about today's training session.

C H A P T E R

3

Exercise Execution Procedures and Instruction

Chapter 2 discussed how to approach teaching and motivating older adults to perform strength training exercises properly and on a regular basis. This chapter begins with a presentation of the scientific basis for movement ranges and speed, breathing sequence, and warm-up and cool-down procedures that we advocate and is followed by suggestions about how to instruct clients in the proper execution of machine, free-weight, and stability ball exercises.

Many older adults have had little or no experience performing specific resistance exercises, so strength training is an unfamiliar activity for them. Although some seniors are relatively fit, most have lost a considerable amount of muscle mass and strength. Many others have physical performance difficulties because of excessive body fat, poor balance, lower- or upper-back pain, various injuries, illnesses, infirmities, and postsurgical complications, as well as motor learning limitations and general frailty. With these issues in mind, we recommend a three-tiered strength training approach for beginning senior exercisers.

1. *Foundational strength training.* Our first objective is to have older adults strengthen their major muscle groups as safely, effectively, and efficiently as possible. We therefore begin with machine exercises that provide supportive structure, body stabilization, and fixed movement patterns. We believe that beginning with machine exercises enhances older participants' training competence and confidence, as well as reduces the risk of injury. We refer to machine exercises as foundational strength training.

2. *Fundamental strength training.* Our second objective is to have older adults perform standard free-weight exercises that require balance, postural control, body stabilization, and coordinated movement patterns. Although some free-weight exercises involve a bench, most are performed from a standing position and require considerable core muscle activation. Because movement possibilities are almost unlimited, free-weight exercises call for greater motor learning and coordinated muscle control. We call free-weight exercises fundamental strength training.

3. *Functional strength training.* Although we believe that machine and free-weight exercises are highly functional for older adults, our next progression is to even less stable forms of strength training and faster movement speeds. We use exercise balls to increase core muscle involvement, and we train with medicine

balls (using various throwing movements) to speed up the muscle actions safely. We believe that these training procedures are productive for enhancing body balance, core stability, and muscle coordination, as well as for activating more fast-twitch motor units. In our opinion, this type of functional strength training should be performed in addition to machine and free-weight exercises.

One aspect of functional strength training that appears to be particularly applicable to older adults is power training. Power is essentially the product of muscle force multiplied by movement speed. Because aging reduces muscle power at a faster rate than it does muscle strength (ACSM 2010), we recommend that seniors perform some power training exercises. We prefer medicine ball power exercises to fast lifting movements with machines or free weights. Unlike a fast-moving weight stack or barbell, the medicine ball can be released at the end of the action with minimum stress on joint structures. Excellent examples of medicine ball exercises can be found in publications by Mediate and Faigenbaum (2004). Another alternative for power training is resistance bands. If elastic band equipment is to be used in power training your clients, you should instruct them to perform the concentric phase of exercises as quickly as possible and then control the eccentric phase back to the starting position. For example in the bench press, instruct clients to push away (concentric phase) from the chest as quickly as possible until the elbows are almost straight, and then to control the speed of the return movement (eccentric phase) back to the starting position at the chest. Because the tension increases as the elastic band lengthens during the concentric movement phase (straightening of the elbows), the speed toward the end of the exercise slows the momentum and therefore decreases the likelihood of injury.

FULL RANGE OF MOVEMENT

The term *full range* implies the performance of an exercise from the position of full muscle stretch to the position of full muscle contraction, assuming that the client is able to do so without pain. Note that when the targeted muscle group (e.g., quadriceps) is fully contracted, the opposing muscle group (e.g., hamstrings) is fully stretched. Therefore, full-range training simultaneously strengthens and stretches the muscle pairs that control joint actions, and it enhances joint flexibility (Westcott 1995). Full-range exercise movements are also necessary for developing full-range muscle strength (Graves et al. 1989; Jones et al. 1988). Researchers at the University of Florida Medical School showed that people with low muscle strength in positions of trunk extension were more likely to experience low-back pain. They also discovered that training the low-back muscles through the full movement range markedly increased trunk extension strength and significantly decreased low-back discomfort (Risch et al. 1993). Performing full-range strength training exercises also may enhance physical performance. Senior golfers who performed full-range strengthening and stretching exercises improved their driving ability (measured by club head speed) by 6 percent after 8 weeks of training, compared with no improvement in those who did not exercise (Westcott et al. 1996). Therefore, such training encourages a good balance of strength across joints, improves flexibility, and helps increase functional movement ranges, which are especially important for older adults who have been physically inactive. For seniors who have been more active, full-range training can contribute to better performance in many sports.

Although full-range training is strongly recommended, there are exceptions. Two cardinal rules apply here: Training should not cause pain during any phase of the exercise movement, and the range of movement should never exceed normal joint limits. Ranges of pain-free movement vary among individuals, especially older adults, many of whom have arthritic conditions. In 2007 the Arthritis Foundation reported that over 46 million adults had some form of arthritis. Great care should be taken to eliminate exercises that produce immediate or delayed discomfort in the joints, or at least abbreviate the range to permit pain-free movement. Older adults should not exceed a comfortable range of movement—an unnecessary effort at best, because continued training typically results in an extended range of pain-free movement. For example, full-depth free-weight squats are not recommended for senior trainees. Chapter 4 provides some helpful suggestions regarding selection and modifications of standard training exercises.

> ### Perform Exercises Through the Full Range of Movement
>
> You should instruct clients to perform all repetitions through a full range of movement, provided that they can accomplish this movement without pain.

CONTROLLED MOVEMENT SPEED

Movement speed refers to the time required to perform each exercise repetition (i.e., to lift and lower the weight or machine arm). Faster repetition speeds generally create more momentum and result in less consistent muscle force production. As momentum increases, so does the loss of movement control and the potential for injury. Conversely, slower movement speeds create less momentum and more consistent muscle tension throughout the range of movement. Performing repetitions in a slow, controlled manner enhances exercise safety and is recommended for strength training programs for older adults. The American College of Sports Medicine (2006), for example, recommended repetition speeds of about 6 seconds, and support for that recommendation comes from many key studies with senior subjects. The Tufts University studies (Frontera 1988; Fiatarone 1990; Nelson 1994) used a 3-second lifting phase and a 3-second lowering phase, whereas the University of Maryland studies (Koffler 1992; Menkes 1993; Pratley 1994) and the South Shore YMCA studies (Westcott and Guy 1996; Westcott et al. 2009) used a 2-second lifting phase and a 4-second lowering phase. Although 6-second repetitions serve as a sensible training guideline, shorter and longer repetition speeds may be equally effective as long as the movements are performed under control. We define controlled speed as a movement (lifting or lowering) in which the client can stop at any point. That is, the exerciser is using muscle force alone and not momentum to complete a repetition. We concur with ACSM's earlier 6-second repetition recommendation and suggest 2 seconds for the more difficult concentric muscle action (typically the lifting movement during which the muscle shortens) and 4 seconds for the less demanding eccentric muscle action (typically the lowering movement during which the muscle lengthens).

Athletes often use fast training speeds to improve their performance in competitive sports. Older adults need not do so unless they are well trained and are seeking to improve their athletic performance. Moving relatively heavy weights at fast speeds places considerable stress on the joint structures at the start and end of each repetition, which increases the risk of injury. When using machines and free weights, make sure that your clients perform every repetition under complete control. Training in this manner increases exercise effectiveness and decreases the risk of injury. A simple way to help trainees determine whether they are moving too fast is to administer the stop test. Ask the client to stop a repetition being performed at a specified point in the movement range. If the client cannot stop, she or he is performing the repetition too quickly.

Although we strongly recommend that older adults perform relatively slow repetitions when using machines and free weights, we believe that it may be appropriate for athletic seniors to incorporate some fast-movement training as well. Research reveals that as we age our muscle fibers decrease in size and strength. This age-related muscle atrophy affects the type II (fast-twitch) fibers more than it does the type I (slow-twitch) fibers, leading to progressive loss of the strength needed in everyday activities that require movement speed and muscle power. To slow the loss of fast-twitch fibers, many fitness experts advocate resistance exercises that feature fast movements to activate these fibers. Power or fast-movement training has been found not only to produce increases in strength and power among older adults but also to be safe and well tolerated. In addition, fast-movement training also has been shown to produce adaptive neuromuscular changes that should reduce the likelihood of falls and disability among older adults (Caserotti 2008). Thus, we suggest that you include some power exercises using medicine balls in programs for older adults who are able to handle at least the average loads presented in chapter 4 (tables 4.1 through 4.4). Our senior subjects who performed a few medicine ball throws following their standard strength workout improved their power performance more than twice as much as those who performed only strength training (Westcott, unpublished data 2008).

Control Movement Speed

Instruct clients to perform each repetition in about 6 seconds, using 2 seconds for the concentric muscle action (lifting phase) and 4 seconds during the eccentric muscle action (lowering phase). Consider adding fast-movement exercises to workouts using medicine balls, if clients can safely perform such exercises.

BREATHING

Older adults must breathe properly during strength training workouts. Regardless of the exercise effort, your clients should never hold their breath (referred to as engaging the Valsalva maneuver) when performing strength training exercises. The Valsalva maneuver produces excessive internal pressure that restricts blood flow back to the heart, contributing to high blood pressure responses and possibly to lightheadedness, dizziness, and even blackouts. By breathing continuously throughout every repetition of an exercise, your clients will avoid these undesirable effects.

Breathe Correctly

Instruct clients to exhale during the more demanding concentric muscle action (lifting phase) and inhale during the less demanding eccentric muscle action (lowering phase) of each repetition. Emphasize that they should never hold their breath during the performance of a strength training exercise.

WARM-UP AND COOL-DOWN

Just as it is important to warm up before aerobic activity and cool down afterward, senior exercisers should do the same when strength training. The few minutes required for these activities is time well spent.

Because strength training is a high-effort physical activity that places significant demands on the musculoskeletal system, you should prepare your clients for each workout with a few minutes of warm-up activity. The purpose of the warm-up is to cause a gradual shift of the muscular and cardiovascular systems from a resting to a working state. Standard warm-up exercises include walking, cycling, and stepping. This activity should be followed by a few calisthenic exercises such as knee bends, side bends, and trunk curls. The warm-up period should typically last for 5 to 10 minutes. If there is any concern regarding the readiness of the targeted muscles and joints for a particular exercise, performing a preliminary set with approximately half the training load provides an excellent exercise-specific warm-up. Clients should complete about 10 standard-speed repetitions with the lighter load (approximately 50 percent of 1RM) before performing the first set with the assigned load.

The cool-down is essentially a warm-up in reverse. It helps the muscular and cardiovascular systems gradually shift from a working to a resting state. The cool-down is particularly important for older adults because blood that accumulates in the lower legs following vigorous exercise can cause undesirable changes in blood pressure that may lead to cardiovascular complications. Five to 10 minutes of cool-down activity facilitates a smooth return to resting circulation and blood flow back to the heart. Recommended cool-down exercises include easy walking and cycling followed by stretching exercises. Although time limitations may tend to crowd

---

Warm Up and Cool Down Properly

Instruct your clients to perform 5 to 10 minutes of light exercise before and after each strength training workout to assist the body's transition between resting and exercise states.

the warm-up and cool-down segments, these important transitional activities should be a standard part of each training session (see figure 3.1, *a–d*).

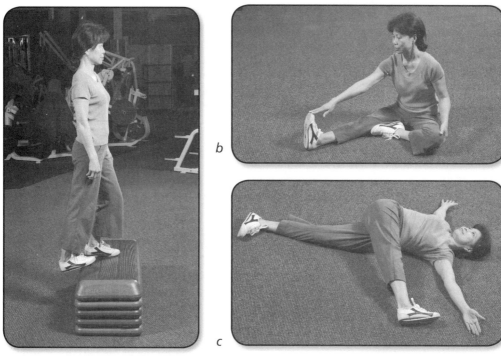

a *b* *c*

Figure 3.1 Stretching exercises during the cool-down segment may include *(a)* the step stretch, *(b)* the number four stretch, *(c)* the letter T stretch, and *(d)* the doorway stretch.

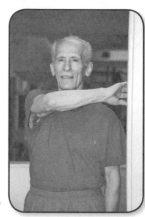

d

Summary of Training Procedures

To enhance training effectiveness and reduce the risk of injury, senior exercisers should perform full-range movements (without experiencing discomfort) using controlled movement speeds (6 seconds per repetition). Instruct clients to breathe continuously throughout each repetition, exhaling during the concentric muscle action and inhaling during the eccentric muscle action. Older adults should begin each strength training session with a few minutes of warm-up activity and should conclude the workout with at least 5 minutes of cool-down exercise.

MACHINE AND FREE-WEIGHT EXERCISE INSTRUCTION

This section of the chapter is designed to provide you with suggestions about what to say to clients when instructing them on the performance of each exercise in this book. Many of the technique recommendations presented can also be found in other books that we have published, such as Baechle and Earle (2008), Westcott and Baechle (2007), Baechle and Earle (2006), Baechle and Earle (2005), Earle and Baechle (2004), Westcott (2003), and Westcott (1995). After providing directions about how to get your clients into the proper position (beginning position) to start an exercise, we provide specific instructional statements that you can use to help them complete the (upward and downward) phases of each of the exercises in this book.

Recommended Reading

Baechle, T., and R. Earle. (2008). *Essentials of Strength Training and Conditioning* (3rd edition). Champaign, IL: Human Kinetics.

Baechle, T., and R. Earle. (2006). *Weight Training: Steps to Success* (3rd edition). Champaign, IL: Human Kinetics.

Baechle, T., and R. Earle. (2005). *Fitness Weight Training* (2nd edition). Champaign, IL: Human Kinetics.

Earle, R.W., and T.R. Baechle. (2004). *Essentials of Personal Training.* Champaign, IL: Human Kinetics.

Girouard, C., and B. Hurley. (1995). Does strength training inhibit gains in range of motion from flexibility training in older adults? *Medicine and Science in Sports and Exercise* 27 (10): 1444–1449.

Golding, L., C. Myers, and W. Sinning. (1989). *Y's Way to Physical Fitness.* Champaign, IL: Human Kinetics.

Mediate, P., and A.D. Faigenbaum. (2004). *Medicine Ball For All Training Handbook.* Montery, CA: Coaches Choice.

Westcott, W.L., and T.R. Baechle. (2006). *Strength Training Past 50* (2nd edition). Champaign, IL: Human Kinetics.

Westcott, W., W. Martin, R. La Rosa Loud, and S. Stoddard. (2008). Research update: Protein and body composition. *Fitness Management* 24 (5): 50–53.

Westcott, W. (1995). Strength training for life: Keeping fit. *Nautilus Magazine* Spring 4 (2): 5–7.

Westcott, W., F. Dolan, and T. Cavicchi. (1996). Golf and strength training are compatible activities. *Strength and Conditioning* 18 (4): 54–56.

Westcott, W. (1994). Strength training for life: Weightloads: Go figure. *Nautilus Magazine* Fall 3 (4): 5–7.

Westcott, W. (1987). *Building Strength at the YMCA.* Champaign, IL: Human Kinetics.

LEG EXTENSION

Muscles most involved: quadriceps

Beginning Position

Help your client adjust the seat so that the knees are in line with the axis of rotation of the machine (where the machine arm pivots). The axis of rotation is indicated by a red dot on most resistance machines. After the seat is adjusted, instruct your client to sit with the back firmly against the seat pad, the ankles behind the roller pad, the knees flexed about 90 degrees, and the hands gripping the handles. Direct your client to complete the exercise in the following manner.

Upward Movement Phase

1. Push the roller pad slowly upward until your knees are extended.
2. Exhale throughout the upward movement.

Downward Movement Phase

1. Return the roller pad slowly to the starting position.
2. Inhale throughout the lowering movement.

Common Errors, Problems, and Modifications

The most common errors in this exercise are arching the back and stopping the lifting action short of the fully extended knee position. Using the attached seatbelt and contracting the abdominal muscles will help prevent back arching. Using a lighter resistance and concentrating on completing the extension movement are effective for attaining full contraction of the quadriceps muscles. If the client experiences knee pain, the exercise should be restricted to the pain-free range of movement.

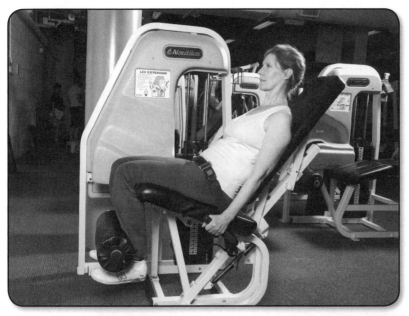

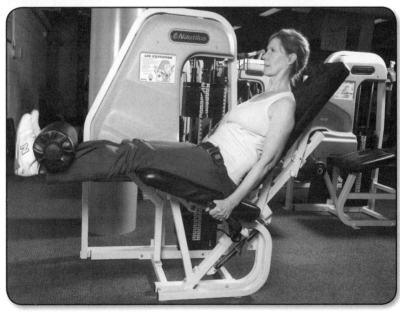

LEG CURL

Muscles most involved: hamstrings

Beginning Position

Help your client adjust the seat so that the knee joints are in line with the axis of rotation of the machine. After the seat is adjusted, instruct your client to sit with the back firmly against the seat pad, to position the lower legs between the roller pads with the knees extended, and to grip the handles. Direct your client to complete the exercise in the following manner.

Backward Movement Phase

1. Pull the roller pad slowly backward until your knees are fully flexed.
2. Exhale throughout the pulling movement.

Forward Movement Phase

1. Allow the roller pads to return slowly to the starting position.
2. Inhale throughout the return movement.

Common Errors, Problems, and Modifications

As with the leg extension, exercisers tend to arch the back and to abbreviate the movement range when performing the leg curl exercise. Consciously contracting the abdominal muscles should enable a better trunk position, and using a lighter resistance will facilitate achieving a full range of movement.

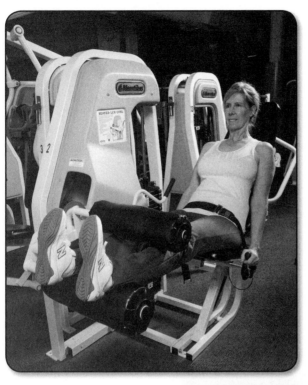

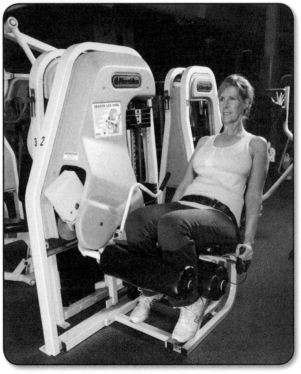

LEG PRESS

Muscles most involved: quadriceps, hamstrings, gluteals

Beginning Position

Help your client adjust the seat so that the knees are flexed to 90 degrees or less. After the seat is adjusted, direct him or her to sit with the back firmly against the seat pad, to place the feet flat on the foot pad in line with the knees and hips, and to grip the handles. Direct your client to complete the exercise in the following manner.

Forward Movement Phase

1. Push the foot pad slowly forward until your knees are almost extended, but not locked.
2. Keep the feet, knees, and hips aligned.
3. Exhale throughout the pushing phase.

Backward Movement Phase

1. Allow the foot pad to return slowly to the starting position.
2. Inhale throughout the return movement.

Common Errors, Problems, and Modifications

The most common mistake in the leg press exercise is not lowering the foot pad to a 90-degree knee angle. This abbreviated movement enables heavier weight loads but limits the training benefits for the hamstrings and gluteus maximus muscles. Each repetition should be performed from a 90-degree knee angle to the almost fully extended leg position.

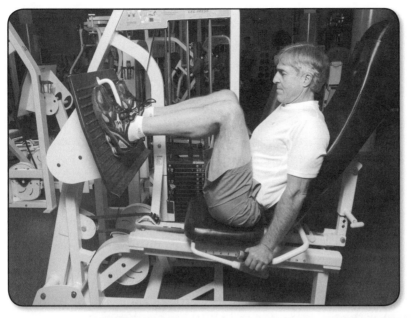

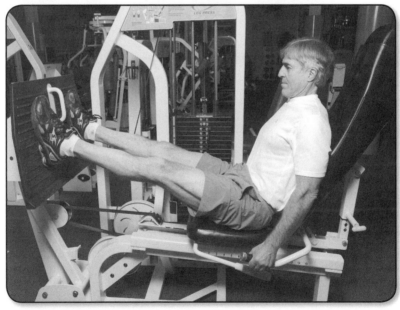

HIP ADDUCTION

Muscles most involved: hip adductors

Beginning Position

Help position your client onto the machine so that the back is firmly against the seat pad. The knees should be positioned outside the movement pads, and the feet should be resting on the supports. After assuming this position, the client should adjust the movement lever to the starting position, place the legs comfortably apart, and grip the handles. Direct your client to complete the exercise in the following manner.

Inward Movement Phase

1. Pull (or squeeze) the movement pads together slowly.
2. Exhale throughout the pulling movement.

Outward Movement Phase

1. Allow the movement pads to return slowly to the starting position with the legs apart.
2. Inhale throughout the return movement.

Common Errors, Problems, and Modifications

Strength performance in hip adduction decreases as the movement range increases, which may result in short outward movements. Establish the appropriate movement range with light resistance and make sure that the same movement range is attained with the training weight loads.

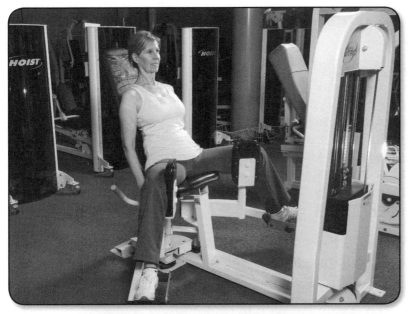

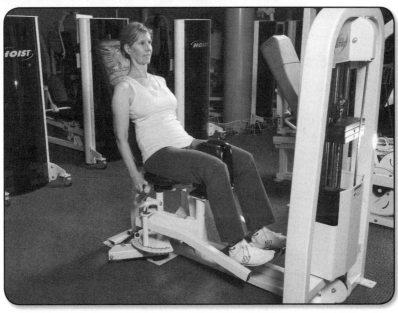

HIP ABDUCTION

Muscles most involved: hip abductors

Beginning Position

Help your client into a position in the machine so that the back is firmly against the seat pad. The knees should be positioned against the inside of the movement pads, and the feet should be resting on the supports. After assuming this position, the client should adjust the movement lever to the starting position, place the legs together, and grip the handles. Direct your client to complete the exercise in the following manner.

Outward Movement Phase

1. Slowly push the movement pads apart as far as is comfortable.
2. Exhale throughout the pushing movement.

Inward Movement Phase

1. Allow the movement pads to return slowly to the starting position with the legs together.
2. Inhale throughout the return movement.

Common Errors, Problems, and Modifications

Many exercisers arch the lower back when performing hip abductions. Although some trunk extension is natural in this exercise, the upper body should be anchored by the hands and a relatively neutral torso position should be maintained during the outward movement phase.

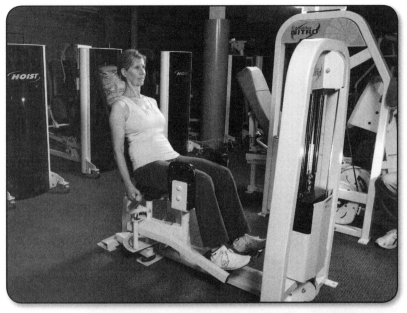

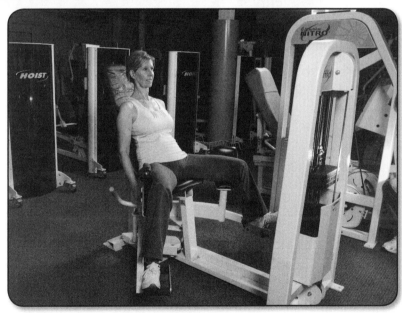

HEEL RAISE

Muscles most involved: gastrocnemius, soleus

Beginning Position

Direct your client to secure the resistance belt around the waist, to place both hands on the support bars, and to stand erect. After the client has assumed this position, instruct him or her to position the balls of the feet on the rear edge of the step and to lower the heels below the step, as far down as is comfortable. Direct your client to complete the exercise in the following manner.

Upward Movement Phase

1. Rise slowly onto the toes to lift the heels upward as high as possible.
2. Keep the knees straight.
3. Exhale throughout the upward movement.

Downward Movement Phase

1. Lower the heels slowly to reach the starting position.
2. Inhale throughout the downward movement.

Common Errors, Problems, and Modifications

The client should maintain a straight body posture when performing the heel raise exercise. Because of the relatively short movement range in the heel raise, a momentary hold in the top position is recommended.

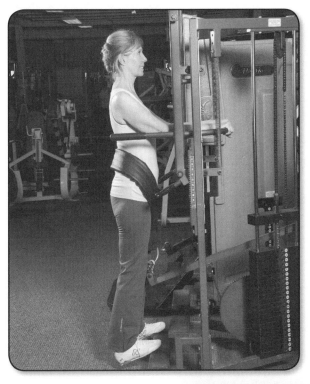

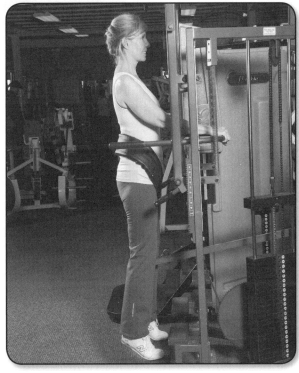

DUMBBELL SQUAT

Muscles most involved: quadriceps, hamstrings, gluteals

Beginning Position

Instruct your client to grasp each dumbbell using an overhand grip and to stand erect with the feet about hip-width apart and parallel to each other. After the client assumes this position, direct him or her to rotate the dumbbells so that the palms face the outside surfaces of the thighs. Direct your client to complete the exercise in the following manner.

Downward Movement Phase

1. Keep the head up, eyes fixed straight ahead, shoulders back, back straight, and weight on the entire foot throughout the upward and downward movement phases of this exercise.
2. Squat down slowly until the thighs are parallel to the floor.
3. Inhale throughout the downward movement.

Upward Movement Phase

1. Begin the upward movement by slowly straightening the knees and hips.
2. Exhale throughout the upward movement.

Common Errors, Problems, and Modifications

The most common problems in the squat exercise are dropping the hips directly downward, moving the knees forward of the feet, and lifting the heels off the floor. This trio of technique errors can lead to various injuries as well as to poor performance. The hips should move backward as they drop downward, the knees should remain over the feet, and the heels should remain firmly planted on the floor. Another common and high-risk form flaw is looking down and rounding the back. The head should be up and the back should be relatively straight throughout the performance of the squat exercise. If balance is an issue, direct your client to position the upper back and buttocks against a wall for support while moving downward and upward (i.e., slide up and down a wall). Instructing the client to think about pushing the heels against the floor while moving upward may also help in maintaining balance.

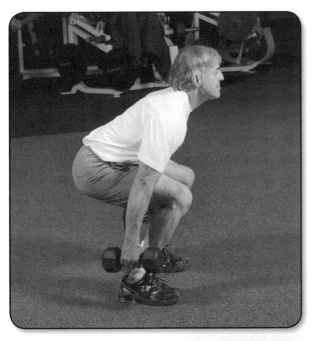

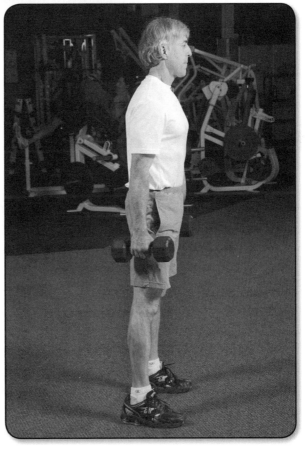

BARBELL SQUAT

Muscles most Involved: quadriceps, hamstrings, gluteals

Beginning Position

Instruct your client to step into the rack and under the bar, to position the feet shoulder-width apart or slightly wider, and to grasp the bar in an overhand grip. After the client assumes this position, direct him or her to move the bar to a position on the shoulders and upper back below the base of the neck. Last, instruct your client to stand erect, to look straight ahead, and to lift the bar out of the rack by straightening the knees. Direct your client to complete the exercise in the following manner.

Downward Movement Phase

1. Keep the head up, eyes fixed straight ahead, shoulders back, back straight, and weight on the entire foot throughout the upward and downward movement phases of this exercise.
2. Squat down slowly until the thighs are parallel to the floor.
3. Inhale throughout the downward movement.

Upward Movement Phase

1. Begin the upward movement by slowly straightening the knees and hips.
2. Exhale throughout the upward movement.
3. Return the bar to the rack carefully after completing the set.

Common Errors, Problems, and Modifications

Besides the common mistakes identified in the dumbbell squat, many exercisers perform the barbell squat with the bar too high on the neck. Be sure that your client places the bar on the trapezius muscles of the upper back and shoulder (just below the seventh cervical vertebra). The barbell squat should not be performed without a competent spotter even when the exercise is executed inside a squat rack.

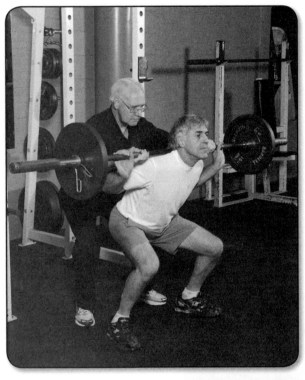

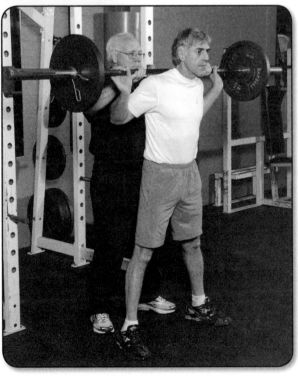

Free-Weight Exercises

DUMBBELL STEP-UP

Muscles most involved: quadriceps, hamstrings, gluteals

Beginning Position

Instruct your client to grasp the dumbbells using an overhand grip and to stand erect with the feet about hip-width apart and parallel to each other. After the client assumes this position, direct him or her to move directly in front of the step (or bench) and to rotate the dumbbells so that the palms are facing the outside surfaces of the thighs. Instruct your client to perform this exercise in the following manner.

Upward Movement Phase

1. Keep your head up, eyes fixed straight ahead, shoulders back, and back straight throughout the performance of this exercise.
2. Place your right foot onto the step (left photo) and then your left foot so that you are standing on the step (right photo).
3. Exhale throughout the upward movement.

Downward Movement Phase

1. Place your right foot on the floor and then your left foot so that you are standing on the floor.
2. Inhale throughout the downward movement.

Common Errors, Problems, and Modifications

The keys to performing dumbbell step-ups safely and effectively are to use a step height that does not cause the knee to be moved higher than the hip and to alternate the lead foot either every repetition or every set, if more than one set is completed.

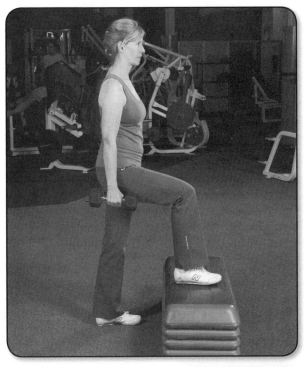

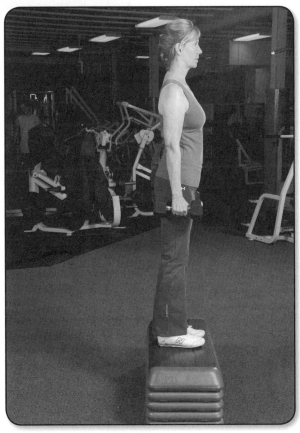

DUMBBELL LUNGE

Muscles most involved: quadriceps, hamstrings, gluteals

Beginning Position

Instruct your client to grasp the dumbbells using an overhand grip, to orient the palms so that they face the outside surfaces of the thighs, and to stand erect with the feet positioned about hip-width apart and parallel to each other. Direct your client to complete the exercise in the following manner.

Downward Movement Phase

1. Keep the head up, eyes fixed straight ahead, shoulders back, and back straight throughout the performance of this exercise.
2. Take a long step forward with your right foot and flex your right knee to a 90-degree angle.
3. Step forward far enough so that your right knee is directly above (not in front of) your right foot.
4. Inhale throughout the downward movement.

Upward Movement Phase

1. Push off the right foot and return to a standing position with the feet parallel to each other.
2. Exhale throughout the upward movement.

Common Errors, Problems, and Modifications

The most important factor in the forward lunge is to prevent the knee from extending farther forward than the foot because this position can place excessive stress on the knee joint. Clients who have difficulty performing the forward lunge properly should substitute the equally effective backward lunge. Instead of stepping forward, the client takes a long step backward. This movement will result in the same lunge position, but the lead knee will always remain directly above the lead foot. For clients with balance challenges, a standing lunge will provide similar benefits without taking either foot off the floor. The client simply assumes a moderate-length lunge position, lowers the hips toward the floor, and returns to the starting position. When performing lunges, the client should alternate the lead foot for each set of the exercise.

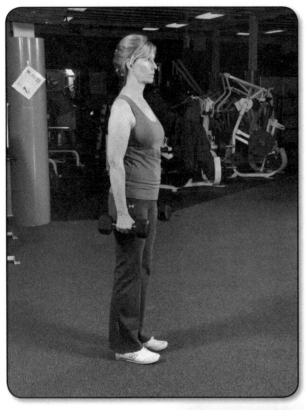

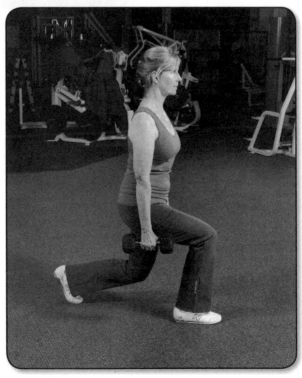

DUMBBELL HEEL RAISE

Muscles most involved: gastrocnemius, soleus

Beginning Position

Instruct your client to grasp the dumbbells with an overhand grip, to orient the palms so that they face the outside surfaces of the thighs, and to stand erect. Next, direct him or her to place the balls of the feet on a stable elevated surface approximately 2 inches (5 cm) high, about hip-width apart and parallel to each other. Direct your client to complete the exercise in the following manner.

Upward Movement Phase

1. Keep the head up, eyes fixed straight ahead, shoulders back, back straight, and weight on the balls of the feet throughout the upward and downward movement phases of this exercise.
2. Rise up slowly onto the toes while keeping the torso erect and the knees straight.
3. Exhale throughout the upward movement.

Downward Movement Phase

1. Lower the heels as far as is comfortable while keeping the torso erect and the knees straight.
2. Inhale throughout the lowering movement.

Common Errors, Problems, and Modifications

Because of the relatively short movement range, the client should hold the fully contracted (highest) position momentarily on each repetition.

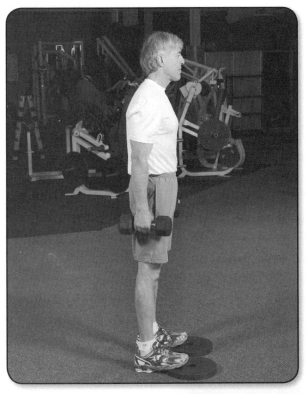

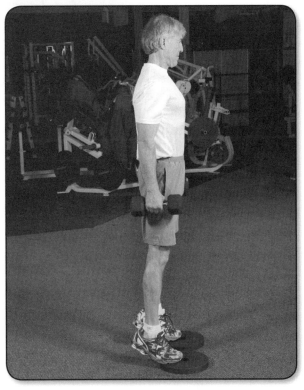

BARBELL HEEL RAISE

Muscles most involved: gastrocnemius, soleus

Beginning Position

Instruct your client to remove the barbell from the rack and assume a position with the bar on the shoulders; then move the bar to the base of the neck (just below the seventh cervical vertebra). After the client assumes this position, direct him or her to place the balls of the feet on a stable elevated surface approximately 2 inches (5 cm) high, about hip-width apart and parallel to each other. Direct your client to complete the exercise in the following manner.

Upward Movement Phase

1. Keep the head up, eyes fixed straight ahead, shoulders back, back straight, and weight on the balls of the feet throughout the upward and downward movement phases of this exercise.
2. Rise up slowly onto the toes while keeping the torso erect and the knees straight.
3. Exhale throughout the upward movement.

Downward Movement Phase

1. Lower the heels as far as is comfortable while keeping the torso erect and the knees straight.
2. Inhale throughout the lowering movement.

Common Errors, Problems, and Modifications

Because of the relatively short movement range, the client should hold the fully contracted (highest) position momentarily on each repetition. This version of the barbell heel raise requires barbell supports, and some clients may need a spotter.

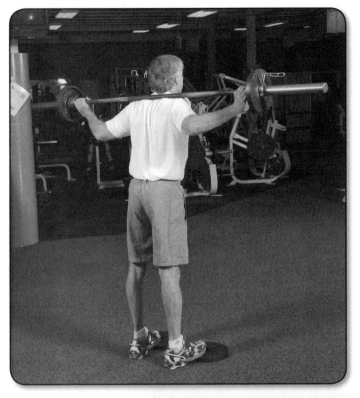

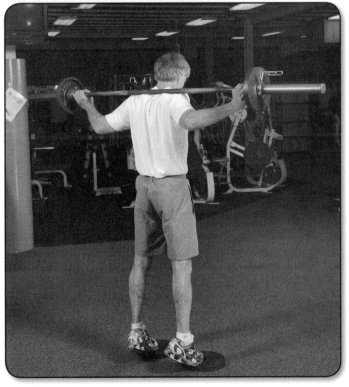

EXERCISE BALL WALL SQUAT

Muscles most involved: quadriceps, hamstrings, gluteals

Beginning Position

Instruct your client to place the exercise ball between the back and the wall with the feet far enough from the wall that the knees are directly over the feet in the down position. Direct your client to complete the exercise in the following manner.

Downward Movement Phase

1. Keep the head up, eyes fixed straight ahead, shoulders back, back straight, and weight on the entire foot throughout the performance of this exercise.
2. Squat down slowly until the thighs are parallel to the floor, rolling the ball between the back and the wall as you descend.
3. Inhale throughout the downward movement.

Upward Movement Phase

1. Begin upward movement by slowly straightening the knees and hips, rolling the ball between the back and the wall as you ascend.
2. Exhale throughout the upward movement.

Common Errors, Problems, and Modifications

Be sure that your client places the feet far enough forward that the knees do not extend beyond the feet at any point in the exercise.

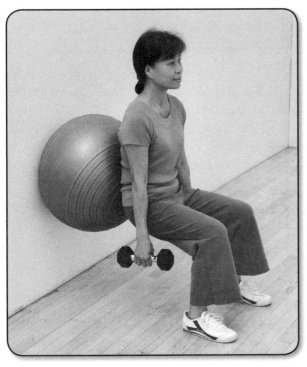

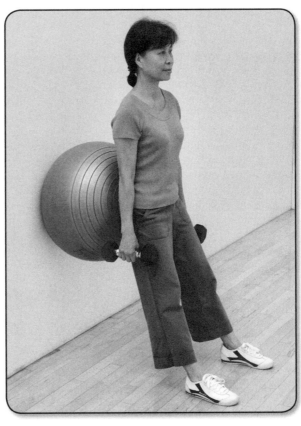

EXERCISE BALL HEEL PULL

Muscles most involved: hamstrings, hip flexors

Beginning Position

Instruct your client to lie face up on the floor with the legs extended and the heels planted firmly on top of the exercise ball, and to place the hands on the floor next to the hips. Direct your client to complete the exercise in the following manner.

Backward Movement Phase

1. Pull the ball slowly toward the hips by flexing the knees toward the chest.
2. Exhale throughout the backward movement.

Forward Movement Phase

1. Return the ball slowly to the extended-leg position.
2. Inhale throughout the forward movement.

Common Errors, Problems, and Modifications

Encourage clients to keep their hips on the floor throughout the performance of this exercise.

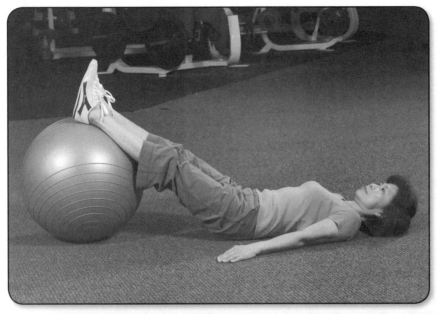

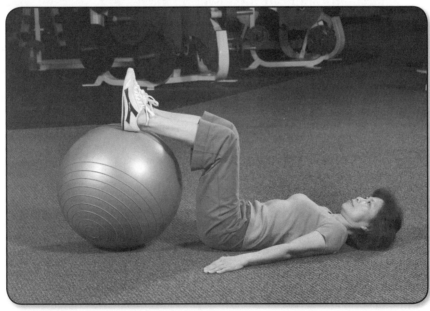

EXERCISE BALL LEG LIFT

**Muscles most involved: quadriceps,
hip flexors, rectus abdominis**

Beginning Position

Instruct your client to lie face up on the floor with the knees flexed, feet pressed against the sides of the exercise ball, and hands placed on the floor next to the hips. Direct your client to complete the exercise in the following manner.

Upward Movement Phase

1. Lift the ball slowly upward by extending the knees until the legs are straight.
2. Exhale throughout the lifting movement.

Downward Movement Phase

1. Lower the ball slowly to the floor by flexing the knees.
2. Inhale throughout the lowering movement.

Common Errors, Problems, and Modifications

Instruct clients to keep the entire back on the floor as they lift and lower the exercise ball.

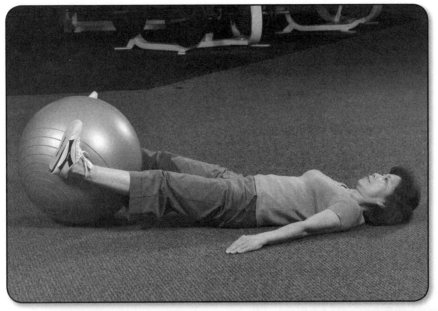

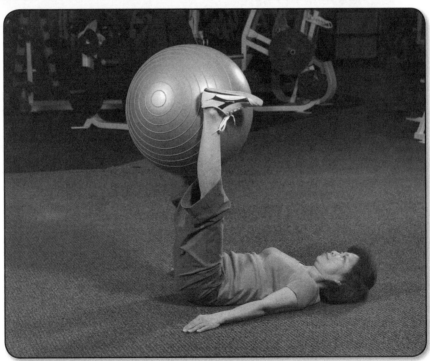

LOW-BACK EXTENSION

Muscles most involved: erector spinae

Beginning Position

Instruct your client to sit all the way back on the seat and adjust the foot pad so that the knees are slightly higher than the hips. After the client assumes this position, direct him or her to secure the seatbelt across the thighs and hips, cross the arms on the chest, and place the upper back firmly against the pad with the trunk flexed forward. Direct your client to complete the exercise in the following manner.

Backward Movement Phase

1. Push the upper back against the pad until the trunk is fully extended.
2. Keep the head in line with the torso.
3. Exhale throughout the extension movement.

Forward Movement Phase

1. Allow the pad to return slowly to the starting position.
2. Inhale throughout the return movement.

Common Errors, Problems, and Modifications

To maximize involvement of the low-back muscles, be sure that the thigh restraining belts are securely tightened. This step reduces the role of the hip extensor muscles and enhances erector spinae development. Do not allow clients to throw the head backward during the trunk extension movement.

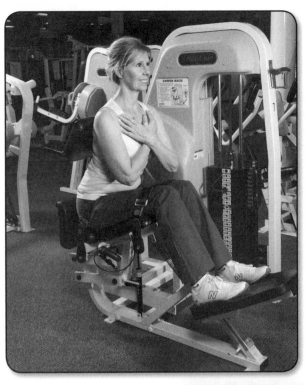

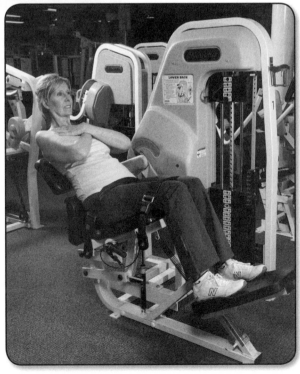

ABDOMINAL FLEXION

Muscles most involved: rectus abdominis

Beginning Position

Instruct your client to adjust the seat so that the navel is aligned with the axis of rotation of the machine, to sit with the upper back firmly pressed against the pad, to place the elbows on the arm pads, and to position the hands on the handles. Direct your client to complete the exercise in the following manner.

Forward Movement Phase

1. Pull the pad forward slowly until the trunk is fully flexed by contracting the abdominal muscles (tightening the abdominal muscles as tight as you can get them).
2. Keep the upper back firmly pressed against the pad.
3. Exhale throughout the forward movement.

Backward Movement Phase

1. Allow the pad to return slowly to the starting position.
2. Inhale throughout the return movement.

Common Errors, Problems, and Modifications

Perhaps the most important consideration for this short-range movement is to concentrate on fully contracting the rectus abdominis muscles and to pause momentarily in the crunched position. Your client's hips should be stationary throughout the performance of this exercise.

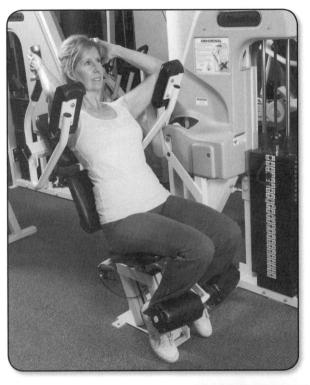

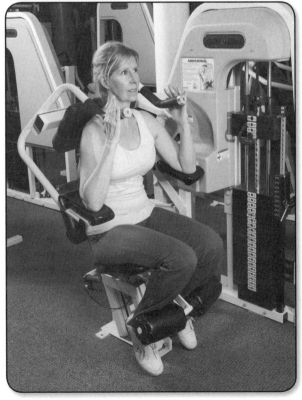

ROTARY TORSO

Muscles most involved: rectus abdominis, external obliques, internal obliques

Beginning Position

Instruct your client to sit all the way back on the seat with the torso erect, to wrap the legs around the seat extension, to position the left upper arm behind the arm pad, and to position the right upper arm against (in front of) the arm pad. Direct your client to complete the exercise in the following manner.

Left Movement Phase

1. Turn the torso slowly to the right, about 60 degrees.
2. Exhale throughout the rotation.

Return Movement Phase

1. Allow the torso to return slowly to the starting position (facing forward).
2. Inhale throughout the return movement.
3. Change the seat position and arm positions, and then repeat the exercise to the left.

Common Errors, Problems, and Modifications

Avoiding excessive torso rotation is important in this exercise, because the oblique muscles have a rather short movement range (about 90 degrees total of clockwise and counterclockwise rotation). Be sure that clients keep the torso erect and the head up throughout the performance of this exercise.

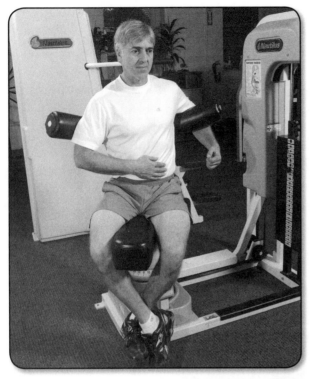

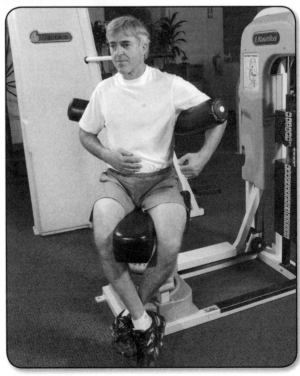

DUMBBELL SIDE BEND

Muscles most involved: obliques, rectus abdominis

Beginning Position

Instruct your client to grasp a dumbbell in the right hand using an overhand grip, to stand erect with the feet about hip-width apart and parallel to each other, and to position the dumbbell with the palm facing the outside surface of the right thigh. Direct your client to complete the exercise in the following manner.

Upward Movement Phase

1. While keeping the shoulders square with the hips and arms straight, lift the dumbbell upward by bending at the waist to the left.
2. Exhale throughout the upward movement.

Downward Movement Phase

1. While keeping the shoulders square with the hips and arms straight, lower the dumbbell downward as far as possible by bending at the waist to the right.
2. Inhale throughout the downward movement.

Common Errors, Problems, and Modifications

This exercise is most effective when done slowly, without moving the arms or leaning forward or backward during the exercise. Your clients should focus their attention on the midsection muscles. After clients complete all the repetitions with the dumbbell in the right hand, direct them to switch the dumbbell to the left hand and repeat the exercise.

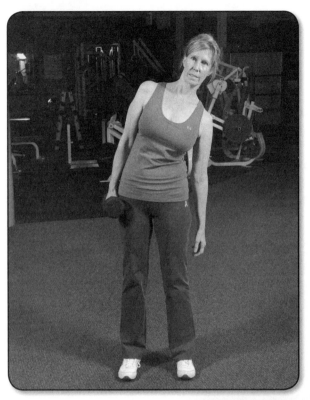

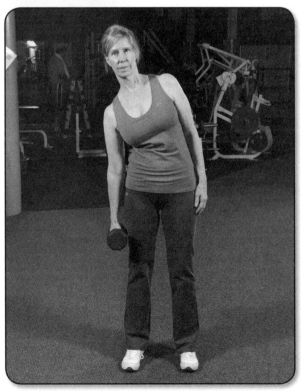

DUMBBELL DEADLIFT

**Muscles most involved: erector spinae,
quadriceps, hamstrings, gluteals**

Beginning Position

Instruct your client to grasp the dumbbells with an overhand grip and to assume a position with the arms straight, feet about hip-width apart, knees and hips flexed, back straight, and head up. After the client assumes this position, direct him or her, while keeping the shoulders square with the hips and arms, to rotate the dumbbells so that the palms face the outside surfaces of the ankles. Direct your client to complete the exercise in the following manner.

Upward Movement Phase

1. Rise slowly to a standing position by extending the knees, hips, and trunk.
2. Exhale throughout the upward movement.

Downward Movement Phase

1. Return slowly to the starting position with the dumbbells on the floor.
2. Inhale throughout the downward movement.

Common Errors, Problems, and Modifications

The most important aspect of the deadlift exercise is to maintain a straight back posture throughout the lifting and lowering movements. Do not let your clients round their backs, especially at the beginning of the exercise. Be sure to emphasize proper leg position. The knees should be over the feet rather than extended forward.

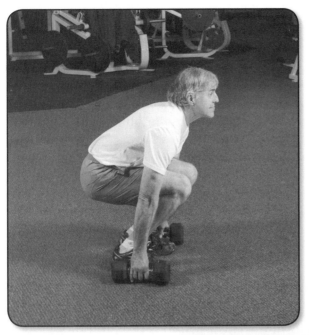

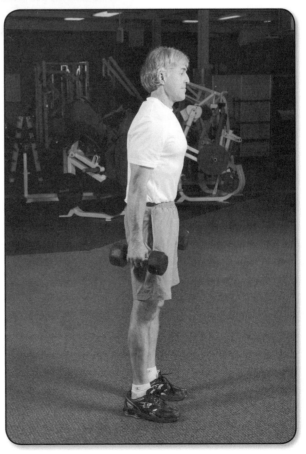

TRUNK EXTENSION

Muscles most involved: erector spinae

Beginning Position

Instruct your client to lie face down on the floor and to place the hands under the chin to maintain a neutral neck position. Direct your client to complete the exercise in the following manner.

Upward Movement Phase

1. Raise the chest slowly about 30 degrees off the floor.
2. Exhale throughout the upward movement.

Downward Movement Phase

1. Lower the chest slowly to the floor.
2. Inhale throughout the downward movement.

Common Errors, Problems, and Modifications

This challenging exercise may require you to secure (hold down) your clients' feet as they perform the chest-lifting action. If they still have difficulty, instruct them to place their hands on the floor and give some assistance (push) with their arms in lifting the trunk upward.

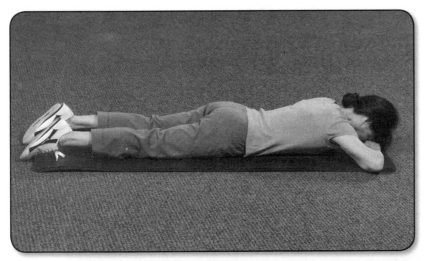

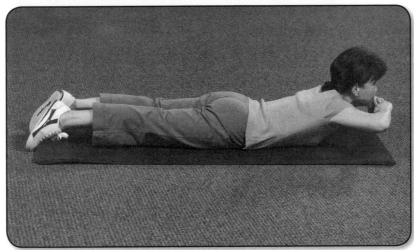

TWISTING TRUNK CURL

Muscles most involved: rectus abdominis, rectus femoris, hip flexors, obliques

Beginning Position

Instruct your client to lie face up on the floor and to place the hands behind the head to maintain a neutral neck position. Direct your client to complete the exercise in the following manner.

Upward Movement Phase

1. Raise the upper back about 30 degrees off the floor and maintain a trunk-curled position throughout the exercise.
2. Lift both legs off the floor with the right leg straight and the left leg flexed.
3. Twist the torso to the left and pull the left leg back until the right elbow touches the left knee.
4. Reverse leg positions and concurrently twist the torso to the right. Pull the right leg back until the left elbow touches the right knee.

Downward Movement Phase

1. Complete as many twisting trunk curls as possible and then lower the legs and upper back to the floor.
2. Breathe continuously throughout the twisting trunk curl exercise.

Common Errors, Problems, and Modifications

The twisting trunk curl is a highly effective abdominal exercise that should be performed in a slow, rhythmic manner for best results. The legs should remain off the floor and alternately flex and extend (like pistons) as your clients alternately turn the torso toward the left knee and then the right knee. Although the goal is to touch opposite elbows and knees, many clients will not be capable of doing this. Just encourage them to twist the torso and pull the knees back as far as possible on each repetition.

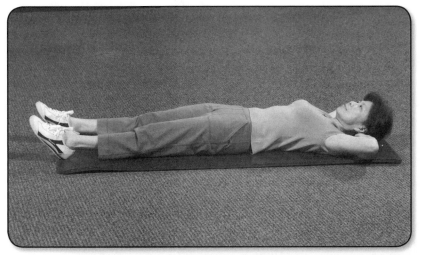

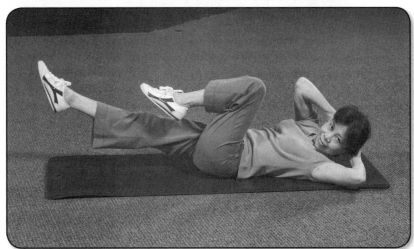

EXERCISE BALL TRUNK CURL

Muscles most involved: rectus abdominis

Beginning Position

Instruct your client to lie face up on the ball, with the feet flat on the floor and the lower back against the ball. After the client assumes this position, direct him or her to place the hands behind the head and to maintain a neutral neck position. Direct your client to complete the exercise in the following manner.

Upward Movement Phase

1. Raise the upper back slowly about 30 degrees off the exercise ball.
2. Exhale throughout the upward movement.

Downward Movement Phase

1. Lower the upper back slowly to full contact with the exercise ball.
2. Inhale throughout the downward movement.

Common Errors, Problems, and Modifications

This exercise is similar to the standard trunk curl, but it extends the movement range and requires more core stabilization from the midsection muscles. Some clients may not feel comfortable bending backward around the exercise ball at first. Allow them to begin from a more horizontal trunk position and gradually increase the range of movement as they become more confident and competent with the exercise performance.

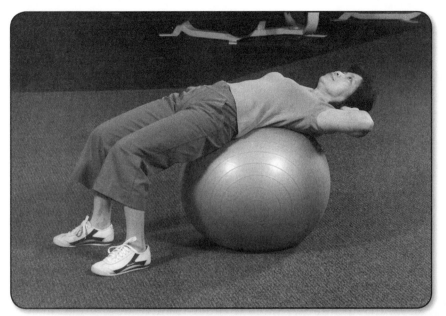

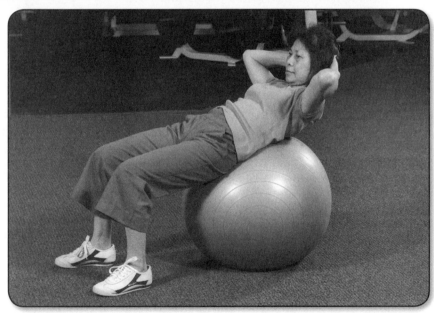

CHEST CROSSOVER

Muscles most involved: pectoralis major, anterior deltoid

Beginning Position

Instruct your client to adjust the seat so that the shoulders are in line with the axis of rotation of the machine and the upper arms are parallel to the floor and in a straight line (180 degrees). After the client assumes this position, direct him or her to sit with the head, shoulders, and back firmly pressed against the seat pad, to grip the handles, and to press the forearms against the arm pads. Direct your client to complete the exercise in the following manner.

Forward Movement Phase

1. Pull the arm pads slowly together, using the arms more than the hands.
2. Keep the wrists straight.
3. Exhale throughout the pulling movement.

Backward Movement Phase

1. Allow the arm pads to return slowly to the starting position.
2. Inhale throughout the return movement.

Common Errors, Problems, and Modifications

For some clients, this exercise may cause discomfort in the shoulder rotator cuff muscles in the arms-stretched position. If this occurs, reduce the movement range, place the forearms lower on the arm pads, or do both.

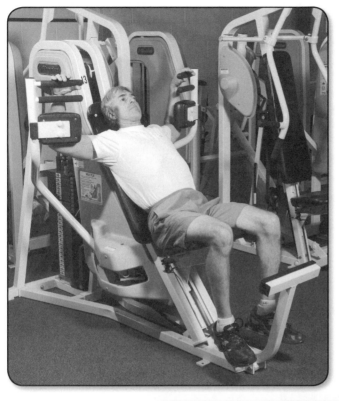

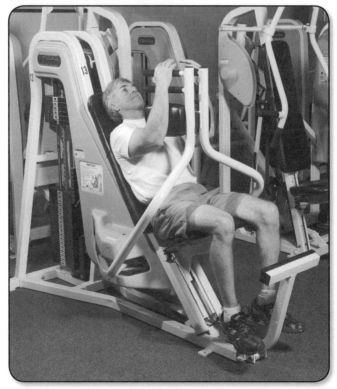

CHEST PRESS

Muscles most involved: pectoralis major, anterior deltoid, triceps

Beginning Position

Instruct your client to adjust the seat so that the handles are about 6 inches below shoulder level; to sit with the head, shoulders, and back pressed against the seat pad; and to grasp the handles so that the palms are facing away. Direct your client to complete the exercise in the following manner.

Forward Movement Phase

1. Push the handles slowly forward until the arms are fully extended.
2. Keep the wrists straight.
3. Exhale throughout the pushing movement.

Backward Movement Phase

1. Allow the handles to return slowly to the starting position.
2. Inhale throughout the return phase.

Common Errors, Problems, and Modifications

Using the horizontal handles is more effective for strengthening the pectoralis major muscles. But if this variation stresses your clients' shoulder (rotator cuff) muscles, have them reduce the movement range, use the vertical handles, or do both. Encourage clients to avoid arching the back during performance of the chest press exercise.

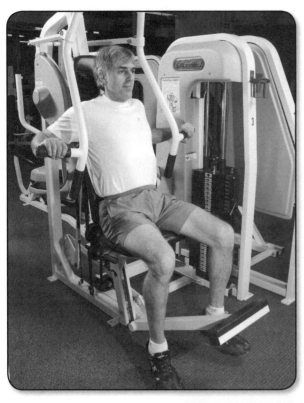

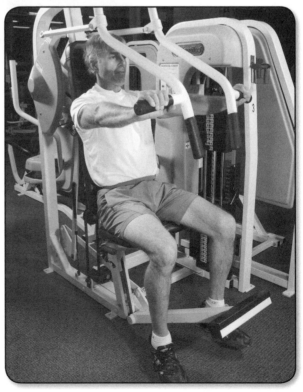

Machine Exercises

INCLINE PRESS

Muscles most involved: pectoralis major, anterior deltoid, triceps

Beginning Position

Instruct your client to adjust the seat so that the handles are below chin level; to sit with the head, shoulders, and back pressed against the seat pad; to place the feet flat on the floor; and to grasp the handles with the palms facing away. Direct your client to complete the exercise in the following manner.

Upward Movement Phase

1. Push the handles slowly upward until the arms are fully extended.
2. Keep the wrists straight.
3. Exhale throughout the pushing movement.

Downward Movement Phase

1. Return the handles slowly to the starting position.
2. Inhale throughout the lowering movement.

Common Errors, Problems, and Modifications

Using the horizontal handles is more effective for strengthening the pectoralis major muscles. But if this variation stresses your clients' shoulder (rotator cuff) muscles, have them reduce the movement range, use the vertical handles, or do both. To reduce the risk of shoulder injuries, have clients stop the downward movement between the chin and clavicles.

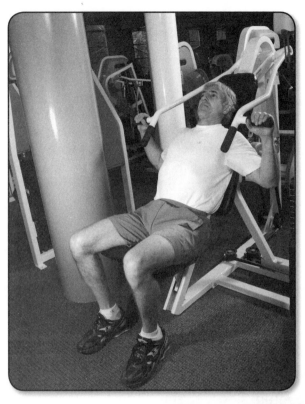

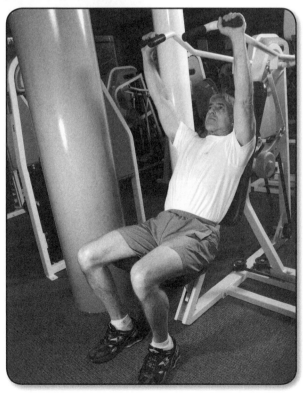

Machine Exercises

LATERAL RAISE

Muscles most involved: deltoids

Beginning Position

Instruct your client to adjust the seat so that the shoulders are in line with the axis of rotation of the machine; to sit with the head, shoulders, and back pressed firmly against the seat pad; and to place the feet flat on the floor. After the client assumes this position, direct him or her to grasp the handles and to press the forearms against the arm pads while the arms are close to the ribs. Direct your client to complete the exercise in the following manner.

Upward Movement Phase

1. Lift the arm pads slowly upward, using the arms more than the hands.
2. Keep the wrists straight.
3. Stop the upward movement when the arms are parallel to the floor.
4. Exhale throughout the lifting movement.

Downward Movement Phase

1. Allow the pads to return slowly to the starting position.
2. Inhale throughout the lowering movement.

Common Errors, Problems, and Modifications

Clients should stop the upward movement of the lateral raise exercise when the arms reach horizontal. Lifting the arms higher may cause shoulder joint impingement in some clients, and further upward movement is not necessary to contract the deltoid muscles fully. Clients should perform this exercise slowly because of the relatively short movement range. Encourage your clients to avoid shrugging their shoulders at the end of the lifting action.

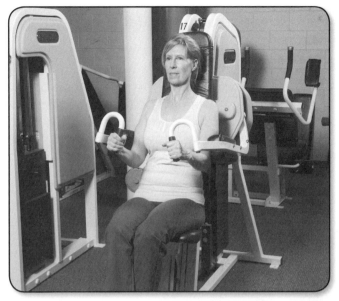

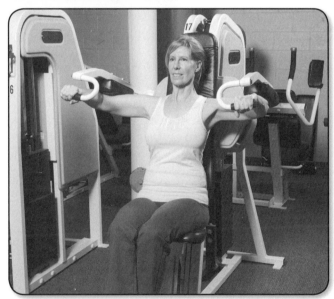

SHOULDER PRESS

Muscles most involved: deltoids, triceps, upper trapezius

Beginning Position

Instruct your client to adjust the seat so that the handles are below chin level; to sit with the head, shoulders, and back pressed against the seat pad; and to place the feet flat on the floor. After assuming this position, instruct him or her to grasp the handles so that the palms are facing away. Direct your client to complete the exercise in the following manner.

Upward Movement Phase

1. Push the handles slowly upward until the arms are fully extended.
2. Keep the wrists straight.
3. Exhale throughout the pushing movement.

Downward Movement Phase

1. Return the handles slowly to the starting position.
2. Inhale throughout the lowering movement.

Common Errors, Problems, and Modifications

Using the horizontal handles is more effective for strengthening the deltoid muscles. But if this variation stresses your clients' shoulder joints, have them reduce the movement range, use the vertical handles, or do both. To reduce the risk of shoulder injuries, have clients stop the downward movement between the chin and clavicles. Encourage clients to maintain an erect torso throughout the performance of this exercise.

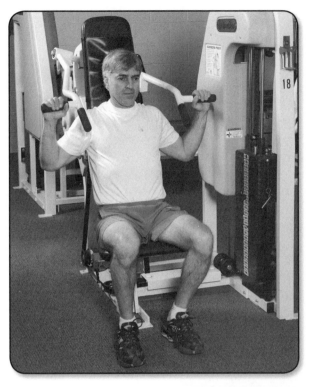

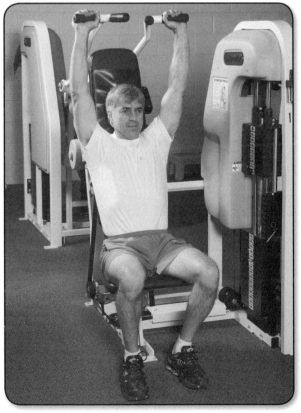

PULLOVER

Muscles most involved: latissimus dorsi

Beginning Position

Instruct your client to adjust the seat so that the shoulders are in line with the axis of rotation of the machine, to sit with the back firmly pressed against the seat pad, and to secure the seatbelt. After the client adjusts the seat, direct him or her to place the feet on the foot lever and press it forward to bring the arm pads into the starting position by the face. After the client assumes this position, instruct him or her to place the hands on the bars, to position the upper arms against the arm pads, and then to release the foot pad. Direct your client to complete the exercise in the following manner.

Downward Movement Phase

1. Pull the arm pads slowly downward, leading with the elbows until the bar touches the body.
2. Keep the wrists straight.
3. Allow the back to round slightly during the downward movement.
4. Exhale throughout the downward movement.

Upward Movement Phase

1. Allow the arm pads to return slowly to the starting position.
2. Inhale throughout the return movement.

Common Errors, Problems, and Modifications

Clients must secure the seatbelt to anchor the body before initiating the pulling action. A key performance factor in the pullover exercise is pulling the movement pads downward with the upper arms rather than pulling the bar with the hands. Encourage clients to flex the trunk at the end of the pulling action so that the lower back contacts the back pad. After they complete the final repetition, have clients place their feet on the foot bar, press the foot bar forward to hold the weight stack, release the hand grips, and slowly lower the weight stack with their legs.

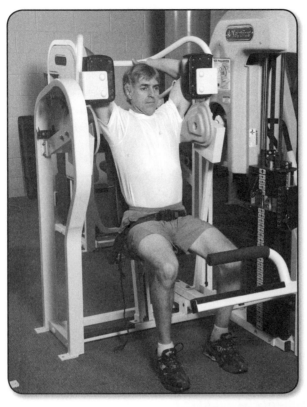

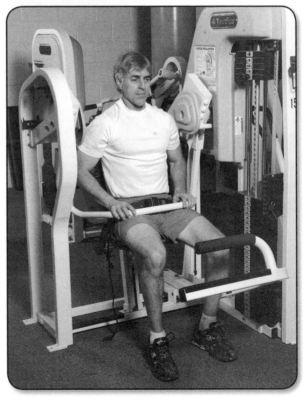

LAT PULL-DOWN

Muscles most involved: latissimus dorsi, biceps

Beginning Position

Instruct your client to place the thighs under the restraining pads, to grip the handles so that the palms face each other about shoulder-width apart, and to hold the elbows straight. Direct your client to complete the exercise in the following manner.

Downward Movement Phase

1. Pull the bar slowly downward below the chin.
2. Exhale throughout the pulling movement.

Upward Movement Phase

1. Allow the bar to return slowly upward until the arms are fully extended.
2. Exhale throughout the upward movement.

Common Errors, Problems, and Modifications

After the legs are secured under the restraining pads, the torso should remain straight throughout the exercise. Alert clients that an unexpected upward pull from the bar may occur during the upward movement phase. Warn clients to avoid overstretching the latissimus dorsi muscles at the top of the upward movement.

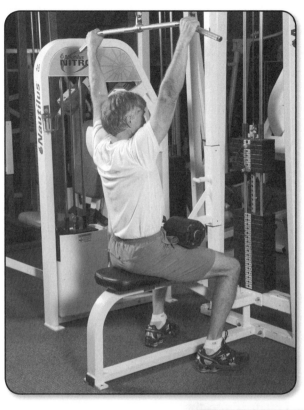

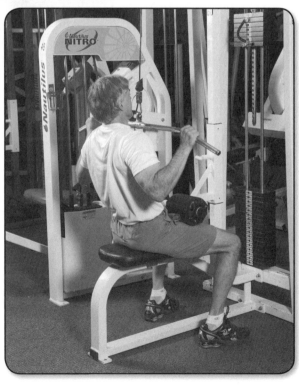

SEATED ROW

**Muscles most involved: latissimus dorsi,
biceps, posterior deltoids**

Beginning Position

Instruct your client to adjust the seat so that the handles are at shoulder level, to sit erect with the chest pressed against the chest pad, and to place the feet flat on the floor. After the client assumes this position, direct him or her to extend the arms fully and to grasp the handles. Direct your client to complete the exercise in the following manner.

Backward Movement Phase

1. Pull the handles slowly back toward the chest.
2. Keep the wrists straight.
3. Exhale throughout the pulling movement.

Forward Movement Phase

1. Allow the handles to return slowly until the arms are fully extended.
2. Inhale throughout the return movement.

Common Errors, Problems, and Modifications

A common problem when performing the seated row exercise is arching the back during the backward pulling action and allowing the trunk to move too far forward and backward. Remind your clients to maintain a flat back and to keep the torso erect (perpendicular to the floor) throughout each repetition of this exercise. Bringing the arms backward in the vertical plane emphasizes the latissimus dorsi muscles, whereas bringing the arms backward in the horizontal plane emphasizes the posterior deltoid muscles.

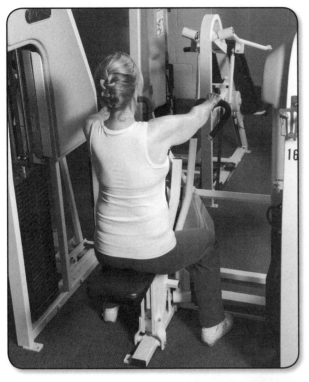

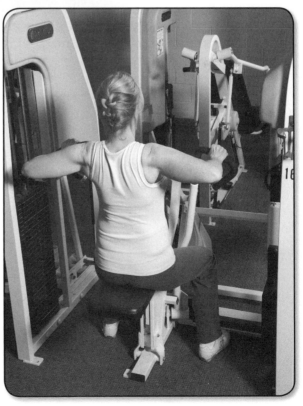

WEIGHT-ASSISTED PULL-UP

Muscles most involved: latissimus dorsi, biceps

Beginning Position

Instruct your client to climb the steps and to grasp the chin bar using an underhand grip. After the client has assumed this position, direct him or her to place the knees on the platform and to descend until the arms are fully extended. Direct your client to complete the exercise in the following manner.

Upward Movement Phase

1. Pull the body upward until the chin is above the chin bar.
2. Keep the wrists and back straight.
3. Exhale throughout the pulling movement.

Downward Movement Phase

1. Return slowly to the starting position (until the arms are fully extended).
2. Inhale throughout the return movement.

Common Errors, Problems, and Modifications

Clients tend to flex the hips during the upward movement, so encourage them to keep a straight body position throughout the performance of this exercise. Keep in mind that adding weight makes this exercise easier because the weight counterbalances your client's bodyweight. Always have clients mount and dismount the apparatus when the platform is at its highest position.

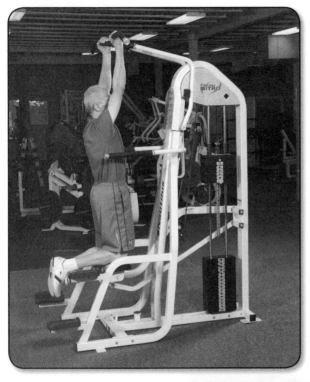

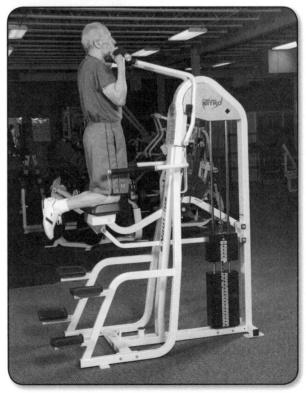

WEIGHT-ASSISTED BAR DIP

Muscles most involved: pectoralis major, triceps

Beginning Position

Instruct your client to climb the steps and to grasp the dip bars using an overhand grip. After the client assumes this position, direct him or her to place the knees on the platform and to descend until the elbows are flexed at 90 degrees. Direct your client to complete the exercise in the following manner.

Upward Movement Phase

1. Push the body slowly upward until the arms are fully extended.
2. Keep the wrists and back straight.
3. Exhale throughout the pushing movement.

Downward Movement Phase

1. Return slowly to the starting position (until the elbows are flexed about 90 degrees).
2. Inhale throughout the return movement.

Common Errors, Problems, and Modifications

The main safety concern with the bar dip exercise is descending too far during the downward movement. Have clients stop the lowering action when the elbows are flexed to 90 degrees and then begin the upward movement. Encourage clients to maintain a straight body position throughout the performance of this exercise. Keep in mind that adding weight makes this exercise easier, because the weight counterbalances the client's bodyweight. Always have clients mount and dismount the apparatus when the platform is at its highest position.

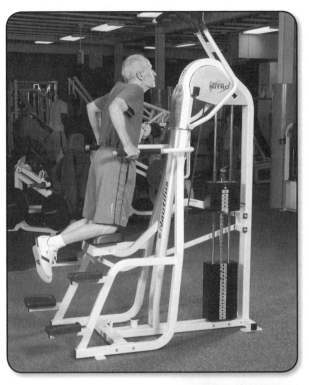

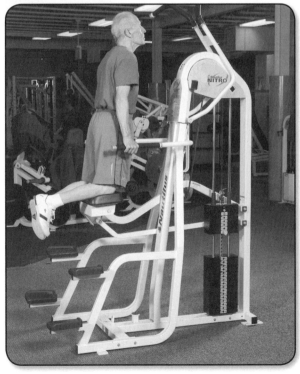

ROWING BACK

Muscles most involved: posterior deltoids, latissimus dorsi, rhomboids

Beginning Position

Instruct your client to adjust the seat so that the upper arms contact the center of the movement pads when they are parallel to the floor. After the client makes this seat adjustment, direct him or her to sit with the head, shoulders, and the back pressed against the seat pad and to place the feet on the foot bar. Direct your client to complete the exercise in the following manner.

Backward Movement Phase

1. Push the movement pads backward as far as possible while maintaining an erect torso position.
2. Exhale throughout the backward movement phase.

Forward Movement Phase

1. Return the movement pads slowly to the starting position.
2. Inhale throughout the return movement phase.

Common Errors, Problems, and Modifications

The most important aspect of this exercise is maintaining an erect torso posture throughout every repetition. Advise clients to use controlled movements rather than try to "throw" the movement pads backward.

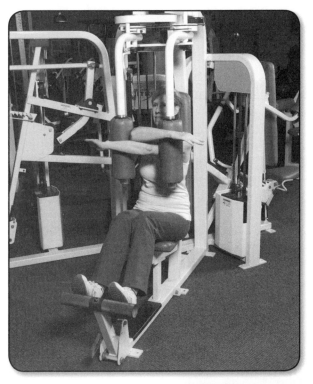

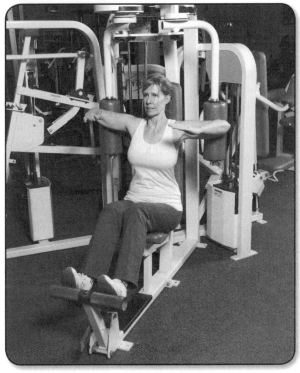

DUMBBELL CHEST FLY

Muscles most involved: pectoralis major, anterior deltoid

Beginning Position

Instruct your client to lie supine with the legs straddling the bench, the knees flexed at 90 degrees, and the feet flat on the floor. After the client assumes this position, direct him or her to grasp the dumbbells so that the palms are facing each other and to press them in unison to a position over the chest until the elbows are almost extended. Direct your client to complete the exercise in the following manner.

Downward Movement Phase

1. Lower the dumbbells slowly and in unison, keeping elbows slightly flexed and perpendicular to the torso until the upper arms are parallel to the floor.
2. Inhale throughout the lowering movement.

Upward Movement Phase

1. Lift the dumbbells upward in unison to the starting position (with the elbows slightly flexed).
2. Exhale throughout the upward movement.

Common Errors, Problems, and Modifications

Care must be taken to keep your client from lowering the dumbbells below chest level, because this action places considerable stress on the shoulder joints and pectoralis major tendons. Clients must keep the head, shoulders, and buttocks in contact with the bench and the feet in contact with the floor throughout the exercise. Be sure to spot clients who are not skilled in this exercise.

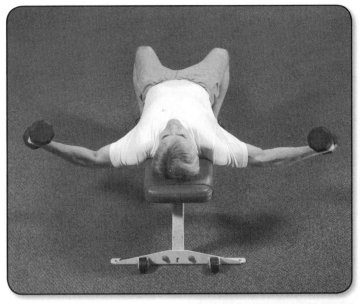

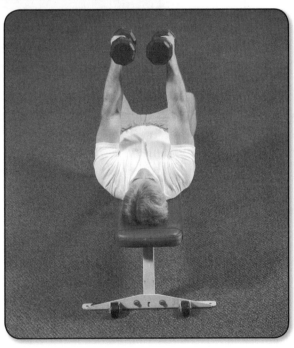

DUMBBELL BENCH PRESS

Muscles most involved: pectoralis major, anterior deltoid, triceps

Beginning Position

Instruct your client to lie supine with the legs straddling the bench, the knees flexed at 90 degrees, and the feet flat on the floor. The client should grasp the dumbbells so that the palms are facing away (thumbs toward each other) and press them in unison to a position over the chest until the elbows are extended. Direct your client to complete the exercise in the following manner.

Downward Movement Phase

1. Lower the dumbbells slowly and evenly to the chest.
2. Inhale throughout the lowering movement.

Upward Movement Phase

1. Press the dumbbells in unison upward until the arms are fully extended.
2. Exhale throughout the upward movement.

Common Errors, Problems, and Modifications

As with the dumbbell chest fly, make sure that your clients do not lower the dumbbells below chest level because this action may cause shoulder injury. The lifting and lowering actions should essentially be vertical movements in line with the thickest part of the chest. Encourage clients to keep the head, shoulders, and buttocks in contact with the bench and the feet in contact with the floor throughout the exercise. Be sure to spot clients who are not skilled in this exercise.

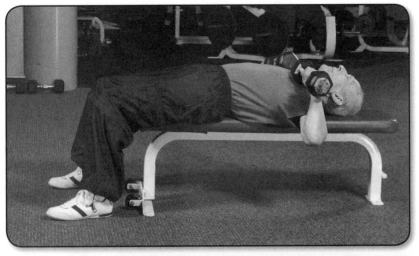

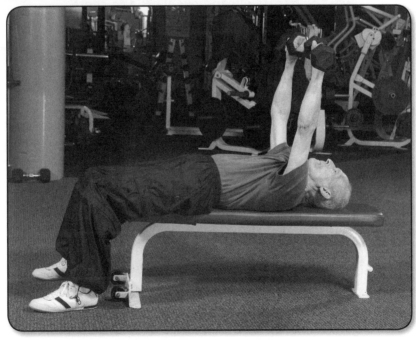

BARBELL BENCH PRESS

Muscles most involved: pectoralis major, anterior deltoid, triceps

Beginning Position

Instruct your client to lie supine with the legs straddling the bench, the knees flexed at 90 degrees, and the feet flat on the floor. After the client assumes this position, direct him or her to grasp the barbell in an overhand grip with the palms facing away (thumbs toward each other) and to press the bar until the arms are fully extended above the chest. Direct your client to complete the exercise in the following manner.

Downward Movement Phase

1. Lower the bar slowly and evenly to the chest.
2. Inhale throughout the lowering movement.

Upward Movement Phase

1. Press the bar upward evenly until the arms are fully extended.
2. Exhale throughout the pressing movement.

Common Errors, Problems, and Modifications

The barbell bench press should be performed only when the bench has secure uprights to hold the bar before and after exercise execution and when a competent spotter is supervising the training set. Instruct clients to keep the head, shoulders, and buttocks in contact with the bench and the feet in contact with the floor throughout the exercise. Do not permit clients to use momentum, bounce the bar off the chest, or press the bar upward in an uneven manner.

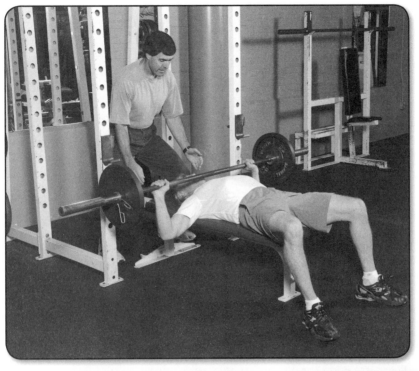

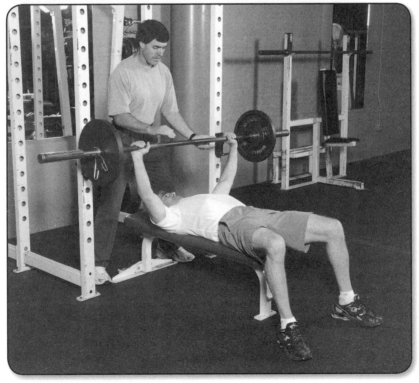

DUMBBELL ONE-ARM ROW

Muscles most involved: latissimus dorsi, biceps

Beginning Position

Instruct your client to grasp the dumbbell with the right hand, to place the left hand and knee on the bench, to place the right foot flat on the floor, and to keep the right leg straight. After the client assumes this position, he or she should extend the right arm, establish and maintain a flat back position, and rotate the dumbbell so that the palm faces the bench. Direct your client to complete the exercise in the following manner.

Upward Movement Phase

1. Pull the dumbbell slowly upward to the chest.
2. Exhale throughout the pulling movement.

Downward Movement Phase

1. Lower the dumbbell slowly to the starting position.
2. Exhale throughout the lowering movement.

Common Errors, Problems, and Modifications

The key to safe and successful performance of this exercise is to maintain a straight (horizontal) back position with support from the arm and leg on the bench. Do not let your client rotate the shoulder upward during lifting movements; emphasize keeping a squared torso throughout exercise execution. After they complete a set with one arm, have clients switch leg positions and repeat the exercise with the opposite arm.

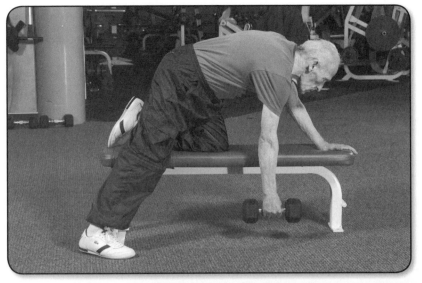

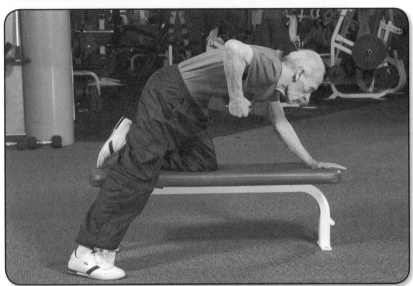

DUMBBELL LATERAL RAISE

Muscles most involved: deltoids

Beginning Position

Instruct your client to grasp the dumbbells in an overhand grip, to flex the elbows slightly, and to stand erect with the feet hip-width apart. After the client assumes this position, direct him or her to rotate the dumbbells so that the palms face the outside of the thighs. Direct your client to complete the exercise in the following manner.

Upward Movement Phase

1. Lift the dumbbells slowly upward and in unison until they are parallel to the floor.
2. Exhale throughout the upward movement.

Downward Movement Phase

1. Lower the dumbbells slowly and in unison to the starting position.
2. Inhale throughout the lowering movement.

Common Errors, Problems, and Modifications

Performing the lateral raise with the arms straight subjects the deltoid muscles to a large range of resistance forces because of unfavorable leverage factors during the lifting movements. Clients must therefore maintain some degree of elbow flexion (about 45 degrees) while performing this exercise. This technique permits a more even application of resistance force throughout the movement range and places less stress on the shoulder and elbow joints. To reduce the risk of shoulder joint impingement, advise clients to stop the upward movement when their arms reach horizontal.

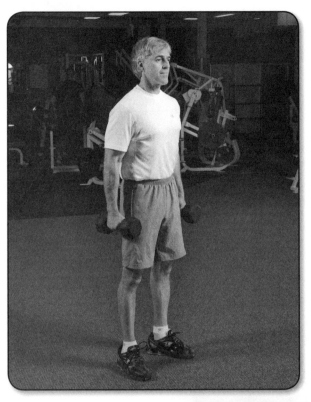

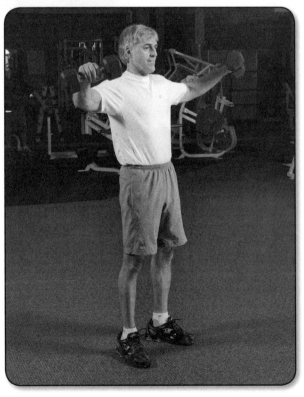

BARBELL INCLINE PRESS

Muscles most involved: pectoralis major, anterior deltoid, triceps

Beginning Position

Instruct your client to sit with the head, shoulders, and back in contact with the incline bench and the feet flat on the floor. After the client assumes this position, direct him or her to grasp the barbell with an overhand grip that is slightly wider than the shoulders and to push the bar upward until the arms are fully extended above the shoulders. Direct your client to complete the exercise in the following manner.

Downward Movement Phase

1. Lower the bar slowly and evenly to chin level.
2. Inhale throughout the lowering movement.

Upward Movement Phase

1. Press the bar upward evenly until the arms are fully extended above the shoulders.
2. Exhale throughout the pressing movement.

Common Errors, Problems, and Modifications

The barbell incline press should be performed only when the bench has secure uprights to hold the bar before and after exercise execution and when a competent spotter is supervising the training set. Most older adults should lower the bar to chin level because lower positions may place excessive stress on the shoulder joints. Advise clients to keep the head, shoulders, and back against the incline bench and the feet flat on the floor throughout this exercise.

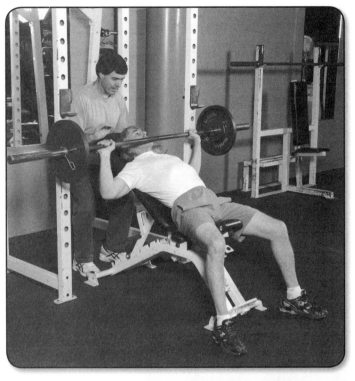

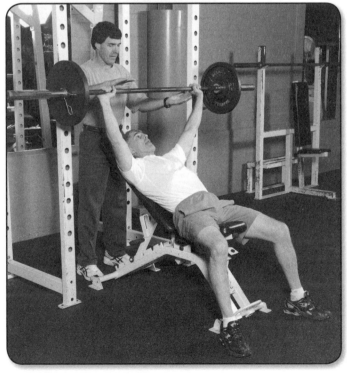

DUMBBELL INCLINE PRESS

Muscles most involved: pectoralis major, anterior deltoid, triceps

Beginning Position

Instruct your client to sit with the head, shoulders, and back in contact with the incline bench and the feet flat on the floor. After the client assumes this position, direct him or her to grasp the dumbbells with an overhand grip and the palms facing forward with the dumbbells positioned slightly wider than the shoulders and to push them upward until the arms are fully extended above the shoulders. Direct your client to complete the exercise in the following manner.

Downward Movement Phase

1. Lower the dumbbells slowly and evenly to chin level.
2. Inhale throughout the lowering movement.

Upward Movement Phase

1. Press the dumbbells upward evenly until the arms are fully extended above the shoulders.
2. Exhale throughout the pressing movement.

Common Errors, Problems, and Modifications

Although the dumbbell incline press does not have the risks associated with the barbell exercise, it is best performed with a spotter to assist with dumbbell placements. As with the barbell incline press, clients should keep the head, shoulders, and back against the incline bench and the feet flat on the floor throughout this exercise. Make sure that clients keep the dumbbells in the vertical plane, pressing them evenly and straight upward above the upper chest.

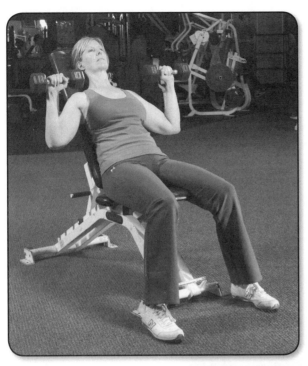

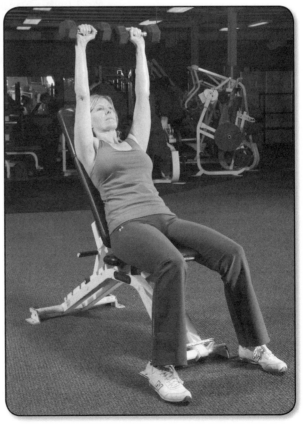

Free-Weight Exercises

DUMBBELL SEATED PRESS

Muscles most involved: deltoids, triceps

Beginning Position

Instruct your client to sit with the legs straddling the bench and the feet in contact with the floor. After the client assumes this position, direct him or her to grasp the dumbbells with an overhand grip and the palms facing forward and to position them at shoulder height. Direct your client to complete the exercise in the following manner.

Upward Movement Phase

1. Push the dumbbells upward slowly and in unison until the arms are fully extended over the shoulders.
2. Exhale throughout the pushing movement.

Downward Movement Phase

1. Lower the dumbbells slowly and in unison to shoulder level.
2. Inhale throughout the lowering movement.

Common Errors, Problems, and Modifications

This exercise is best performed using an upright or adjustable bench that enables clients to keep the head and back supported throughout the exercise. If a flat bench is used, make sure that clients maintain an erect torso throughout the lifting and lowering movements. If clients experience shoulder discomfort, have them perform alternating pressing actions (right arm followed by left arm), a technique that allows more freedom of movement in the shoulder girdle.

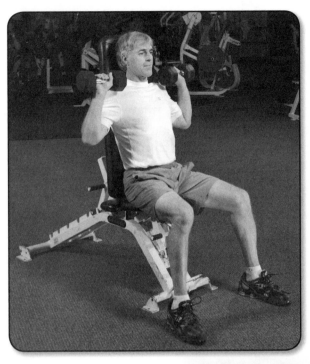

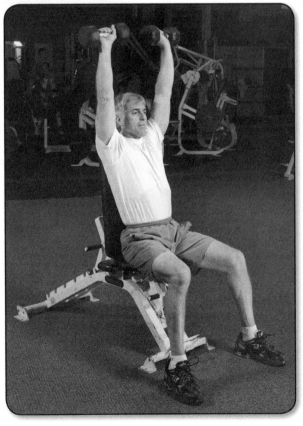

DUMBBELL ALTERNATING SHOULDER PRESS

Muscles most involved: deltoids, triceps, upper trapezius

Beginning Position

Instruct your client to stand with the feet about shoulder-width apart and the torso erect. After the client assumes this position, direct him or her to grasp the dumbbells with an overhand grip and to position them at shoulder height. Direct your client to complete the exercise in the following manner.

Upward and Downward Movement Phases

1. Extend the left arm overhead slowly without moving the right arm.
2. Lower the left arm slowly to the starting position.
3. Extend the right arm overhead slowly without moving the left arm.
4. Lower the right arm slowly to the starting position.
5. Continue alternating the left- and right-arm pressing movements.
6. Exhale during each pressing action and inhale during each lowering movement.

Common Errors, Problems, and Modifications

Clients with poor balance or postural control should perform the seated version of the shoulder press exercise. Best results are attained when the alternating pressing movements are performed at a moderate or slow speed in a rhythmic manner. Instruct clients to maintain an erect posture throughout the exercise, making certain not to lean backward at any time. Be sure to spot clients who are not skilled in this exercise.

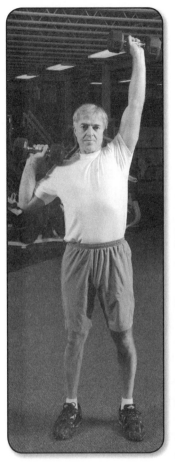

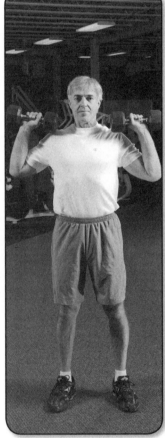

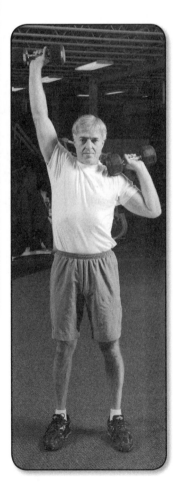

EXERCISE BALL PUSH-UP

**Muscles most involved: pectoralis major,
deltoids, triceps, rectus abdominis**

Beginning Position

Instruct your client to establish the standard push-up position with the hands on the floor, slightly wider than shoulder-width apart. After the client assumes this position, direct him or her to place the toes on top of the exercise ball and to establish a straight body position, angled slightly downward. Direct your client to complete the exercise in the following manner.

Downward Movement Phase

1. Lower the chest toward the floor while maintaining the straight body position.
2. Inhale throughout the lowering movement.

Upward Movement Phase

1. Press the body upward until the arms are fully extended.
2. Exhale throughout the pressing movement.

Common Errors, Problems, and Modifications

This exercise is similar to standard push-ups, but it involves additional core stabilization from the midsection muscles and a slightly higher percentage of bodyweight resistance. Encourage clients to concentrate on abdominal muscle contraction to maintain a straight body position throughout each exercise repetition.

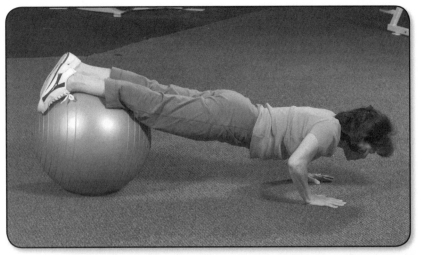

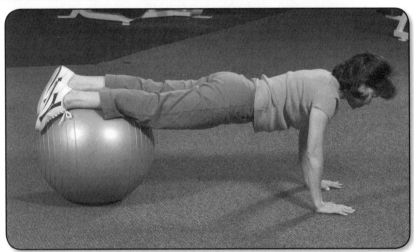

PULL-UP

Muscles most involved: latissimus dorsi, biceps

Beginning Position

Instruct your client to grasp the chin bar with an underhand shoulder-width grip and to establish a fully extended arm position. Direct your client to complete the exercise in the following manner.

Upward Movement Phase

1. Lift the body upward until the chin is above the chin bar.
2. Exhale throughout the upward movement.

Downward Movement Phase

1. Lower the body slowly until the arms are fully extended.
2. Inhale throughout the downward movement.

Common Errors, Problems, and Modifications

This exercise is challenging for most older adults, and some may have to perform the lowering movement first. Have clients stand on a step to begin in the up position (chin above the bar) and slowly lower to the arms-extended position. This movement is possible because muscle force output is approximately 40 percent greater in eccentric muscle actions. After clients can perform several controlled lowering repetitions, they should be capable of doing a few full pull-ups. Remind clients to maintain a straight body position throughout the performance of this exercise and to breathe out as they pull up.

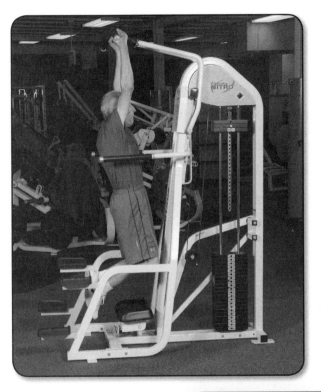

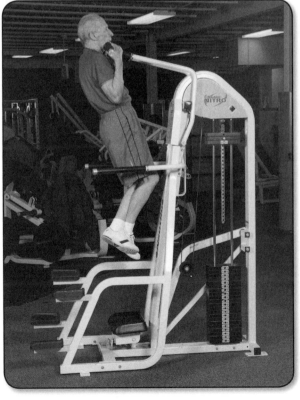

Ball and Bodyweight Exercises

BAR DIP

Muscles most involved: pectoralis major, anterior deltoid, triceps

Beginning Position

Instruct your client to grasp the dip bars with an overhand grip and to push to a fully extended arm position. Direct your client to complete the exercise in the following manner.

Downward Movement Phase

1. Lower the body slowly until the elbows are flexed to 90 degrees.
2. Inhale throughout the downward movement.

Upward Movement Phase

1. Press the body upward until the arms are extended.
2. Exhale throughout the upward movement.

Common Errors, Problems, and Modifications

Like pull-ups, bar dips are highly challenging for most older adults, and some may have to perform the lowering movement first. Have clients stand on a step to begin in the up position (arms fully extended) and slowly lower until the elbows are flexed to 90 degrees. This movement is possible because muscle force output is approximately 40 percent greater in eccentric muscle actions. After clients can perform several controlled lowering repetitions, they should be capable of doing a few full bar dips. Remind clients to maintain the straight body position throughout the performance of this exercise.

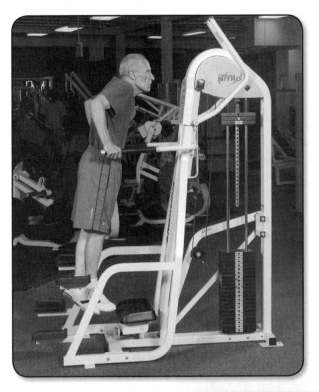

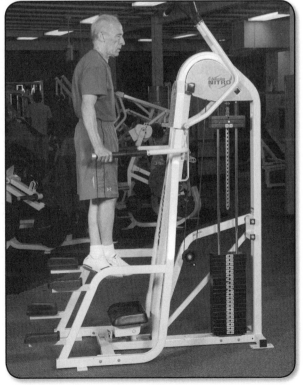

Ball and Bodyweight Exercises

BICEPS CURL

Muscles most involved: biceps

Beginning Position

Help your client adjust the seat so that the elbows are in line with the axis of rotation of the machine and the upper arms are fully on the pads. After the client has adjusted the seat, direct him or her to sit erect and to grasp the handles with an underhand grip, with the elbows slightly flexed. Direct your client to complete the exercise in the following manner.

Upward Movement Phase

1. Pull or curl the handles slowly upward until the elbows are fully flexed.
2. Keep the wrists straight.
3. Exhale throughout the lifting movement.

Downward Movement Phase

1. Allow the handles to return slowly to the starting position.
2. Inhale throughout the lowering movement.

Common Errors, Problems, and Modifications

The most important aspect of performing the machine biceps curl is to position the elbows in line with the axis of rotation of the machine. After clients accomplish this, encourage them to use slow or moderate movement speeds to maximize the cam effect of the machine to match resistance force to muscle force throughout each repetition. A momentary pause in the fully contracted biceps position is highly recommended.

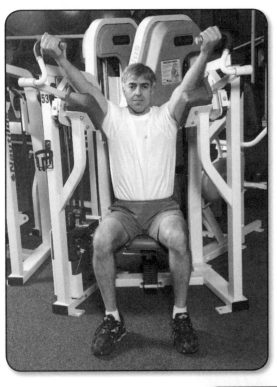

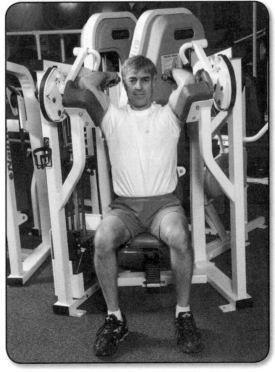

Machine Exercises

133

TRICEPS EXTENSION

Muscles most involved: triceps

Beginning Position

Help your client adjust the seat so that the elbows are in line with the axis of rotation of the machine and the upper arms are fully on the pads. After the client has adjusted the seat, direct him or her to sit with the back firmly against the seat pad and to place the side of the hands against the hand pads. Direct your client to complete the exercise in the following manner.

Forward Movement Phase

1. Push the handles slowly forward until the arms are fully extended.
2. Keep the wrists straight.
3. Exhale throughout the forward movement.

Backward Movement Phase

1. Allow the handles to return slowly to the starting position.
2. Inhale throughout the return movement.

Common Errors, Problems, and Modifications

As with the biceps curl, the most important aspect of performing the machine triceps extension is to position the elbows in line with the axis of rotation of the machine. After your clients accomplish this, encourage them to use slow or moderate movement speeds to maximize the cam effect of the machine to match resistance force to muscle force throughout each repetition. A momentary pause in the fully contracted triceps position is highly recommended. Instruct your clients to stand and remove the hands from the hand pads for easy exit from the seat following the last repetition.

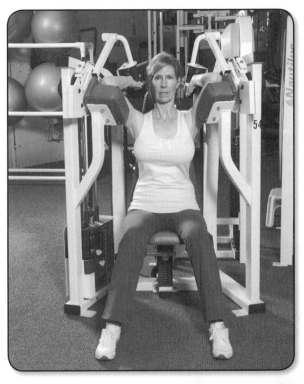

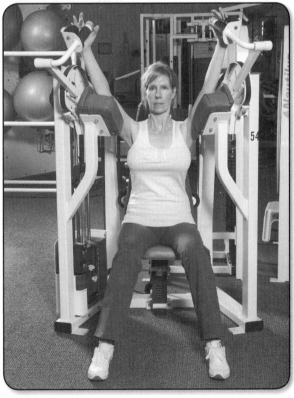

TRICEPS PRESS

**Muscles most involved: triceps,
pectoralis major, anterior deltoid**

Beginning Position

Help your client adjust the seat so that when he or she is sitting erect, the elbows are at 90-degree angles and the hands are grasping the handles directly below the shoulders. After the client assumes this position, direct him or her to secure the seatbelt. Direct your client to complete the exercise in the following manner.

Downward Movement Phase

1. Push the handles downward until the arms are fully extended.
2. Keep the wrists straight.
3. Exhale throughout the pushing movement.

Upward Movement Phase

1. Return the handles slowly to the starting position.
2. Inhale throughout the return movement.

Common Errors, Problems, and Modifications

The triceps press is a highly effective exercise for the upper-body "pushing" muscles, but it should be performed within a low-risk movement range of 90 degrees (from elbows flexed at 90 degrees to elbows straight at 180 degrees). Flexing the elbows more than a right angle may place excessive stress on the shoulder joint and is therefore not recommended. Clients must anchor the body with the seatbelt before performing triceps presses.

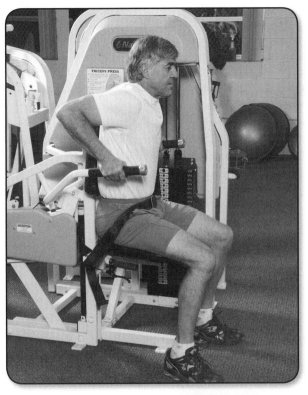

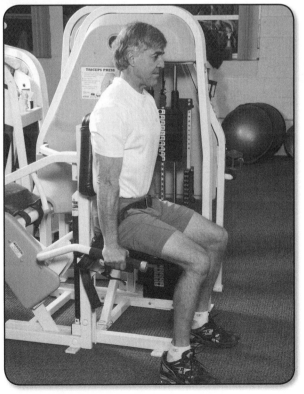

TRICEPS PRESS-DOWN

Muscles most involved: triceps

Beginning Position

Instruct the client to stand erect with the feet hip-width apart and the knees slightly flexed. After the client assumes this position, direct him or her to grasp the bar with an overhand grip and push the bar down until the upper arms are perpendicular with the floor and touching the ribs. The bar should be at upper-chest level. Direct your client to complete the exercise in the following manner.

Downward Movement Phase

1. Push the bar downward until the arms are fully extended.
2. Exhale throughout the pushing movement.

Upward Movement Phase

1. Return the bar slowly to the starting position.
2. Inhale throughout the upward movement.

Common Errors, Problems, and Modifications

The key to productive triceps press-down performance is isolating the triceps muscles. This goal is best achieved by keeping the elbows "riveted" to the ribs and stopping the upward movement at upper-chest level. Allowing the bar to rise higher allows other muscle groups (such as the latissimus dorsi) to initiate the downward movement. Make sure that clients maintain a straight body position throughout performance of this exercise. Alert clients that an unexpected upward pull from the bar may occur at the beginning of the upward movement phase.

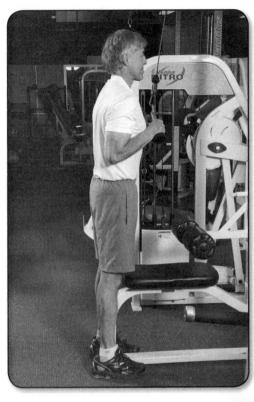

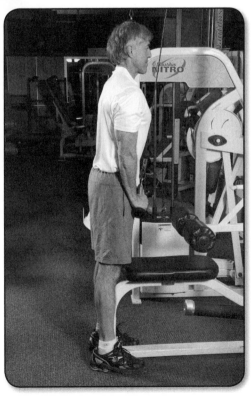

BARBELL CURL

Muscles most involved: biceps

Beginning Position

Instruct your client to grasp the bar with an underhand grip and to stand erect with the feet hip-width apart and parallel to each other. Direct your client to complete the exercise in the following manner.

Upward Movement Phase

1. While keeping the upper arms against the ribs and perpendicular to the floor, curl the barbell slowly upward toward the shoulders.
2. Exhale throughout the curling movement.

Downward Movement Phase

1. Lower the barbell slowly until the arms are fully extended.
2. Inhale throughout the lowering movement.

Common Errors, Problems, and Modifications

The barbell curl must be performed with proper technique to produce the best results and lower the risk of injury. Make sure that clients maintain an erect posture (no back arching) and that their elbows are fully extended before the upward curling motion is initiated. Also, impress upon clients the importance of keeping their upper arms perpendicular to the floor and "riveted" to their ribs throughout this exercise.

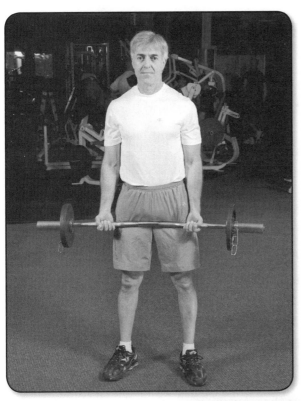

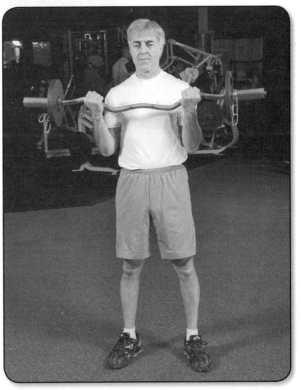

DUMBBELL STANDING CURL

Muscles most involved: biceps

Beginning Position

Instruct your client to grasp the dumbbells with an underhand grip and to stand erect with the feet hip-width apart and parallel to each other. Direct your client to complete the exercise in the following manner.

Upward Movement Phase

1. While keeping the upper arms against the ribs and perpendicular to the floor, curl the dumbbells upward slowly and in unison toward the shoulders with the palms toward the face.
2. Exhale throughout the upward movement.

Downward Movement Phase

1. Lower the dumbbells slowly and in unison to the starting position.
2. Inhale throughout the lowering movement.

Common Errors, Problems, and Modifications

Just like the barbell curl, the dumbbell standing curl should be performed with an erect posture (no back arching) and the elbows should be fully extended before the upward curling motion is initiated. The upper arms should be kept perpendicular to the floor and "riveted" to the ribs throughout this exercise. We recommend that older adult clients perform unison dumbbell curls rather than alternating dumbbell curls.

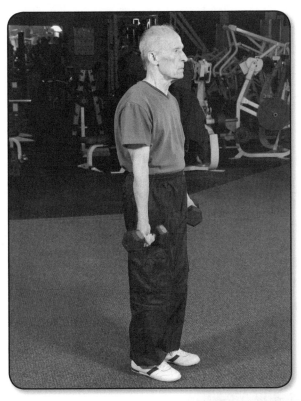

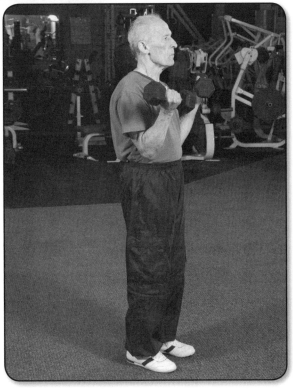

DUMBBELL INCLINE CURL

Muscles most involved: biceps

Beginning Position

Instruct your client to establish a seated position on the incline bench with the shoulders and back against the seat pad and the feet flat on the floor. After the client assumes this position, direct him or her to grasp the dumbbells with an underhand grip and to position the arms perpendicular to the floor. Direct your client to complete the exercise in the following manner.

Upward Movement Phase

1. While keeping the upper arms against the ribs and stationary, curl the dumbbells upward slowly and in unison until the elbows are fully flexed.
2. Exhale throughout the upward movement.

Downward Movement Phase

1. Lower the dumbbells slowly and in unison to the starting position.
2. Inhale throughout the lowering movement.

Common Errors, Problems, and Modifications

The major advantage of dumbbell incline curls is the stretched biceps position at the start of each repetition. This position makes the exercise more challenging and effective. Consequently, clients must lower the dumbbells to the fully stretched, straight-arm position on every repetition. The upper arms should remain perpendicular to the floor throughout each set of dumbbell incline curls.

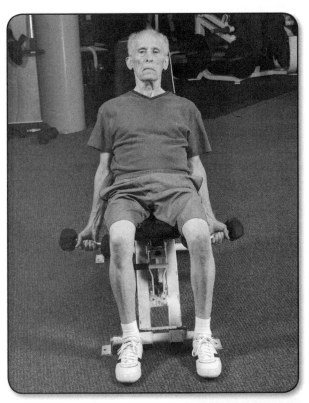

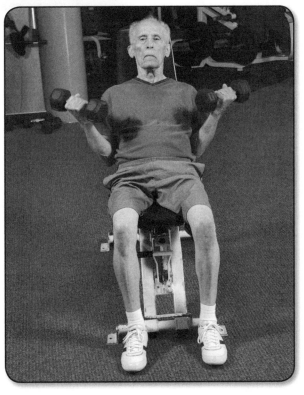

DUMBBELL PREACHER CURL

Muscles most involved: biceps

Beginning Position

Instruct your client to sit on the preacher bench with the upper arms supported on the diagonal arm pad and the feet flat on the floor. After the client assumes this position, direct him or her to grasp the dumbbells with an underhand grip and to rest the arms on the arm pad with the elbows extended. Direct your client to complete the exercise in the following manner.

Upward Movement Phase

1. Curl the dumbbells upward slowly and in unison until the elbows are fully flexed.
2. Exhale throughout the upward movement.

Downward Movement Phase

1. Lower the dumbbells slowly and in unison to the starting position.
2. Inhale throughout the lowering movement.

Common Errors, Problems, and Modifications

Make sure that your clients adjust the seat so that their upper arms are fully supported by the arm pad before they perform dumbbell preacher curls. To avoid potential wrist and elbow problems, they should lower the dumbbells to a position about 30 degrees short of full arm extension on each repetition.

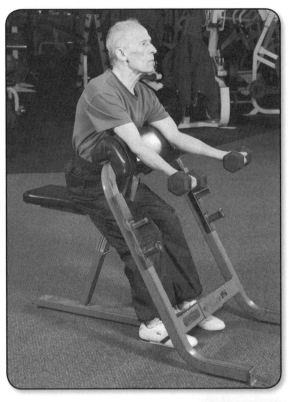

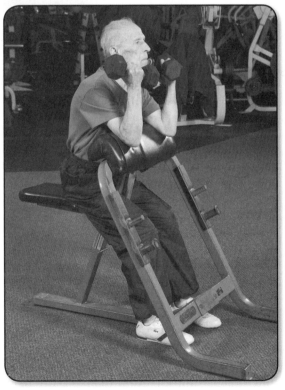

DUMBBELL CONCENTRATION CURL

Muscles most involved: biceps

Beginning Position

Instruct your client to sit on a bench, to position the feet shoulder-width apart, and to grasp a dumbbell in the right hand using an underhand grip. Next, direct him or her to position the right elbow against the right inner thigh to serve as a brace for the right arm. After your client assumes this position, instruct him or her to lean forward and straighten the right arm. Direct your client to complete the exercise in the following manner.

Upward Movement Phase

1. Curl the dumbbell slowly toward the chin.
2. Keep the upper arm firmly braced against the thigh.
3. Exhale throughout the curling movement.

Downward Movement Phase

1. Lower the dumbbell slowly back to the starting position.
2. Keep the upper arm firmly braced against the thigh.
3. Inhale throughout the lowering movement.
4. Direct your client to repeat the same procedures using the left arm.

Common Errors, Problems, and Modifications

Clients should provide a firm and supportive elbow brace with the inner thigh so that the upper arm does not move during performance of the exercise. Make sure that clients do not lean or jerk the torso backward during the lifting movements or lean forward during the lowering movements.

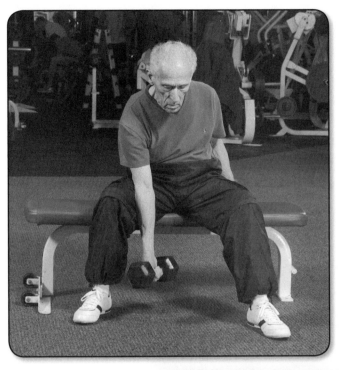

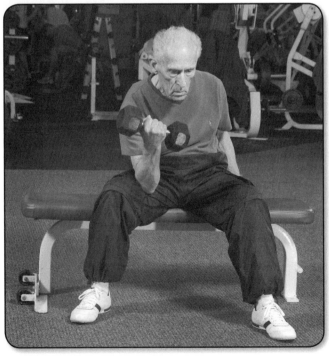

DUMBBELL OVERHEAD TRICEPS EXTENSION

Muscles most involved: triceps

Beginning Position

Instruct your client to position the feet in a hip-width stance, grasp a dumbbell with both hands, and stand erect. After the client assumes this position, direct him or her to push the dumbbell upward until the arms are fully extended, directly above the head. Direct your client to complete the exercise in the following manner.

Downward Movement Phase

1. While keeping the upper arms perpendicular to the floor, slowly lower the dumbbell behind the head toward the base of the neck.
2. Inhale throughout the lowering movement.

Upward Movement Phase

1. While keeping the upper arms perpendicular to the floor, lift the dumbbell slowly upward until the arms are fully extended.
2. Exhale throughout the lifting movement.

Common Errors, Problems, and Modifications

The key to performing this exercise properly is for clients to maintain an erect torso with strong core stabilization. Make sure that clients do not move their upper arms forward but keep them vertical throughout the exercise. Clients should lower the dumbbell only as far as is comfortable on the downward movement.

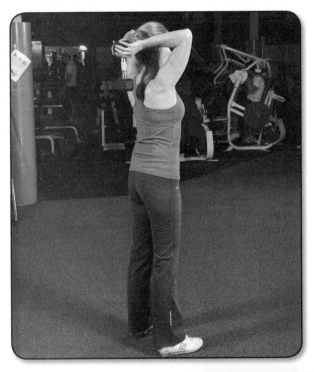

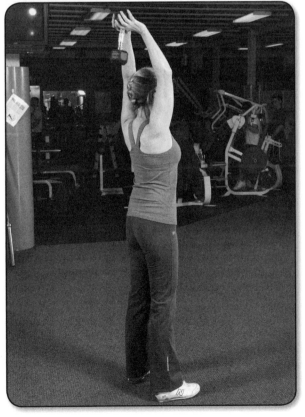

DUMBBELL LYING TRICEPS EXTENSION

Muscles most involved: triceps

Beginning Position

Instruct your client to lie face up on a flat bench with the feet flat on the floor and a dumbbell in each hand. After the client assumes this position, direct him or her to lift the dumbbells upward until the arms are fully extended directly above the shoulders. The upper arms should remain perpendicular to the floor throughout the upward and downward movements. Direct your client to complete the exercise in the following manner.

Downward Movement Phase

1. Lower the dumbbells slowly and in unison until they are next to the ears.
2. Inhale throughout the lowering movement.

Upward Movement Phase

1. Lift the dumbbells upward slowly and in unison until the arms are fully extended above the shoulders.
2. Exhale throughout the upward movement.

Common Errors, Problems, and Modifications

Instruct clients to keep their upper arms perpendicular to the floor and stationary throughout every repetition, moving only their forearms slowly as they perform the dumbbell lying triceps extension. Be sure to spot clients who are not skilled in this exercise.

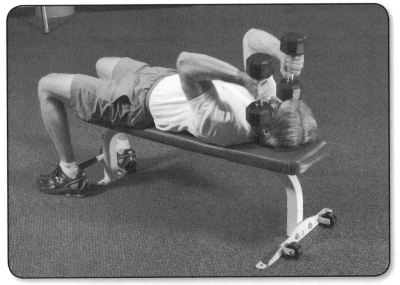

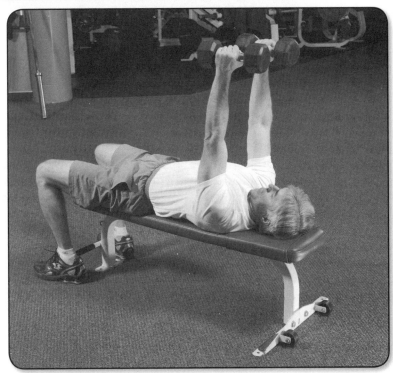

EXERCISE BALL BENCH DIP

**Muscles most involved: triceps,
pectoralis major, anterior deltoid**

Beginning Position

Instruct your client to place the heels of the hands on the bench with the arms extended, the heels of the feet on the exercise ball, and the legs extended so that the hips are in front of the bench. Direct your client to complete the exercise in the following manner.

Downward Movement Phase

1. While maintaining an "L" body position, slowly lower the hips toward the floor until the arms form a 90-degree angle at the elbows.
2. Inhale throughout the downward movement.

Upward Movement Phase

1. While maintaining an "L" body position, press the body slowly upward until the arms are fully extended.
2. Exhale throughout the upward movement.

Common Errors, Problems, and Modifications

This exercise is similar to standard bench dips, but it requires more core stabilization from the midsection muscles. Encourage clients not to flex their elbows more than 90 degrees in the bottom position, because greater elbow flexion may place excessive stress on the shoulder joints.

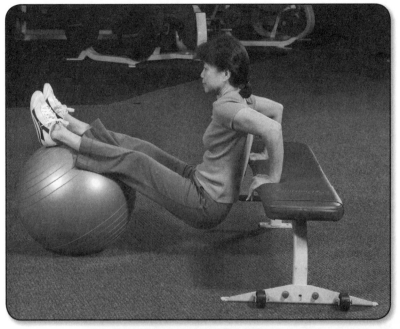

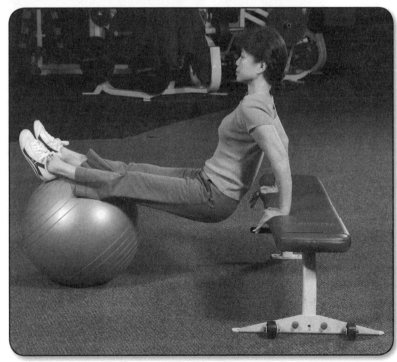

EXERCISE BALL WALK-OUT

Muscles most involved: triceps, pectoralis major, anterior deltoid

Beginning Position

Instruct your client to assume a standard push-up position with the hands on the floor and slightly wider than shoulder-width apart. After the client assumes this position, direct him or her to place the ankles on top of the exercise ball and to establish a straight body position, parallel to the floor. Direct your client to complete the exercise in the following manner.

Backward Movement Phase

1. While maintaining a straight body position, walk the hands backward toward the exercise ball, allowing the legs to roll backward over the ball.
2. Breathe continuously throughout the backward movement.

Forward Movement Phase

1. While maintaining a straight body position, walk the hands forward away from the exercise ball, allowing the legs to roll forward over the ball.
2. Breathe continuously throughout the forward movement.

Common Errors, Problems, and Modifications

This exercise is similar to a walking push-up and is more physically challenging than it may appear. Encourage your clients to use controlled and deliberate arm movements during the performance of exercise ball walk-outs.

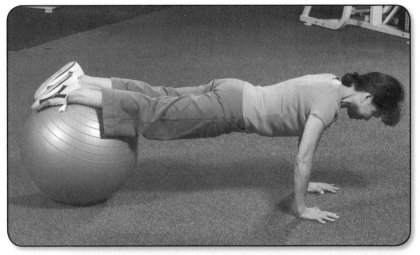

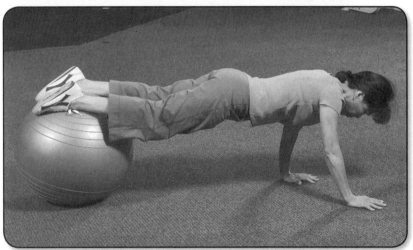

NECK EXTENSION

Muscles most involved: neck extensors

Beginning Position

Help your client adjust the seat so that the back of the head fits comfortably in the head pad and then adjust the torso pad so that an erect posture can be established. After the client has made the seat adjustment, direct him or her to place the back of the head against the head pad with the head angled slightly forward and to grasp the handles. Direct your client to complete the exercise in the following manner.

Backward Movement Phase

1. Push the head pad slowly backward until the neck is comfortably extended.
2. Keep the torso straight.
3. Exhale throughout the backward movement.

Forward Movement Phase

1. Allow the head pad to return slowly to the starting position, with the head angled slightly forward.
2. Inhale throughout the return movement.

Common Errors, Problems, and Modifications

This exercise must be performed slowly with complete control, and proper form may require relatively light weight loads (at first). If clients experience any neck discomfort, have them train only in a pain-free range of movement.

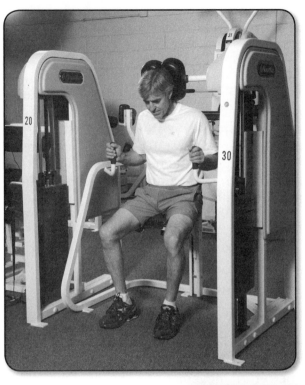

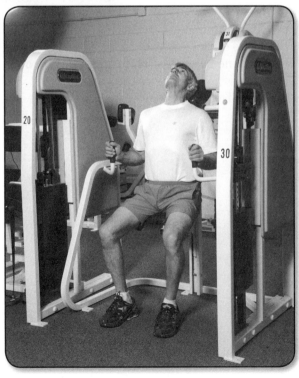

NECK FLEXION

Muscles most involved: neck flexors

Beginning Position

Help your client adjust the seat so that the face fits comfortably against the head pad while the nose is parallel to the crossbar and then adjust the torso pad so that an erect posture can be established. After the client has made the seat adjustment, direct him or her to place the forehead and cheeks against the head pad with the head angled slightly backward and to grasp the handles. Direct your client to complete the exercise in the following manner.

Forward Movement Phase

1. Push the head pad slowly forward until the neck is fully flexed.
2. Keep the torso straight.
3. Exhale throughout the forward movement.

Backward Movement Phase

1. Allow the head pad to return slowly to the starting position, with the head angled slightly backward.
2. Inhale throughout the return movement.

Common Errors, Problems, and Modifications

Like its neck extension counterpart, the neck flexion exercise must be performed slowly with complete control, and proper form may require relatively light weight loads (at first). If clients experience any neck discomfort, have them train only in the pain-free range of movement.

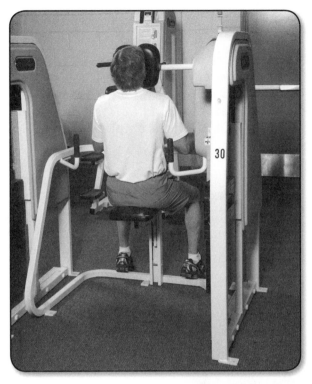

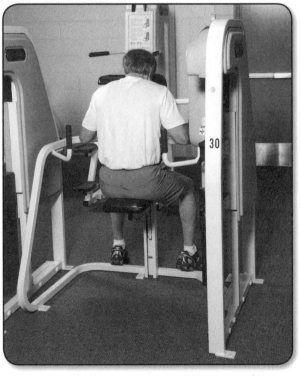

DUMBBELL SHRUG

Muscles most involved: upper trapezius

Beginning Position

Instruct your client to grasp the dumbbells with an overhand grip, with the arms at the sides and fully extended, and to stand erect with the feet hip-width apart. Direct your client to complete the exercise in the following manner.

Upward Movement Phase

1. While keeping the arms straight, elevate (shrug) the shoulders in unison toward the ears, as high as possible.
2. Exhale throughout the shrugging movement.

Downward Movement Phase

1. While keeping the arms straight, lower the dumbbells slowly and in unison to the starting position.
2. Exhale throughout the lowering movement.

Common Errors, Problems, and Modifications

We do not recommend that clients roll their shoulders during the shrug exercise. Simply have clients raise their shoulders as high as is comfortable and pause momentarily in the top position before returning to the starting position. Make sure that clients maintain an erect torso (not leaning forward or backward) during performance of this exercise.

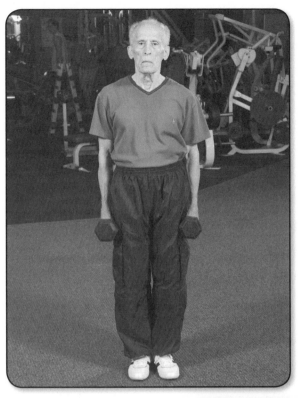

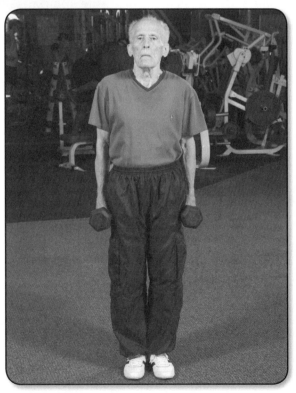

BARBELL SHRUG

Muscles most involved: upper trapezius

Beginning Position

Instruct your client to grasp the barbell with an overhand grip, with the arms at the sides and fully extended, and to stand erect with the feet hip-width apart. Direct your client to complete the exercise in the following manner.

Upward Movement Phase

1. While keeping the arms straight, elevate (shrug) the shoulders toward the ears, as high as possible.
2. Exhale throughout the shrugging movement.

Downward Movement Phase

1. While keeping the arms straight, slowly lower the barbell to the starting position.
2. Inhale throughout the lowering movement.

Common Errors, Problems, and Modifications

As with the dumbbell shrug, we advise against rolling the shoulders during the barbell shrug exercise. Simply have clients raise their shoulders as high as is comfortable and pause momentarily in the top position before returning to the starting position. Make sure that clients maintain an erect torso (not leaning forward or backward) during performance of this exercise.

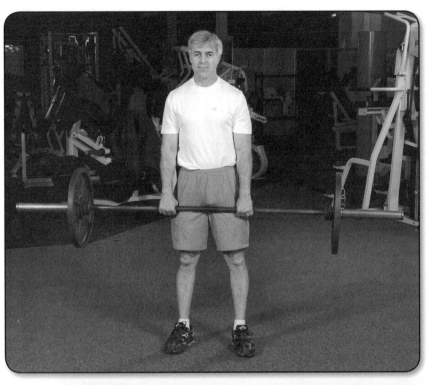

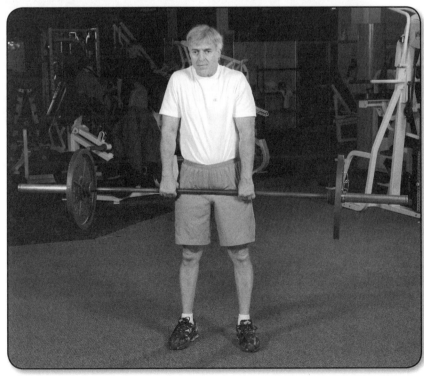

4

Basic Workout Programs

Based on the training principles and teaching strategies outlined in chapter 2 and the exercises presented in chapter 3, we have designed beginner, intermediate, and advanced strength training workouts for men and women in their 50s, 60s, or 70s. The exercises use equipment typically found in fitness facilities, and the programs feature appropriate loads and repetitions for healthy older adults. Chapter 6 discusses alternative equipment such as elastic bands, and chapter 8 suggests modifications for older adults with various medical conditions.

We have included exercises for both machine and free-weight equipment, so you can choose a workout program that best suits your situation. If your clients have strength trained previously or demonstrate above-average strength fitness, you can move more quickly to the intermediate or advanced programs presented later in this book. We strongly suggest that you follow the beginner workout progressions with untrained clients as well as those with experience but below-average strength fitness.

RECOMMENDED LOAD ASSIGNMENTS

To assign appropriate training loads, you must consider age, gender, previous strength training experience, current level of strength fitness, and underlying medical conditions. The load selection tables in this chapter suggest starting loads for clients who will be following the beginner, intermediate, or advanced workouts and who are performing exercises presented here for the first time.

The suggested starting loads for the machine exercises (table 4.1 for men, table 4.2 for women) are based on data from more than 200 older adults who trained on machines (Westcott 1994). Although the suggested loads should result in about 8 to 12 repetitions, adjustments may be necessary, especially if your clients use machines made by a different manufacturer.

The starting loads for the free-weight exercises (table 4.3 for men, table 4.4 for women) are based on the authors' training experiences with many older clients. These loads should also result in 8 to 12 repetitions. You will find other options for determining loads in the discussion of intermediate and advanced programs (chapter 5).

Figure 4.1 (see page 171) shows how to fill out the training log in the appendix, using information from tables 4.1 through 4.4 to assign loads. First determine the type of equipment to be used and the appropriate age category; then adjust

TABLE 4.1

Machine Training—Men

Exercises	Muscle group	SUGGESTED STARTING LOADS IN LB (KG)		
		50–59 years	60–69 years	70–79 years
EXERCISES FOR WEEKS 1 AND 2				
Leg press	Quadriceps Hamstrings	110.0 (49.9)	100.0 (45.4)	90.0 (40.8)
Chest press	Pectoralis major Anterior deltoids Triceps	50.0 (22.7)	45.0 (20.4)	40.0 (18.1)
Seated row	Latissimus dorsi Posterior deltoids Biceps	70.0 (31.7)	62.5 (28.3)	55.0 (24.9)
Lateral raise	Deltoids	47.5 (21.5)	45.0 (20.4)	42.5 (19.3)
Trunk curl	Rectus abdominis	55.0 (24.9)	50.0 (22.7)	45.0 (20.4)
Trunk extension	Erector spinae	55.0 (24.9)	50.0 (22.7)	45.0 (20.4)
ADDITIONAL EXERCISES FOR WEEKS 3 AND 4				
Hip adduction	Hip adductors	65.0 (29.5)	60.0 (27.2)	55.0 (24.9)
Hip abduction	Hip abductors	55.0 (24.9)	50.0 (22.7)	45.0 (20.4)
ADDITIONAL EXERCISES FOR WEEKS 5 AND 6				
Triceps extension	Triceps	45.0 (20.4)	40.0 (18.1)	35.0 (15.9)
Biceps curl	Biceps	45.0 (20.4)	40.0 (18.1)	35.0 (15.9)
ADDITIONAL EXERCISES FOR WEEKS 7 AND 8				
Chest crossover	Pectoralis major	52.5 (23.8)	50.0 (22.7)	47.5 (21.6)
Super pullover	Latissimus dorsi	57.5 (26.1)	55.0 (24.9)	52.5 (23.8)
ADDITIONAL EXERCISES FOR WEEKS 9 AND 10				
Leg curl	Hamstrings	55.0 (24.9)	50.0 (22.7)	45.0 (20.4)
Leg extension	Quadriceps	55.0 (24.9)	50.0 (22.7)	45.0 (20.4)

TABLE 4.2

Machine Training—Women

Exercises	Muscle group	SUGGESTED STARTING LOADS IN LB (KG)		
		50–59 years	60–69 years	70–79 years
EXERCISES FOR WEEKS 1 AND 2				
Leg press	Quadriceps Hamstrings	75.0 (34.0)	67.5 (30.6)	60.0 (27.2)
Chest Press	Pectoralis major Anterior deltoids Triceps	32.5 (14.7)	30.0 (13.6)	27.5 (12.5)
Seated row	Latissimus dorsi Posterior deltoids Biceps	47.5 (21.6)	42.5 (19.3)	37.5 (17.0)

Exercises	Muscle group	50–59 years	60–69 years	70–79 years
EXERCISES FOR WEEKS 1 AND 2 *(continued)*				
Lateral raise	Deltoids	27.5 (12.5)	25.0 (11.3)	22.5 (10.2)
Trunk curl	Rectus abdominis	37.5 (17.0)	35.0 (15.9)	32.5 (14.7)
Trunk extension	Erector spinae	37.5 (17.0)	35.0 (15.9)	32.5 (14.7)
ADDITIONAL EXERCISES FOR WEEKS 3 AND 4				
Hip adduction	Hip adductors	47.5 (21.6)	45.0 (20.4)	42.5 (19.3)
Hip abduction	Hip abductors	37.5 (17.0)	35.0 (15.9)	32.5 (14.7)
ADDITIONAL EXERCISES FOR WEEKS 5 AND 6				
Triceps extension	Triceps	25.0 (11.3)	22.5 (10.2)	20.0 (9.1)
Biceps curl	Biceps	25.0 (11.3)	22.5 (10.2)	20.0 (9.1)
ADDITIONAL EXERCISES FOR WEEKS 7 AND 8				
Leg curl	Hamstrings	35.0 (15.9)	30.0 (13.6)	25.0 (11.3)
Leg extension	Quadriceps	35.0 (15.9)	30.0 (13.6)	25.0 (11.3)
ADDITIONAL EXERCISES FOR WEEKS 9 AND 10				
Chest crossover	Pectoralis major	30.0 (13.6)	27.5 (12.5)	25.0 (11.3)
Super pullover	Latissimus dorsi	32.5 (14.7)	30.0 (11.3)	27.5 (12.5)

TABLE 4.3

Free-Weight Training—Men

Exercises	Muscle group	SUGGESTED STARTING LOADS IN LB (KG)		
		50–59 years	60–69 years	70–79 years
EXERCISES FOR WEEKS 1 AND 2				
Dumbbell squat	Quadriceps Hamstrings	25.0 (11.3)	20.0 (9.1)	15.0 (6.8)
Dumbbell bench press	Pectoralis major Anterior deltoids Triceps	25.0 (11.3)	20.0 (9.1)	15.0 (6.8)
Dumbbell one-arm row	Latissimus dorsi Posterior deltoids Biceps	25.0 (11.3)	20.0 (9.1)	15.0 (6.8)
Dumbbell seated press	Deltoids Triceps	20.0 (9.1)	15.0 (6.8)	10.0 (4.5)
Trunk curl	Rectus abdominis	20 reps	15 reps	10 reps
Trunk extension	Erector spinae	15 reps	10 reps	5 reps
ADDITIONAL EXERCISES FOR WEEKS 3 AND 4				
Dumbbell standing curl	Biceps	15.0 (6.8)	12.5 (5.7)	10.0 (4.5)
Dumbbell overhead triceps extension	Triceps	15.0 (6.8)	12.5 (5.7)	10.0 (4.5)

(continued)

ADDITIONAL EXERCISES FOR WEEKS 5 AND 6 *(continued)*				
Dumbbell shrug	Upper trapezius	25.0 (11.3)	20.0 (9.1)	15.0 (6.8)
Dumbbell heel raise	Gastrocnemius and soleus	25.0 (11.3)	20.0 (9.1)	15.0 (6.8)
ADDITIONAL EXERCISE FOR WEEKS 7 AND 8				
Dumbbell chest fly	Pectoralis major	15.0 (6.8)	12.5 (5.7)	10.0 (4.5)
ADDITIONAL EXERCISE FOR WEEKS 9 AND 10				
Lat pull-down	Latissimus dorsi Biceps	60.0 (27.2)	50.0 (22.7)	40.0 (18.1)

TABLE 4.4

Free-Weight Training—Women

		SUGGESTED STARTING LOADS IN LB (KG)		
Exercises	**Muscle group**	**50–59 years**	**60–69 years**	**70–79 years**
EXERCISES FOR WEEKS 1 AND 2				
Dumbbell squat	Quadriceps Hamstrings	15.0 (6.8)	12.5 (5.7)	10.0 (4.5)
Dumbbell bench press	Pectoralis major Anterior deltoids Triceps	12.5 (5.7)	10.0 (4.5)	7.5 (3.4)
Dumbbell one-arm row	Latissimus dorsi Posterior deltoids Biceps	12.5 (5.7)	10.0 (4.5)	7.5 (3.4)
Dumbbell seated press	Deltoids Triceps	12.5 (5.7)	10.0 (4.5)	7.5 (3.4)
Trunk curl	Rectus abdominis	15 reps	10 reps	5 reps
Trunk extension	Erector spinae	12 reps	8 reps	4 reps
ADDITIONAL EXERCISES FOR WEEKS 3 AND 4				
Dumbbell Standing curl	Biceps	10.0 (4.5)	7.5 (3.4)	5.0 (2.3)
Dumbbell overhead triceps extension	Triceps	7.5 (3.4)	5.0 (2.3)	2.5 (1.1)
ADDITIONAL EXERCISES FOR WEEKS 5 AND 6				
Dumbbell shrug	Upper trapezius	15.0 (6.8)	12.5 (5.7)	10.0 (4.5)
Dumbbell heel raise	Gastrocnemius and soleus	15.0 (6.8)	12.5 (5.7)	10.0 (4.5)
ADDITIONAL EXERCISE FOR WEEKS 7 AND 8				
Dumbbell chest fly	Pectoralis major	10.0 (4.5)	7.5 (3.4)	5.0 (2.3)
ADDITIONAL EXERCISE FOR WEEKS 9 AND 10				
Lat pull-down	Latissimus dorsi Biceps	40.0 (18.1)	35.0 (15.9)	30.0 (13.6)

Training Log

Write in goal for number of reps to perform here

Order	Exercise	Sets		Day 1			Day 2			Day 3		
Name				Week #								
		Reps		Set 1	Set 2	Set 3	Set 1	Set 2	Set 3	Set 1	Set 2	Set 3
1	Leg press	1	Weight	100								
		10	Reps	10								
2	Chest press	1	Weight	45								
		10	Reps	9								
3	Seated row	1	Weight	62								
		10	Reps	10								
4	Lateral raise	1	Weight	45								
		10	Reps	8								
5	Trunk curl	1	Weight	50								
		10	Reps	6								
6	Trunk extension	1	Weight	50								
		10	Reps	8								
7			Weight									
			Reps									
8			Weight									
			Reps									
9			Weight									
			Reps									
10			Weight									
			Reps									
11			Weight									
			Reps									
12			Weight									
			Reps									
13			Weight									
			Reps									
14			Weight									
			Reps									
Bodyweight												
Date												
Comments												

Record actual weight used here

Record actual reps completed here

Write in goal for number of sets to perform here

Figure 4.1 How to record workout information in the training log.

the loads for each exercise according to your client's strength fitness level (see the first part of chapter 7, especially table 7.1). Figure 4.1 also shows how to transfer load and "goal" repetition information to your clients' training log and where to record dates and reps completed. (Weeks 1 and 2 of the beginner program are used as an example.) Follow the same procedure to record information for intermediate or advanced workouts. If you intend to have clients complete all three of the 4-week training cycles, make 12 copies of the training log before writing in training information. (A blank copy of the training log may be found in the appendix; copy the training log at 120 percent if you want an 8.5-inch-by-11-inch log.)

As a rule, clients with below-average strength fitness should reduce the recommended exercise loads in tables 4.1 through 4.4 by about 10 to 20 percent; those who are above average should increase the loads by about 10 to 20 percent. Reduce the resistance if a client cannot complete at least eight repetitions with good form; increase the load if he or she can perform more than 12 reps. Use table 4.5 to calculate changes in load.

Beginner Workout Program

The beginner workout program includes five 2-week segments. It begins with six exercises that involve most of the major muscle groups and adds new exercises every 2 weeks.

TABLE 4.5

Load Adjustment Guidelines for Repetitions Completed

Goal reps	Below goal subtract lb (kg)	Above goal add lb (kg)
1	2.5 (1.1)	2.5 (1.1)
2	5.0 (2.3)	5.0 (2.3)
3	7.5 (3.4)	7.5 (3.4)
4	10.0 (4.5)	10.0 (4.5)
5	12.5 (5.7)	12.5 (5.7)
6	15.0 (6.8)	15.0 (6.8)

In the left-hand column identify the number of reps that your client performed below or above the "Goal reps" listed in the training log for a particular exercise. Subtract the weight listed in the "Below goal" column from the current load if your client performed too few reps. Add the weight in the "Above goal" column if your client performed too many reps.

WEEKS 1 AND 2

For machine equipment, the exercises for weeks 1 and 2 of the beginner program (refer to tables 4.1 and 4.2 for training loads) are performed in this order:

1. Leg press
2. Chest press
3. Seated row
4. Lateral raise
5. Trunk curl
6. Trunk extension

For free-weight equipment, exercises for weeks 1 and 2 (refer to tables 4.3 and 4.4 for training loads) are performed in this order:

1. Dumbbell squat
2. Dumbbell bench press
3. Dumbbell one-arm row
4. Dumbbell seated press
5. Trunk curl
6. Trunk extension

Copy the training log in the appendix for your clients' use (copy at 120 percent for an 8.5-inch-by-11-inch log). If you have questions about how to fill out the training log, study figure 4.1. Be sure that your clients perform these exercises in the order in which they are listed. As you add exercises to beginner workouts in weeks 3, 5, 7, and 9, refer to tables 4.1 through 4.4 for appropriate load assignments. Instruct beginning clients to perform 8 to 12 repetitions in all exercises except the trunk curl and trunk extension, in which they should perform 20 to 30 repetitions. In all other exercises, as soon as your client is able to perform 12 repetitions with good form during two consecutive workouts, increase the load by 1.25 to 2.5 pounds (0.57 to 1.1 kg).

WEEKS 3 AND 4

At this point your clients are strengthening most of their major muscle groups, and the exercise movement patterns should be second nature. Because many older adults are concerned about hip function, we suggest that you add two exercises to the machine training program if the machines are available—the hip adduction machine for the hip adductor muscles and the hip abduction machine for the hip abductor muscles. Insert these exercises between the leg press and chest press exercises.

For a free-weight program, the squat exercise that is already included is an excellent hip strengthener, so you need not add other lower-body exercises at this time. Instead, complement the basic workout with dumbbell curls for the biceps muscles and dumbbell overhead triceps extensions for the triceps muscles. These two new exercises should be done after the dumbbell press and before the trunk curls.

For a machine exercise program, then, the exercises during weeks 3 and 4 (again, refer to tables 4.1 and 4.2 for training loads for new exercises) are performed in this order:

1. Leg press
2. Hip adductor
3. Hip abductor
4. Chest press

5. Seated row
6. Lateral raise
7. Trunk curl
8. Trunk extension

For a free-weight program, the exercises during weeks 3 and 4 (refer to tables 4.3 and 4.4 for training loads for new exercises) are performed in this order:

1. Dumbbell squat
2. Dumbbell bench press
3. Dumbbell one-arm row
4. Dumbbell seated press

5. Dumbbell standing curl
6. Dumbbell overhead triceps extension
7. Trunk curl
8. Trunk extension

Record either the machine or free-weight exercises, in the order presented, onto a training log (see page 307) and label this training log "Weeks 3 and 4."

WEEKS 5 AND 6

The machine training program involves three exercises for the legs, two for the trunk, and three for the upper body. Although the arms are involved in both the chest press and the seated row exercises, triceps extensions and biceps curls will train these muscles more directly. The triceps extension machine targets the triceps muscles, and the biceps curl machine targets the biceps muscles. Add these two exercises between the lateral raise and trunk curl exercises.

If your client is training with free weights, add the dumbbell shrug for the upper trapezius and the dumbbell heel raise for the gastrocnemius and soleus muscles. These new exercises should follow all the other exercises.

The machine exercise program during weeks 5 and 6 (refer to tables 4.1 and 4.2 for training loads for new exercises) comprises the following exercises to be performed in this order:

1. Leg press
2. Hip adduction
3. Hip abduction
4. Chest press
5. Seated row
6. Lateral raise
7. Triceps extension
8. Biceps curl
9. Trunk curl
10. Trunk extension

For weeks 5 and 6 of a free-weight program (refer to tables 4.3 and 4.4 for training loads for new exercises), your clients should perform the following exercises in this order:

1. Dumbbell squat
2. Dumbbell bench press
3. Dumbbell one-arm row
4. Dumbbell seated press
5. Dumbbell standing curl
6. Dumbbell overhead triceps extension
7. Trunk curl
8. Trunk extension
9. Dumbbell shrug
10. Dumbbell heel raise

Record either the machine or free-weight exercises, in the order presented, onto a training log (see page 307) and label this training log "Weeks 5 and 6."

WEEKS 7 AND 8

After 6 weeks of regular strength training, your clients should have more muscle and less fat, and should feel stronger than when they entered the program. At this point you may want to spend a little time explaining some of the adaptations that the muscles are making because of regular strength training (chapter 1). If your client is using machines, follow the chest press with the chest crossover and the seated row with the super pullover. This pattern provides two sequential exercises for the large pectoralis major and latissimus dorsi muscles.

If your client is using free weights, complement the dumbbell bench press exercise with the dumbbell chest fly exercise to emphasize chest development.

This exercise better isolates the pectoralis major muscle and should be performed after the dumbbell bench press.

Thus, in a machine exercise program, the exercises for weeks 7 and 8 (refer to tables 4.1 and 4.2 for training loads for new exercises) are performed in this order:

1. Leg press
2. Hip adduction
3. Hip abduction
4. Chest press
5. Chest crossover
6. Seated row
7. Super pullover
8. Lateral raise
9. Triceps extension
10. Biceps curl
11. Trunk curl
12. Trunk extension

In a free-weight exercise program, the exercises for weeks 7 and 8 (refer to tables 4.3 and 4.4 for training loads for new exercises) are performed in this order:

1. Dumbbell squat
2. Dumbbell bench press
3. Dumbbell chest fly
4. Dumbbell one-arm row
5. Dumbbell seated press
6. Dumbbell standing curl
7. Dumbbell overhead triceps extension
8. Trunk curl
9. Trunk extension
10. Dumbbell shrug
11. Dumbbell heel raise

Record either the machine or free-weight exercises in the order presented onto a training log (see page 307) and label this training log "Weeks 7 and 8."

WEEKS 9 AND 10

Just as you added two upper-body machine exercises to target the chest and upper-back muscles, you can now better address your clients' leg muscles. Follow the leg press with the leg curl and leg extension exercises. The leg curl specifically works the hamstring muscles, and the leg extension specifically works the quadriceps muscles.

If clients following a free-weight program have access to a pulley apparatus on which they can perform lat pull-downs, consider adding this exercise after the dumbbell one-arm row. The lat pull-down works the latissimus dorsi and biceps muscles. This pulley exercise provides excellent training for these muscle groups and adds variety to the workout program.

For a machine exercise program in weeks 9 and 10 (refer to tables 4.1 and 4.2 for training loads for new exercises), the exercises are performed in this order:

1. Leg press
2. Leg curl
3. Leg extension
4. Hip adduction
5. Hip abduction
6. Chest press
7. Chest crossover
8. Seated row
9. Super pullover
10. Lateral raise
11. Triceps extension
12. Biceps curl
13. Trunk curl
14. Trunk extension

For a free-weight exercise program, the exercises for weeks 9 and 10 (refer to tables 4.3 and 4.4 for training loads for new exercises) are performed in this order:

1. Dumbbell squat
2. Dumbbell bench press
3. Dumbbell chest fly
4. Dumbbell one-arm row
5. Lat pull-down
6. Dumbbell seated press
7. Dumbbell standing curl
8. Dumbbell overhead triceps extension
9. Trunk curl
10. Trunk extension
11. Dumbbell shrug
12. Dumbbell heel raise

Record either the machine or free-weight exercises in the order presented onto a training log (see page 307) and label this training log "Weeks 9 and 10."

What Next?

Your clients have now completed 10 weeks of regular strength training exercises, working almost all their major muscle groups productively and progressively. The results should be obvious. At this point you have many options for continuing or changing their strength training program. For example, you can alternate different exercises for the target muscles, thereby increasing the training variety and the developmental stimulus. You can also combine machine and free-weight training exercises.

C H A P T E R

5

Intermediate and Advanced Workout Programs

If your clients have the time and desire to expand their strength training workouts, they may perform more sets of each exercise or additional exercises for each major muscle group. You can also use different training protocols to emphasize larger muscle size, greater muscle strength, or more muscle endurance. This chapter will help you design such programs.

The 10-week beginner training program (in chapter 4) provided a sensible progression of strength training exercises and starting training loads for completing 8 to 12 repetitions. The systematic integration of these exercises enabled your clients to master the performance techniques and to adapt physiologically to the training program. As your clients near the end of the 10-week program, they may ask what they should do next. You may want them to continue their current workouts because they have experienced excellent improvements in muscle strength and body composition. If so, be sure to vary the exercises periodically and increase the training resistance progressively as your clients become stronger.

You may also decide to introduce a capable client to more challenging workouts. This can be an exciting time! Their muscle strength should be sufficient to handle heavier loads, and their muscle endurance should enable them to complete longer and more demanding workouts. Obviously, the purpose of more comprehensive workouts is to produce even greater strength gains and muscle development. Just be sensible in the approach that you take. Always keep your clients' ability levels in mind; reinforce the importance of proper form; and add exercises, increase sets, and increase loads gradually.

INTERMEDIATE TRAINING CONSIDERATIONS

For further strength training, you can choose from three intermediate programs included in this chapter. Each is designed with a specific training outcome in mind. One emphasizes muscle size increases, another emphasizes muscle strength increases, and the third emphasizes muscle endurance as a training outcome.

After you have decided which outcome best meets your clients' needs, refer to the appropriate sample training program in this chapter. These workouts offer the option of using free weights or machines, or a combination of both.

Be sure to apply the training principles and teaching strategies presented in chapter 2 and the exercise execution procedures and instruction recommendations presented in chapter 3.

The intermediate training options presented here build on the 10-week program of exercises in the beginner workouts. To reduce the chance of setbacks caused by doing too much too soon, each program starts with a 4-week transition period. Following the transition period is a less intense training week followed by a 4-week program of greater intensity. A less intense week occurs again and is followed by another 4-week program of more intense training time. The 4-week programs described here are referred to as training cycles. Each training cycle presents workouts that are more intense than the preceding one.

As the workouts become more demanding, the time required to complete them increases. To help you schedule your clients' training sessions, we have listed the approximate amount of time necessary for completing workouts at the end of each program. We have kept the workouts as brief as possible without sacrificing effectiveness. If clients can devote only a limited amount of time to train, use the transition period workouts (weeks 1–4) for their standard training program because these require less time than the more comprehensive programs do (weeks 6–9 and 11–14).

The following directions should help you adapt the 10-week basic program to the more intense training cycles presented next. Consider the equipment requirements for the program selected before deciding which workouts you will have your clients follow. Also note that certain free-weight exercises require a spotter, such as the barbell squat, heel raise, and bench press exercises.

Whichever program you choose for your clients, be sure to do the following:

- Record exercises, training loads, and goal reps onto the training log (page 307).
- Teach clients how to record dates and the number of repetitions completed for each workout (suggestion: Use figure 4.1).
- Remind clients to perform exercises in the order in which they are listed.
- Encourage clients to perform the number of repetitions indicated, expecting that the number of reps completed in the second and third sets will be fewer than those in the preceding set.

Recording Workout Information in the Training Logs

After you have decided which program (muscle size, muscle strength, or muscle endurance) and which type of equipment (machines, free weights) that your client will be following, the next step is to record his or her training information onto the appropriate training log. Make 12 copies of the training log in the appendix if your client will be completing all three 4-week training cycles (enlarge at 120 percent for 8.5-inch-by-11-inch forms). If necessary, refer to figure 4.1 in the last chapter for a review of how to transfer information regarding "goal reps," number of sets to perform, and training loads. This figure also shows where to record training dates, the number of reps completed, and comments about the workout.

- When clients are performing more than one set of an exercise and exceed the specified number of reps in the final set on two successive workouts, increase the training load as indicated in table 4.5. If clients cannot complete the desired number of repetitions, decrease the training load as recommended in table 4.5.
- If your clients have been training with dumbbells and you change to barbell exercises, you will need to increase training loads. A good rule of thumb is to double the dumbbell weight (weight of one dumbbell) that you are using in the same exercise.
- If you decide to add exercises or ask your clients to perform additional sets, and especially if you decide to do both, consider the 4-day-a-week program described in the advanced programs section of this chapter.

MUSCLE SIZE

Modify the 10-week beginner program (chapter 4) in the following ways to emphasize muscle size improvements:

- Prescribe 8 to 12 repetitions per exercise, which should require an increased training load (see tables 5.1 and 5.2). Adding about 5 pounds

TABLE 5.1

Intermediate Machine Program for Muscle Size Development (Three Nonconsecutive Days)

| | | | TRAINING CYCLES | | |
| | | | Weeks 1-4 | Weeks 6-9 | Weeks 11-14 |
Order	Exercise	Reps	Sets	Sets	Sets
1	Leg press	8-12	2	3	3
2	Leg curl	8-12	2	3	3
3	Leg extension	8-12	2	2	3
4	Chest crossover	8-12	2	3	3
5	Chest press	8-12	2	2	3
6	Seated row	8-12	2	2	3
7	Super pullover	8-12	2	2	3
8	Lateral raise	8-12	1	2	3
9	Triceps extension	8-12	2	3	3
10	Biceps curl	8-12	2	3	3
11	Bar dip	8-12	1	2	2
12	Pull-up	8-12	1	2	2
13	Trunk extension	8-12	1	2	2
14	Trunk curl	8-12	1	2	2
Estimated time requirements (min)			45	65	70

Note: Weeks 4, 9, and 14 should be followed with a less intense week of training in which loads are reduced by 10 pounds (4.5 kg) and only one set of each exercise is performed.

TABLE 5.2

Intermediate Free-Weight Program for Muscle Size Development (Three Nonconsecutive Days)

			TRAINING CYCLES		
			Weeks 1-4	Weeks 6-9	Weeks 11-14
Order	Exercise	Reps	Sets	Sets	Sets
1	Dumbbell or barbell squat	8-12	2	3	3
2	Dumbbell or barbell bench press	8-12	2	3	3
3	Dumbbell chest fly	8-12	1	2	2
4	Dumbbell one-arm row	8-12	2	2	3
5	Lat pull-down	8-12	2	2	2
6	Dumbbell lateral raise	8-12	1	2	2
7	Dumbbell or barbell curl	8-12	2	3	
8	Dumbbell concentration curl	8-12	1	2	2
9	Dumbbell overhead triceps extension	8-12	1	2	2
10	Triceps press down	8-12	1	2	2
11	Barbell shrug	8-12	1	2	2
12	Trunk curl	30-50	1	2	2
13	Trunk extension	10-15	1	2	2
Estimated time requirements (min)			40	60	65

Note: Weeks 4, 9, and 14 should be followed with a less intense week of training in which loads are reduced by 10 pounds (4.5 kg) and only one set of each exercise is performed.

(2.3 kg) to the exercises in the beginner program should reduce the number of repetitions to the lower end of the 8-to-12 rep range. The 10 weeks of training leading up to these workouts should have prepared the muscles for these heavier loads. But if you are not confident about increasing your clients' training loads by 5 pounds (2.3 kg) at a time, you may add 2.5 (1.1 kg) pounds in week 1 and another 2.5 pounds in week 2.

- In the free-weight training program, you have the option of using either barbells or dumbbells; we have also added a new biceps exercise, the dumbbell concentration curl. Remember that your client should use a little less than half of the barbell curl load to perform the dumbbell concentration curl. We have added the weight-assisted pull-up and bar dip exercises to the machine training program—try using 40 percent of bodyweight for male clients and 60 percent for female clients. The load used in these exercises is designed to counterbalance bodyweight, so adding weight makes them easier to perform. Again, refer to table 4.5 if load adjustments are needed. You may want to add different exercises if your client expresses a desire to emphasize a muscle area other than the arms.

- Increase the number of sets in certain exercises to two for the first 4 weeks and then to three in the last 4 weeks. In other exercises, the number of sets increases to two during the second 4-week cycle and remains at two in the third cycle (see tables 5.1 and 5.2).

- Rest periods recommended for the basic program in chapter 4 should be shortened to 1 minute unless you believe that a client would benefit from more complete muscle recovery.

- Set a goal of 30 reps in both sets of the trunk curl exercises during weeks 1 through 4, 40 reps in weeks 6 through 9, and 50 reps in weeks 11 through 14.

- After each training cycle, your clients should benefit from a week of less intense training. This break from the mental repetitiveness of the training program will allow muscles to gain some needed rest, rebuild tissue, and become stronger. At this point, have clients perform only one set of 8 to 12 reps of each exercise with loads reduced by 10 pounds (4.5 kg), except the trunk curl and trunk extension. Keep the reps in these exercises the same. After week 15, resume the workout program performed in weeks 1 to 4 (table 5.1 or 5.2), adjusting loads appropriately as indicated in table 4.5. Thereafter, plan a less intense week of training after the 4th week of every training cycle. This protocol (including a week of less intense training) is also important to implement if you intend to have clients follow one of the more advanced programs offered at the end of this chapter.

MUSCLE STRENGTH

To emphasize muscular strength as a training outcome, modify the 10-week beginner program (chapter 4) in the following ways:

- In the exercises marked with an asterisk (see tables 5.3 and 5.4), gradually increase the training load so that the number of repetitions decreases— from 8 to 12 down to 6 to 8—during weeks 1 and 2. To put your clients in the range of 6 to 8 repetitions for these exercises, add about 10 pounds (4.5 kg) to the present training loads. If adding 10 pounds fails to achieve the rep range of 6 to 8, make appropriate load adjustments using table 4.5 as a guide. But if you are not confident about increasing a client's load by 10 pounds (4.5 kg) all at once, add 5 pounds (2.3 kg) in week 1, another 2.5 pounds (1.1 kg) in week 2, and 2.5 more pounds during week 3. Whenever your client is able to complete 2 or more repetitions beyond the goal in the final set during two consecutive workouts, increase the training load by 2.5 pounds (1.1 kg).

- For exercises without an asterisk, instruct clients to perform 8 to 12 repetitions, again referring to table 4.5 if load adjustments are needed. When clients are able to complete 12 or more repetitions in the last exercise set on two consecutive occasions, increase the load by 2.5 pounds (1.1 kg).

- For exercises in the range of 6 to 8 reps, increase the number of sets from one to two during the second 4-week cycle, and to three during the

TABLE 5.3

Intermediate Machine Program for Strength Development
(Three Nonconsecutive Days)

| | | | TRAINING CYCLES | | |
| | | | Weeks 1-4 | Weeks 6-9 | Weeks 11-14 |
Order	Exercise	Reps	Sets	Sets	Sets
1	*Leg press	6-8	1	2	3
2	Heel raise	8-12	2	2	2
3	*Chest press	6-8	1	2	3
4	*Seated row	6-8	1	2	3
5	Lateral raise	8-12	2	2	2
6	Triceps extension	8-12	2	2	2
7	Biceps curl	8-12	2	2	2
8	Trunk extension	8-12	2	2	2
9	Trunk curl	8-12	2	2	2
Estimated time requirements (min)			45	60	70

*In the exercises marked with an asterisk, gradually increase loads, which will reduce the number of repetitions—from 8 to 12 down to 6 to 8—during weeks 1 through 2.

Note: Weeks 4, 9, and 14 should be followed with a less intense week of training in which loads are reduced by 10 pounds (4.5 kg) and only one set of each exercise is performed.

TABLE 5.4

Intermediate Free-Weight Program for Strength Development
(Three Nonconsecutive Days)

| | | | TRAINING CYCLES | | |
| | | | Weeks 1-4 | Weeks 6-9 | Weeks 11-14 |
Order	Exercise	Reps	Sets	Sets	Sets
1	*Dumbbell or barbell squat	6-8	1	2	3
2	Dumbbell or barbell heel raise	8-12	2	2	2
3	*Dumbbell or barbell bench press	6-8	1	2	3
4	*Dumbbell one-arm row	6-8	1	2	3
5	Dumbbell lateral raise	8-12	2	2	2
6	Dumbbell or barbell curl	8-12	2	2	2
7	Dumbbell overhead triceps extension	8-12	2	2	2
8	Trunk curl	30-50	2	2	2
9	Trunk extension	10-15	2	2	2
Estimated time requirements (min)			45	60	70

*In the exercises marked with an asterisk, gradually increase loads, which will reduce the number of repetitions—from 8 to 12 down to 6 to 8—during weeks 1 through 2.

Note: Weeks 4, 9, and 14 should be followed with a less intense week of training in which loads are reduced by 10 pounds (4.5 kg) and only one set of each exercise is performed.

last 4-week cycle. In exercises in the range of 8 to 12 reps, the number of sets increases to two during the first 4-week cycle and remains at two throughout the second and third cycles (see tables 5.3 and 5.4).

- Increase the length of the rest periods between sets to 2 to 3 minutes. Longer rest periods allow more time for the muscles to recover, enabling the use of heavier training loads in succeeding sets.

- After each training cycle, your clients will benefit from a week of less intense training. Have them perform only one set of each exercise with loads reduced by 10 pounds (4.5 kg), performing the same number of reps (6–8 or 8–12) listed for each exercise. After week 15, they may resume the workout that they were doing in weeks 1 to 4, with appropriate load adjustments as indicated in table 4.5. Thereafter, plan a less intense week of training after the 4th week of every training cycle. This procedure is also recommended if your clients follow one of the more advanced programs at the end of this chapter. For a more detailed explanation of how and why to vary exercise intensity over time to maximize strength gains, refer to the books by Baechle and Earle (2004, 2005, 2006, 2008).

MUSCLE ENDURANCE

To emphasize muscle endurance as a training outcome, modify the beginner 10-week training program as follows:

- Progressively increase your clients' reps to 15 (see tables 5.5 and 5.6) while using the same training load. After they are able to complete 15 or more repetitions in the last set on two consecutive occasions, increase the load by 2.5 pounds (1.1 kg).

- Increase the number of sets in certain exercises to two in the first 4-week cycle and then to three during the last 4-week cycle. In other exercises, increase the number of sets to two for both the second and third 4-week cycles (see tables 5.5 and 5.6).

- Rest periods of 1 minute should be continued, even when multiple sets are performed.

- Encourage your clients to perform 30 reps in both sets of the trunk curl during weeks 1 through 4, 40 reps in weeks 6 through 9; and 50 reps in weeks 11 through 14.

- After each training cycle, your clients will benefit from a week of less intense training for the reasons mentioned on page 181. Reduce training loads by 10 pounds (4.5 kg) and prescribe only one set of 15 reps in each exercise. After week 15, your clients should resume the workouts that they were performing in weeks 1 to 4 (table 5.5 or 5.6), making appropriate load adjustments as indicated in table 4.5. Thereafter, plan a less intense week of training after the 4th week of every training cycle. Also, if you intend to have clients perform one of the more intense training programs at the end of this chapter, prescribe a less intense week of training just before initiating the more advanced program.

TABLE 5.5

Intermediate Machine Program for Muscle Endurance Development (Three Nonconsecutive Days)

| | | | TRAINING CYCLES | | |
| | | | Weeks 1-4 | Weeks 6-9 | Weeks 11-14 |
Order	Exercise	Reps	Sets	Sets	Sets
1	Leg extension	12-15	2	2	3
2	Leg curl	12-15	2	2	3
3	Hip abduction	12-15	1	2	2
4	Hip adduction	12-15	1	2	2
5	Chest crossover	12-15	2	2	3
6	Super pullover	12-15	2	2	3
7	Lateral raise	12-15	2	2	3
8	Triceps extension	12-15	2	2	3
9	Biceps curl	12-15	2	2	3
10	Rotary torso	12-15	1	2	2
Estimated time requirements (min)			35	40	55

Note: Weeks 4, 9, and 14 should be followed with a less intense week of training in which loads are reduced by 10 pounds (4.5 kg) and only one set of each exercise is performed.

TABLE 5.6

Intermediate Free-Weight Program for Muscle Endurance Development (Three Nonconsecutive Days)

| | | | TRAINING CYCLES | | |
| | | | Weeks 1-4 | Weeks 6–9 | Weeks 11-14 |
Order	Exercise	Reps	Sets	Sets	Sets
1	Dumbbell or barbell squat	12-15	2	2	3
2	Dumbbell or barbell heel raise	12-15	1	2	2
3	Dumbbell or barbell bench press	12-15	2	2	3
4	Dumbbell chest fly	12-15	1	2	2
5	Dumbbell one-arm row	12-15	2	2	3
6	Dumbbell seated press	12-15	2	2	3
7	Dumbbell or barbell biceps curl	12-15	2	2	3
8	Dumbbell overhead triceps extension	12-15	2	2	3
9	Barbell shrug	12-15	1	2	2
10	Trunk curl	30-50	2	2	2
11	Trunk extension	10-15	2	2	2
Estimated time requirements (min)			40	45	55

Note: Weeks 4, 9, and 14 should be followed with a less intense week of training in which loads are reduced by 10 pounds (4.5 kg) and only one set of each exercise is performed.

If body reproportioning is the primary goal of a client, it is likely that he or she has too much fat, too little muscle, or both. Consider one or all of these actions to help the client improve his or her body composition:

- Follow the muscle size program described earlier in this chapter to increase muscle mass.

- Encourage clients to select foods more carefully (refer to chapter 10 for relevant nutrition information), and emphasize the importance of reducing fat and calorie intake. You should strongly encourage clients interested in improving their body composition to include aerobic training along with strength training, ideally using a circuit training approach.

- Design an aerobic (endurance) program to help burn more calories. For additional guidance in this area, refer to the texts *Fitness Weight Training* by Baechle and Earle (2005) and *Building Strength and Stamina* by Westcott (2003).

Recording Workout Information in the Training Logs

After you have decided which program (muscle size, muscle strength, or muscle endurance) and which type of equipment (machines, free weights) your client will be following, the next step is to record the training information onto the appropriate training log. Make 12 copies of the training log in the appendix if your client will be completing all three 4-week training cycles (enlarge at 120 percent for 8.5-inch-by-11-inch forms). If necessary, refer to figure 4.1 for a review of how to transfer information regarding "goal reps," number of sets to perform, and training loads. This figure also shows where to record training dates, the number of reps completed, and comments about the workout.

ADVANCED TRAINING CONSIDERATIONS

The advanced training workouts, like the intermediate workouts, permit you to emphasize specific training outcomes (muscle size, strength, or endurance). Each program consists of two 4 week schedules with a less intense week of training between them; therefore, each is 9 weeks in length. Presented first are the workouts that emphasize muscle size. Next are programs designed to enhance muscle strength. Finally, programs that focus on muscle endurance are presented. Unlike the intermediate workouts, the muscle size and strength workouts involve what is referred to as the split system of training. This advanced training method splits up the exercises according to body parts, working some muscles 2 days a week and other muscles on 2 different days of the week. This type of training protocol enables you to spread your clients' exercises over 4 days instead of 3, reducing the amount of time needed to complete each workout. This arrangement also offers the opportunity to add more exercises and sets while keeping the length of each workout reasonable. Because your clients can perform a wider variety

> ### Training Days for Muscle Endurance
>
> As explained in chapter 2, your clients should not work the same muscle groups on 2 consecutive days or allow more than 3 days to go by between training sessions. For muscle endurance workouts, therefore, we suggest that you have clients follow a Monday–Wednesday–Friday schedule or a Tuesday–Thursday–Saturday schedule.

of exercises each session, they are able to emphasize muscle size and strength development in specific muscle groups. Examples of such an arrangement are presented later. The disadvantage of the split training approach is that your clients must add an extra training day to their week.

Split training programs require four workouts a week. Choose a program that best fits your client's schedule and make four copies of the training log. Each of the following protocols includes two upper-body and two lower-body workouts per week and provides sufficient rest days between weight training days for the same muscle groups:

1. Mondays, Thursdays—upper body; Tuesdays, Fridays—lower body.
2. Sundays, Wednesdays—upper body; Mondays, Thursdays—lower body.
3. Tuesdays, Fridays—upper body; Wednesdays, Saturdays—lower body.

Advanced Workout: Muscle Size

The 4-week advanced muscle size program shown in table 5.7 includes four workouts each week—2 training days for the upper body and 2 for the lower body. The upper-body workouts include two exercises for the chest and back, and one each for the shoulders, biceps, and triceps. The lower-body workouts include two for the combined thigh muscles and one each for the hamstrings, quadriceps, calves, lower back, and abdominal muscles.

Have clients perform 10 to 12 reps of the seven upper-body and seven lower-body exercises listed. During the 5th week reduce their training loads by 10 pounds (4.5 kg) and have them perform only one set of each exercise during each workout. The reduced training load and number of sets will permit the muscles to recover and become stronger. For weeks 6 through 9, instruct clients to increase the number of sets in the exercises as shown in table 5.8 and to make needed load increases as indicated in table 4.5. For week 10, have clients follow the directions given for week 5. If they want to engage in more intense split training workouts, and if you believe that it would be safe for them to do so, refer your clients to the more advance workout section in the book *Fitness Weight Training* by Baechle and Earle (2005).

Advanced Workout: Muscle Strength

The 4-week advanced muscle strength program described in table 5.9 includes two upper-body and two lower-body workouts each week. Your clients will perform two or three sets of 8 to 10 reps in most exercises during the first 2 weeks and then 6 to 8 reps during weeks 3 and 4 in exercises marked with an

TABLE 5.7

Advanced Muscle Size Program: Weeks 1-4 (First Cycle)

Order	Muscle group	Reps	Sets	Free weight	Machine
			UPPER-BODY EXERCISES: 30 MIN		
1	Chest	10-12	2	Bench press	Chest press
2	Chest	10-12	2	Dumbbell fly	Chest crossover
3	Upper back	10-12	2	Dumbbell one-arm row	Seated row
4	Shoulder	10-12	2	Dumbbell alternating shoulder press	Shoulder press
5	Upper back	10-12	2	Lat pull-down	Pull-down or pullover
6	Triceps	10-12	2	Dumbbell lying triceps extension	Triceps extension
7	Biceps	10-12	2	Barbell curl	Biceps curl
			LOWER-BODY EXERCISES: 30 MIN		
1	Thigh	10-12	2	Squat	Double-leg press
2	Thigh	10-12	2	Lunge	Single-leg press
3	Hamstrings	10-12	2	Squat	Leg curl
4	Quadriceps	10-12	2	Lunge	Leg extension
5	Calf	10-12	2	Heel raise	Heel raise
6	Abdomen	30-40	2	Trunk curl	
		10-12	2		Abdominal flexion
7	Low back	10-15	2	Trunk extension	
		10-12	2		Low-back extension

Note: Week 4 should be followed with a less intense week of training in which loads are reduced by 10 pounds (4.5 kg) and only one set of each exercise is performed.

TABLE 5.8

Advanced Muscle Size Program: Weeks 6-9 (Second Cycle)

Order	Muscle group	Reps	Sets	Free weight	Machine
			UPPER-BODY EXERCISES: 35 MIN		
1	Chest	10-12	3	Bench press	Chest press
2	Chest	10-12	2	Dumbbell fly	Chest crossover
3	Upper back	10-12	2	Dumbbell one-arm row	Seated row
4	Shoulder	10-12	3	Dumbbell lateral raise	Shoulder press
5	Upper back	10-12	2	Lat pull-down	Pull-down or pullover
6	Triceps	10-12	2	Dumbbell lying triceps extension	Triceps extension
7	Biceps	10-12	3	Barbell curl	Biceps curl
			LOWER-BODY EXERCISES: 40 MIN		
1	Thigh	10-12	3	Squat	Double-leg press
2	Thigh	10-12	2	Lunge	Single-leg press
3	Hamstrings	10-12	2	Squat	Leg curl

(continued)

Table 5.8 *(continued)*

Order	Muscle group	Reps	Sets	Free weight	Machine
				LOWER-BODY EXERCISES: 40 MIN	
4	Quadriceps	10-12	2	Lunge	Leg extension
5	Calf	10-12	2	Heel raise	Heel raise
6	Abdomen	40-50	3	Trunk curl	
		10-12	2		Abdominal flexion
7	Low back	15-20	3	Trunk extension	
		10-12	3		Low-back extension

Note: Week 9 should be followed with a less intense week of training in which loads are reduced by 10 pounds (4.5 kg) and only one set of each exercise is performed.

TABLE 5.9

Advanced Muscle Strength Program: Weeks 1-4 (First Cycle)

Order	Muscle group	Reps	Sets	Free weight	Machine
				UPPER-BODY EXERCISES: 35 MIN	
1	Chest	6-10	3	Bench press	Chest press
2	Chest	8-10	2	Dumbbell fly	Chest crossover
3	*Upper back	6-10	2	Dumbbell one-arm row	Seated row
4	*Shoulder	6-10	3	Dumbbell alternating shoulder press	Shoulder press
5	Upper back	8-10	2	Lat pull-down	Pull-down or pullover
6	Triceps	10	2	Dumbbell lying triceps extension	Triceps extension
7	Biceps	10	2	Barbell curl	Biceps curl
				LOWER-BODY EXERCISES: 40 MIN	
1	*Thigh	6-10	3	Squat	Double-leg press
2	*Thigh	6-10	3	Lunge	Single-leg press
3	Hamstrings	8-10	2	Squat	Leg curl
4	Quadriceps	8-10	2	Lunge	Leg extension
5	Calf	8-10	2	Heel raise	Heel raise
6	Abdomen	30-40	3	Trunk curl	
		8-10	3		Abdominal flexion
7	Low back	10-15	3	Trunk extension	
		8-10	3		Low-back extension

*In the exercises marked with an asterisk gradually increase loads, which will reduce the number of repetitions—from 8 to 10 down to 6 to 8—during weeks 3 through 4.

Note: Week 4 should be followed with a less intense week of training in which loads are reduced by 10 pounds (4.5 kg) and only one set of each exercise is performed.

asterisk. The exercises are similar to those in the muscle size program. Reduce the training load by 10 pounds (4.5 kg) in these exercises during the 5th week and have clients perform only one set each training day. The lighter effort during week 5 provides an opportunity for the muscles to recover, adapt, and become stronger. As shown in table 5.10, the strength development exercises remain the same for the second 4-week cycle. But clients' training loads should increase enough to limit the number of repetitions to those shown in table 5.10. All the exercises are performed for three sets. During the 10th week, instruct clients to follow the directions given for week 5.

If your clients want more intense split training workouts, refer to the books *Fitness Weight Training* (2005) and *Essentials of Personal Training* (2004) by Baechle and Earle.

TABLE 5.10

Advanced Muscle Strength Program: Weeks 6-9 (Second Cycle)

Order	Muscle group	Reps	Sets	Free weight	Machine
UPPER-BODY EXERCISES: 45 MIN					
1	Chest	5	3	Bench press	Chest press
2	Chest	8-10	3	Dumbbell fly	Chest crossover
3	Upper back	5	3	Dumbbell one-arm row	Seated row
4	Shoulder	5	3	Dumbbell alternating shoulder press	Shoulder press
5	Upper back	8-10	3	Lat pull-down	Pull-down or pullover
6	Triceps	10	3	Dumbbell lying triceps extension	Triceps extension
7	Biceps	10	3	Barbell curl	Biceps curl
LOWER-BODY EXERCISES: 50 MIN					
1	Thigh	5	3	Squat	Double-leg press
2	Thigh	5	3	Lunge	Single-leg press
3	Hamstrings	8-10	3	Squat	Leg curl
4	Quadriceps	8-10	3	Lunge	Leg extension
5	Calf	8-10	3	Heel raise	Heel raise
6	Abdomen	40-50	3	Trunk curl	
		8-10	3		Abdominal flexion
7	Low back	15-20	3	Trunk extension	
		8-10	3		Low-back extension

Note: Week 9 should be followed with a less intense week of training in which loads are reduced by 10 pounds (4.5 kg) and only one set of each exercise is performed.

Advanced Workout: Muscle Endurance

The first 4 weeks of the advanced muscle endurance program in table 5.11 include three sets of 15 reps in seven exercises for three workouts a week. One exercise targets each of the eight major muscle areas: chest, back, shoulders,

TABLE 5.11

Advanced Muscle Endurance Program: Weeks 1-4 (First Cycle)

Order	Muscle group	Reps	Sets	Free weight	Machine
			ALL EXERCISES: 31 MIN		
1	Chest	15-20	3	Bench press	Chest press
2	Back	15-20	3	Dumbbell one-arm row	Seated row
3	Shoulder	15-20	3	Dumbbell alternating shoulder press	Shoulder press
4	Biceps	15-20	3	Biceps curl	Biceps curl
5	Triceps	15-20	3	Dumbbell lying triceps extension	Triceps extension
6	Thigh	15-20	3	Lunge	Double-leg press
7	Abdomen	30-40	3	Trunk curl	
		15-20	3		Abdominal flexion
8	Low back	10-15	3	Trunk extension	
		8-10	3		Low-back extension

TABLE 5.12

Advanced Muscle Endurance Program: Weeks 6–9 (Second Cycle)

Order	Muscle group	Reps	Sets	Free weight	Machine
			ALL EXERCISES: 34 MIN		
1	Chest	15-20	3	Bench press	Chest press
2	Chest	15-20	1	Dumbbell fly	Chest crossover
3	Back	15-20	3	Dumbbell one-arm row	Seated row
4	Shoulder	15-20	3	Dumbbell alternating shoulder press	Shoulder press
5	Back	15-20	1	Lat pull-down	Pull-down or pullover
6	Triceps	15-20	3	Dumbbell lying triceps extension	Triceps extension
7	Biceps	15-20	3	Barbell curl	Biceps curl
8	Thigh	15-20	3	Lunge	Double-leg press
9	Calf	15-20	3	Heel raise	Heel raise
10	Abdomen	40-50	3	Trunk curl	
		15-20	3		Abdominal flexion
11	Low back	15-20	3	Trunk extension	
		8-10	3		Low-back extension

biceps, triceps, thighs, lower back, and abdomen. During week 5, reduce your client's training load by 10 pounds (4.5 kg) and the number of sets to one, thus allowing the muscles to recover, adapt, and become stronger. Weeks 6 through 9 include three additional exercises—one each for the chest, back, and calves (see table 5.12). During weeks 6 through 9, progressively increase the number of repetitions to 20. After week 9, repeat the protocol described for week 5.

Determining Training Loads for New Exercises

To determine loads for new exercises, follow these guidelines:

1. Show your client how to perform exercises with the lightest weight-stack plate (machine exercises), the lightest dumbbell (dumbbell exercises), or with a dowel stick or unloaded bar (barbell exercises) and follow the teaching strategies described in chapter 2.

2. Identify a load that you believe will permit 15 repetitions and ask your client to perform 15 reps.

3. Observe your client's level of effort in performing the number of repetitions completed.

4. Use table 4.5 as a guide for decreasing or increasing loads selected.

6

Alternative Exercises and Programs

Although machine training and free-weight training offer certain advantages, other forms of resistance equipment can produce excellent results as well. Weight training equipment intimidates some older adults. For others, budget constraints make membership in a fitness facility or the purchase of strength training equipment impractical. The exercise procedures described in this chapter should enhance your clients' strength training experiences and reduce the likelihood of injury, and they are inexpensive. These alternatives to free-weight and machine exercises will be especially helpful to instructors who value resistance training for older clients but have limited access to expensive equipment. Many exercise options are available to enthusiastic and creative instructors who realize that resistance training can significantly improve the quality of life for senior men and women.

PLANNING YOUR PROGRAM

We have grouped both the bodyweight and the elastic band exercises by muscle areas worked and have arranged them from the less challenging to the more challenging. Instruct your clients to move through the ranges of joint movement shown in the exercises and to perform them in a slow, controlled manner. If some individuals initially cannot perform the entire range of movement, encourage them to move gradually toward the full range, unless doing so will aggravate an existing joint or muscle condition.

Because people vary widely in strength, no specific prescription—for number of reps or thickness of elastic bands—applies to all clients. Before prescribing an exercise, consider the potential difficulty that your client will have in performing the exercise, as well as the resistance that he or she must overcome. Table 6.1 provides some helpful guidelines for tailoring the exercises to each client.

GUIDELINES FOR REPS, SETS, AND REST PERIODS

For clients with the lowest strength levels, try to identify which exercises they can perform correctly for at least 5 repetitions (see table 6.1). For average individuals,

TABLE 6.1

Bodyweight and Elastic Resistance Training Guidelines

	FITNESS LEVEL		
	Low	Average	High
Exercise or resistance	Permits 5 reps	Permits 10 reps	Permits 15-20 reps
Starting number of sets	1	1	2
Increase sets when reps completed equals	10	15	20-25
Increase sets to	2	2-3	3-4
Rest periods between sets	3 min	2-3 min	1-2 min

identify which exercises they can perform correctly for no more than 10 repetitions. And for those who are most fit, identify exercises that result in fatigue after about 15 or 20 reps. If you are using elastic resistance exercises, select a band or thickness that will accommodate the number of repetitions recommended for the various strength levels in table 6.1. Unless joint or muscle problems preclude certain exercises, try to include at least one exercise for the upper body, one for the lower body, and one for the midsection from among those presented later in this chapter. Low-strength clients, using a bodyweight program, can use the push-away (wall) for the chest and triceps, the quarter (depth) knee bend for the quadriceps and hamstrings, and the assisted flexed-knee trunk curl for the abdominal muscles. If clients will be using elastic bands or tubing, they can perform the chest press for the chest and triceps, the squat for the quadriceps and hamstrings, and the trunk curl for the abdominal muscles.

Depending on your clients' strength levels and goals for training, start out less-fit clients with one set and more-fit clients with two sets. If the goal for training is to develop endurance, muscle size, or muscle strength, assign rest periods of 30 seconds to 1 minute, 1 1/2 minutes, and 2 or more minutes, respectively, between sets. Table 6.1 provides guidelines for progressively increasing the number of sets.

BODYWEIGHT EXERCISES

Each of the following exercises uses only bodyweight, thereby offering considerable training versatility at no cost. One drawback of bodyweight exercises is that matching the appropriate resistance to different strength levels is difficult. This chapter includes some variations of traditional exercises that can make bodyweight exercises more practical and productive no matter what your clients' fitness levels are. Whichever variations your clients use, be sure that they perform all exercises through the proper range, in a slow and controlled manner (without pain).

PUSH-UP AND PUSH-UP VARIATIONS

Muscles most involved:
pectoralis major, anterior deltoid, triceps

The basic push-up and its variations are excellent exercises for developing the pectoralis major, anterior deltoid, and triceps muscles. These exercises are good for seniors who find standard push-ups too difficult, because they recruit essentially the same muscle groups. Instruct your clients to keep the back straight during the basic push-up and its variations, shown below and through page 198. Note that in all push-up exercises (including the push-away), clients should exhale during pushing movements and inhale on return movements.

PUSH-AWAY (WALL)

1. Instruct clients to assume a position in which the feet are about 2 to 3 feet from a wall, the hands are on the wall slightly wider than shoulder-width apart, and the elbows are almost fully extended.

2. They should move the chest toward the wall by flexing the elbows, pausing briefly, and then pushing back to the starting position.

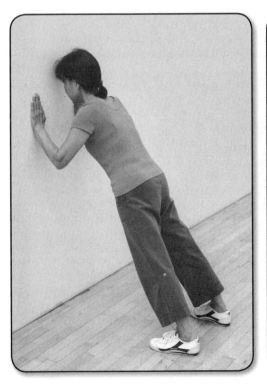 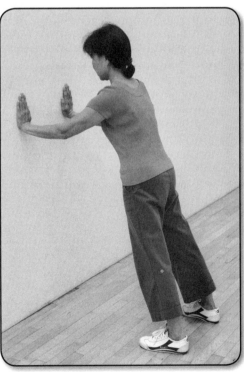

TABLE PUSH-UP

1. Make sure that the table is stable or braced against a wall.
2. Instruct clients to stand about 4 feet from the table and place the hands slightly more than shoulder-width apart on the edge of the table.
3. They should slowly lower the torso until the chest is near the table.
4. After a momentary pause, they should push back to the starting position.

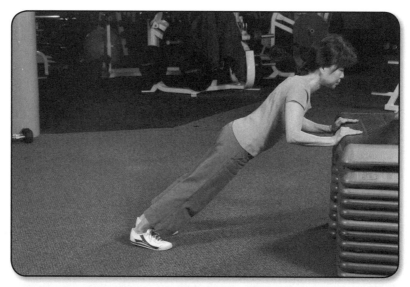

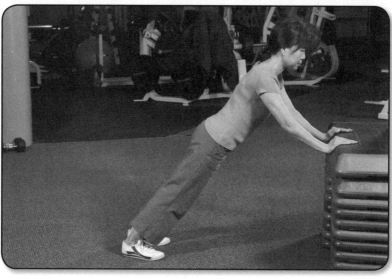

FLOOR PUSH-UP

1. While lying on the abdomen, your clients should place the hands slightly more than shoulder-width apart on the floor while maintaining a straight body posture.

2. They should push up to the starting position, pause momentarily, and then lower the torso slowly until the chest nears the floor.

3. If the straight body position makes it too difficult for clients to complete at least five repetitions, have them do the push-ups from the knees to reduce the resistance.

4. By instructing them to vary the hand position, you can emphasize different muscles. Placing the hands farther apart puts more stress on the pectoral muscles, whereas putting the hands closer together stresses the triceps.

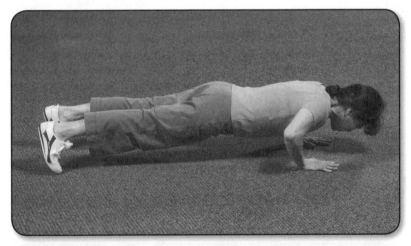

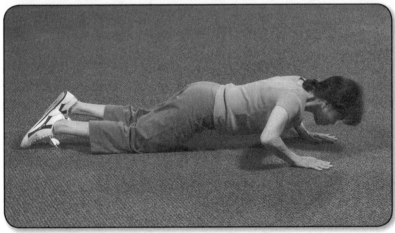

CHAIR PUSH-UP

1. When clients are able to complete 15 controlled floor push-ups, you can increase the difficulty by having them put the feet on a stable chair or bench.
2. With the hands slightly wider than shoulder-width apart on the floor and the body straight, they should slowly lower the torso until the chest almost touches the floor.
3. After a momentary pause, they should push back up to the starting position.

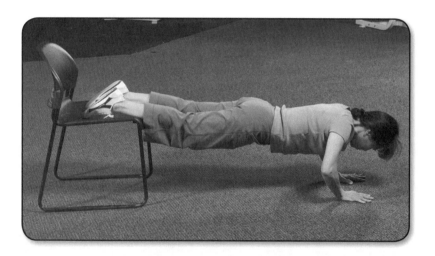

TRUNK CURL

Muscles most involved:
rectus abdominis, external and internal obliques

Properly performed trunk curls strengthen the abdominal muscles in the front and sides of the midsection. Proper breathing technique during all the trunk curl exercises involves exhaling during upward movements and inhaling during downward movements. Variations of the trunk curl follow on pages 199 through 201.

ASSISTED FLEXED-KNEE TRUNK CURL

1. Instruct clients to assume a supine position on a mat with the arms at the sides and the elbows, forearms, and palms in contact with the mat.

2. The knees should be in a flexed position, and the heels should be close to the buttocks.

3. Have your clients initiate the upward curling movement by flexing the trunk and pushing against the mat with the forearms.

4. When the upper back reaches a 30-degree angle, clients should pause momentarily before returning to the starting position.

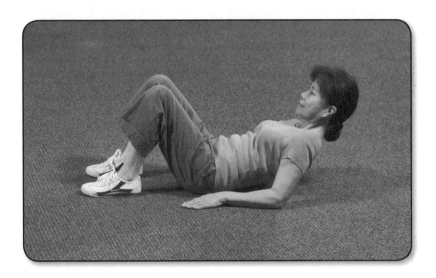

TRUNK CURL WITH FLEXED KNEES

1. Have clients assume the position described in the assisted flexed-knee trunk curl but to place the hands loosely on the sides of the head to help keep the head and neck in a neutral position.

2. Instruct clients to curl the shoulders and upper back slowly off the floor until the lower back is pressed firmly against the floor.

3. They should pause momentarily before returning to the starting position.

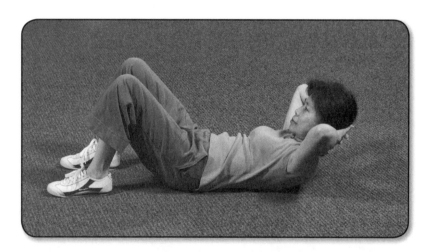

TRUNK CURL WITH KNEE PULL

1. This exercise is similar to the basic trunk curl, with one additional component: As the trunk curls upward, the exerciser pulls back the left knee in an effort to touch the left elbow.

2. Clients should pause momentarily before returning to the starting position.

3. The next repetition involves the right knee and right elbow in the same manner.

4. Have your clients alternate the knee-to-elbow action throughout the exercise.

5. The trunk curl with knee pull provides resistance from both the upper and lower body, placing more stress on the abdominal and hip flexor muscles.

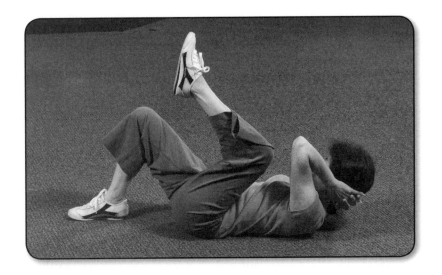

TWISTING TRUNK CURL WITH LEGS ON CHAIR

1. Instruct clients to place the legs on a stable chair or bench as shown and then curl the shoulders upward off the floor until the lower back is pressed firmly against the floor. They then rotate the trunk to the left or right, pausing momentarily before returning to the starting position.

2. They should alternate the direction of the trunk rotation on each repetition.

3. The alternating twists emphasize the muscles on the sides of the midsection (obliques) as well as the rectus abdominis.

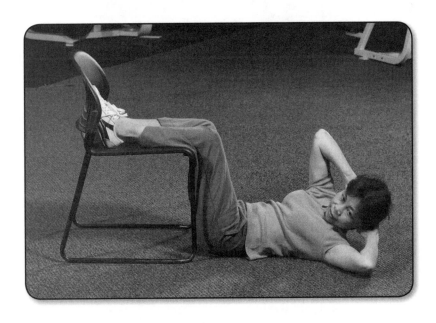

KNEE BEND

Muscles most involved:
quadriceps, hamstrings, gluteal muscle groups

Exhalation in these exercises should occur during upward movement, and inhalation should occur during downward movement. Variations of knee bends are shown below and through page 204.

QUARTER KNEE BEND

1. With the feet slightly more than shoulder-width apart and the torso erect, clients should lower the hips downward and backward to a one-quarter flexed-knee position.
2. They should pause momentarily before returning to the starting position.
3. If maintaining balance is a problem, instruct clients to place one or both hands on a fixed object such as a chair or table.
4. The heels will tend to come up as the hips are lowered, but the feet should remain flat on the floor throughout the exercise.

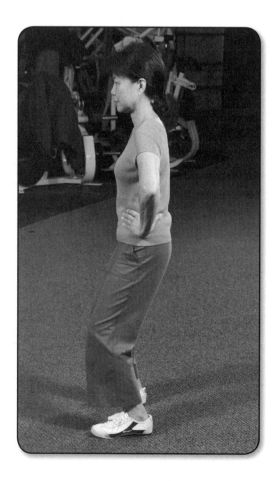

HALF KNEE BEND

1. This exercise is identical to the quarter knee bend except that the hips are lowered downward and backward to a one-half flexed-knee position.
2. The heels will tend to come up as the hips are lowered, but the feet should remain flat on the floor throughout the exercise.

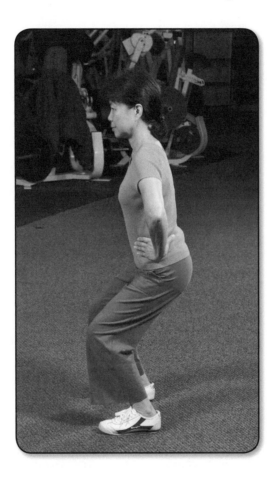

THREE-QUARTER KNEE BEND

1. This exercise is simply a more demanding version of the half knee bend because the hips need to be lowered to a three-quarter depth position.
2. This figure illustrates the bottom position of the three-quarter knee bend exercise.

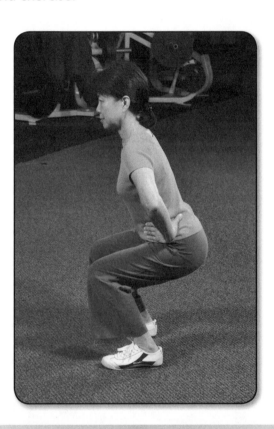

PULL-UP

**Muscles most involved:
latissimus dorsi, biceps**

Many people cannot pull up their full bodyweight, but because muscles are stronger in lowering than in lifting movements, almost everyone is able to perform some variation of this exercise. In all pull-up exercises, have your clients use an underhand grip, keep the back straight, and look straight ahead. Variations of pull-ups follow on pages 205 through 207.

PARTIAL PULL-UP

1. Have your clients stand on a box so that the chin is above the bar. They grasp the bar with the palms facing the shoulders, about shoulder-width apart.
2. They slowly lower the body until the elbows are one-quarter extended, pause momentarily, and then pull back up to the starting position.
3. Clients should inhale during the lowering movement and exhale during the upward movement.
4. As clients become stronger, you may want to instruct them to lower the body until the elbows are halfway extended.
5. The next step is to have them try three-quarter depth repetitions. The final stage is to perform a full-range pull-up.

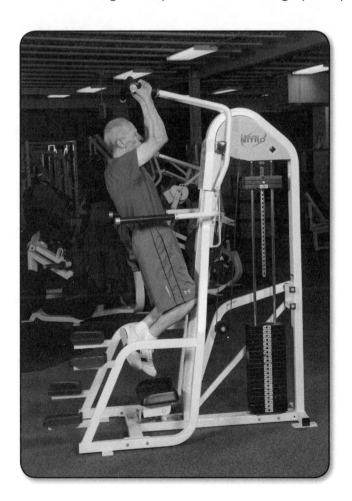

1. Skilled clients should step onto the box so that the chin is above the bar. They grasp it with the palms facing the shoulders, about shoulder-width apart.

2. They slowly lower the body until the elbows are fully extended.

3. As soon as the arms are straight, they should return to the starting position by stepping onto the box again.

4. In this exercise, have your clients exhale during the lowering phase and inhale when stepping back onto the box.

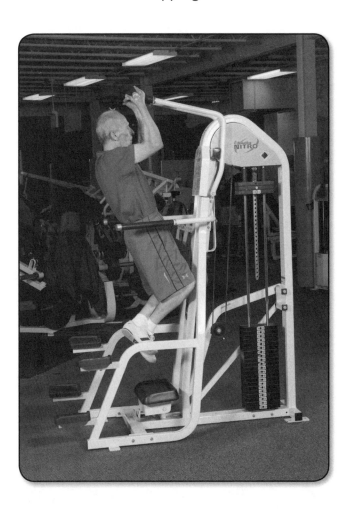

STEP BOX PULL-UP—LEG ASSIST

1. Skilled clients should step onto the box and grasp the bar with the palms facing the shoulders, about shoulder-width apart.
2. They then flex the knees so that the elbows are nearly extended.
3. They should use the legs to help lift the body during the upward pull-up phase but not during the lowering phase.
4. They should exhale during the upward movement and inhale during the downward movement.

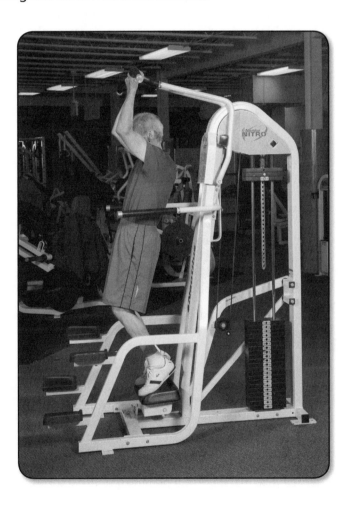

ELASTIC RESISTANCE EXERCISES

Another inexpensive and versatile alternative to traditional strength training equipment is resistance bands or tubing. Bands have some limitations, the first being the difficulty of assigning which lengths and thicknesses of tubing to use. Because no standardized system is in place for classifying resistance levels for length and thickness, you must simply use your best judgment to determine what your client needs at a given stage. Doing this may not be as difficult as it sounds; through careful observation of your clients, you can gauge pretty well when they are ready to progress to shorter lengths or greater thicknesses. The main drawback of elastic resistance exercise is that measuring progress is less objective and observable than it is with free weights and weight-stack machines. One method suggested for helping clients grasp the band or tubing at the same point so that the resistance is similar from day to day is to mark the elastic band or tubing at 6-inch (15 cm) intervals. Improvements in strength are also easier to recognize as clients move toward the lower markings while maintaining the same repetition range. Another limitation is the lack of uniform resistance throughout the movement range; resistance is low at the start of an exercise and increases at the end when the elastic is stretched the most.

On a positive note, because the bands come in many thicknesses, they offer progressive levels of resistance. You can purchase elastic tubing of various diameters (easily distinguished by different colors) in either precut sections or a roll. We recommend rolls, which you can cut to whatever length you need. You should probably purchase a variety of elastic equipment, from thin flat bands to thicker round tubing, to accommodate smaller and larger muscle groups, as well as various strength levels. These variations enable you to increase your clients' training intensity progressively in a systematic manner. Elastic equipment offers an excellent training option, especially for training large exercise groups or in small exercise areas.

Technique Pointers

Along with teaching your clients when to inhale and exhale and how to perform repetitions in a controlled manner, you also should instruct them to perform elastic resistance exercises in the proper plane of movement (Purvis 1997). By doing so, they will apply resistance to the muscle groups for which the specific exercises are designed and will avoid placing inappropriate stress on ligaments and joints.

You may have difficulty determining where to anchor the elastic so that the movement pattern will be in the correct plane. Figures 6.1 through 6.3 illustrate correct and incorrect planes of movement for several exercises. These examples should help you position your client and the anchoring end of the elastic so that the exercise is performed in the proper movement pattern.

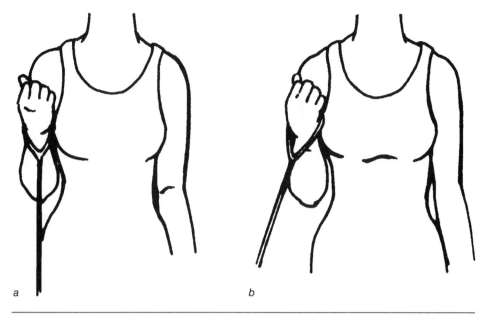

Figure 6.1 *(a)* Correct, *(b)* incorrect.

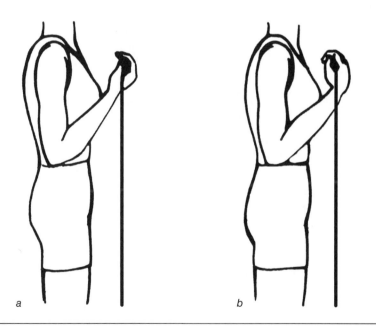

Figure 6.2 *(a)* Correct, *(b)* incorrect.

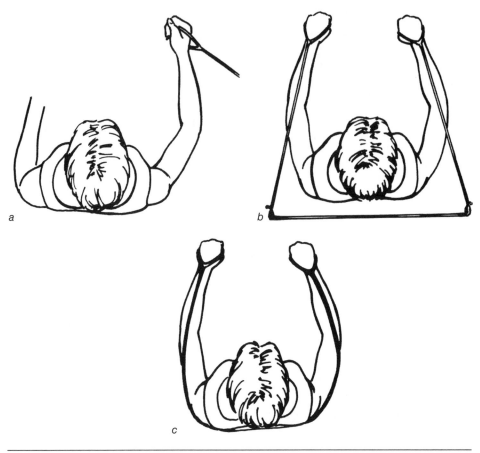

Figure 6.3 *(a)* Correct, *(b)* correct, and *(c)* incorrect.

Safety Precautions

Figuring out how to anchor the elastic is also a challenge. Take great care to ensure that the anchor is secure! Try installing hooks in strategic locations in the stud of a wall or in a platform. Only as a last resort should you assign a partner to hold the anchoring end. Because of the skill required of both persons to balance the opposing pulling actions, partner exercises with elastic bands increase injury risk.

Consider the type and shape of the handle needed for the moving end of the elastic band. Before you purchase or design equipment, analyze the grip requirements of the planned exercises as well as the limitations (e.g., arthritis) of your older adult clients. Purvis (1997) has suggested the use of webbing or mesh that is long enough to fit over the ball of the foot. The same concept can be adapted to almost any situation in which your client is unable to grip or otherwise hold onto the end of the elastic band. The four elastic resistance exercises that follow address most of the major muscle groups. When used with the previously described training guidelines, they should provide a good basic workout.

ELASTIC RESISTANCE BAND SQUAT

Muscles most involved:
quadriceps, hamstrings, gluteal muscles

1. Instruct your clients to establish a stance slightly wider than shoulder width with the feet squarely on the resistance band.
2. They should grasp the handles of the bands so that the bands are taut when your clients are at the three-quarter knee bend position.
3. From this depth, clients should extend the knees and hips until they are standing upright.
4. After a momentary pause, they should return slowly to the starting position shown in the figure.
5. Have your clients exhale during the upward movement and inhale during the downward movement.

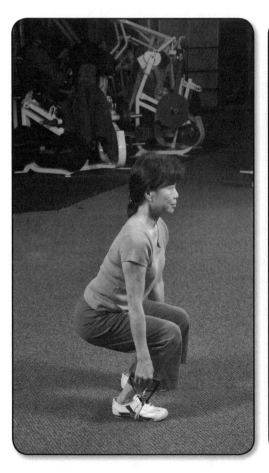
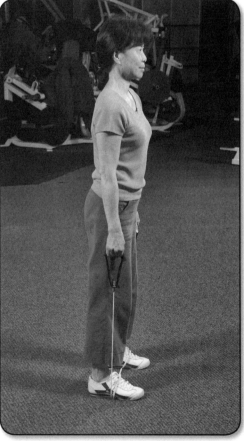

ELASTIC RESISTANCE BAND BENCH PRESS

Muscles most involved:
pectoralis major, anterior deltoid, triceps

1. Have clients sit or stand in an upright position with the resistance band or tubing at chest height.

2. The tubing should be attached to a wall hook, although it may be secured adequately to a chair back or a stationary piece of equipment.

3. A less preferred option is to instruct clients to position the band around the back at a level parallel to the chest.

4. Instruct clients to hold the handles so that the bands are taut while near the chest before pushing the hands forward.

5. They should push the hands forward until the elbows are almost fully extended, pause momentarily, and then return slowly to the starting position.

6. They should exhale during the pushing phase and inhale during the return movement.

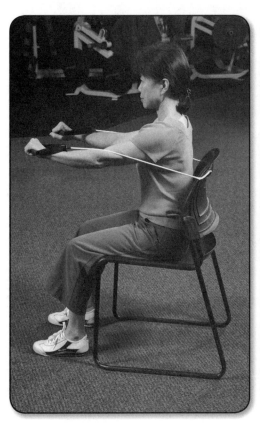 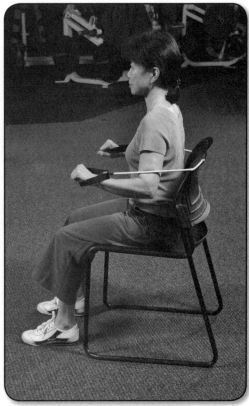

ELASTIC RESISTANCE BAND SEATED ROW

Muscles most involved: latissimus dorsi, rhomboid muscles of the upper back, biceps

1. Have clients sit on the floor with the legs almost straight and the torso erect.
2. Secure the tubing to a stationary piece of equipment or to hooks on a wall, or wrap the band securely around the soles of the feet.
3. They should grasp the handles so that the tubing is taut when the arms are extended straight in front.
4. While maintaining an erect torso, clients should pull the handles to the chest, pause momentarily, and then return slowly to the starting position.
5. Instruct clients to exhale during the pulling phase and inhale during the return movement.

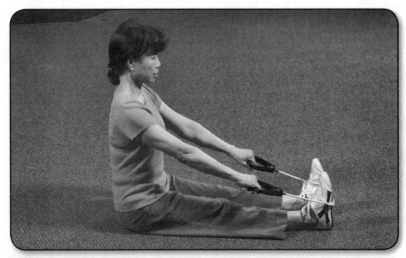

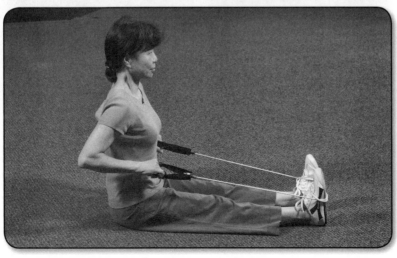

ELASTIC RESISTANCE BICEPS CURL

Muscles most involved:
biceps, brachialis muscle

1. Have clients anchor the band or tubing beneath the feet or onto a floor platform hook and position the feet so that the band or tubing is correctly aligned in the upper position as shown in figure 6.1a.

2. The exercise begins from the straight-elbow position and ends in the position shown in the figure.

3. Exhalation should occur during the upward movement, and inhalation should occur during the downward movement.

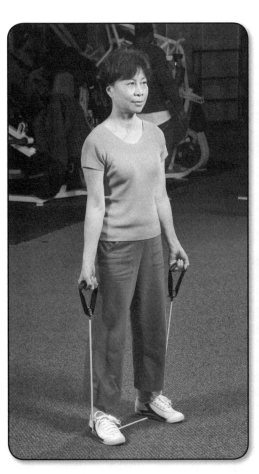
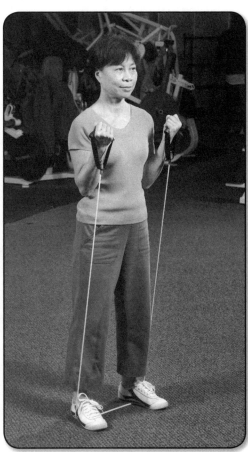

Progress Assessment

Experiencing personal progress is a great motivator, especially for older adults who continue strength training and witness a lot of personal success. Informal progress assessments—such as noting load increases on their training logs, recognizing their ability to climb stairs with less effort, or observing a more fit appearance in the mirror—are strong motivators. Others may appreciate formal assessments of their training progress, as well as the use of normative standards against which to evaluate their strength, flexibility, body composition, and mental outlook or personal perceptions. In this chapter we provide some normative standards that can be used to assess and monitor changes in strength, flexibility, and personal perceptions among seniors, keeping in mind that reliable progress assessments depend on precise testing procedures that are performed in exactly the same manner before and after the training program.

MUSCLE STRENGTH

Of course, we expect trained muscles to be stronger than untrained muscles, and improvements in strength can be estimated easily by comparing exercise loads before and after a training program. Many clients, however, also want to know how their strength compares with others in their category of age and sex. For this reason, we have determined normative strength data for men and women between 20 and 80 years of age.

Age and Sex Comparisons

Table 7.1 presents normative information on 245 men and women in their 20s through 70s who were assessed for muscle strength on 13 standard weight-stack machines (Westcott 1994). Although loads may vary among different machines, the normative data presented here should be applicable to most standard weight-stack machines. For example, the 100-pound (45 kg) selection on one manufacturer's leg extension machine should be similar to a 100-pound selection on another leg extension machine. The numbers in table 7.1 represent the average exercise loads that the subjects could perform for 10 repetitions (10RM) with good form after 2 months of regular strength training.

These data show that the 10-repetition maximum loads generally decreased between 5 and 10 percent every decade, demonstrating a progressive loss of muscle strength throughout the adult years. Also, within each age category,

TABLE 7.1

Average Exercise Loads on Common Machines (*n* = 245)

Exercises	AGE GROUPS					
	20-29	30-39	40-49	50-59	60-69	70-79
LEG EXTENSION						
Males lb	112.5	105.0	97.5	90.0	82.5	75.0
kg	51.0	47.6	44.2	40.8	37.4	34.0
Females lb	67.5	65.0	62.5	60.0	57.5	55.0
kg	30.6	29.5	28.3	27.2	26.1	24.9
LEG CURL						
Males lb	112.5	105.0	97.5	90.0	82.5	75.0
kg	51.0	47.6	44.2	40.8	37.4	34.0
Females lb	67.5	65.0	62.5	60.0	57.5	55.0
kg	30.6	29.5	28.3	27.2	26.1	24.9
LEG PRESS						
Males lb	240.0	220.0	200.0	180.0	160.0	140.0
kg	108.9	99.8	90.7	81.6	72.6	63.5
Females lb	165.0	150.0	135.0	120.0	110.0	100.0
kg	74.8	68.0	61.2	54.4	49.9	45.4
CHEST CROSSOVER						
Males lb	100.0	95.0	90.0	85.0	80.0	70.0
kg	45.4	43.1	40.8	38.6	36.3	31.8
Females lb	57.5	55.0	52.5	50.0	47.5	45.0
kg	26.1	24.9	23.8	22.7	21.6	20.4
CHEST PRESS						
Males lb	110.0	102.5	95.0	87.5	80.0	72.5
kg	49.9	46.5	43.1	39.7	36.3	32.9
Females lb	57.5	55.0	52.5	50.0	47.5	45.0
kg	26.1	24.9	23.8	22.7	21.6	20.4
SEATED ROW						
Males lb	140.0	132.5	125.0	117.5	110.0	102.5
kg	63.5	60.1	56.7	53.3	49.9	46.5
Females lb	85.0	82.5	80.0	77.5	75.0	70.0
kg	38.6	37.4	36.3	35.2	34.0	31.8
SHOULDER PRESS						
Males lb	105.0	97.5	90.0	82.5	72.5	62.5
kg	47.6	44.2	40.8	37.4	32.9	28.3
Females lb	50.0	47.5	45.0	42.5	40.0	37.5
kg	22.7	21.6	20.4	19.3	18.1	17.0
BICEPS CURL						
Males lb	90.0	85.0	80.0	75.0	70.0	60.0
kg	40.8	38.6	36.3	34.0	31.8	27.2
Females lb	50.0	47.5	45.0	42.5	40.0	37.5
kg	22.7	21.6	20.4	19.3	18.1	17.0

	AGE GROUPS					
Exercises	**20-29**	**30-39**	**40-49**	**50-59**	**60-69**	**70-79**
TRICEPS EXTENSION						
Males lb kg	90.0 40.8	85.0 38.6	80.0 36.3	75.0 34.0	70.0 31.8	60.0 27.2
Females lb kg	50.0 22.7	47.5 21.6	45.0 20.4	42.5 19.3	40.0 18.1	37.5 17.0
LOW-BACK EXTENSION						
Males lb kg	110.0 49.9	105.0 47.6	100.0 45.4	95.0 43.1	90.0 40.8	85.0 38.6
Females lb kg	80.0 36.3	77.5 35.2	75.0 34.0	72.5 32.9	67.5 30.6	65.0 29.5
TRUNK CURL						
Males lb kg	110.0 49.9	105.0 47.6	100.0 45.4	95.0 43.1	90.0 40.8	80.0 36.3
Females lb kg	65.0 29.5	62.5 28.3	60.0 27.2	57.5 26.1	55.0 24.9	52.5 23.8
NECK FLEXION						
Males lb kg	70.0 31.8	67.5 30.6	65.0 29.5	62.5 28.3	60.0 27.2	55.0 24.9
Females lb kg	45.0 20.4	42.5 19.3	40.0 18.1	37.5 17.0	35.0 15.9	32.5 14.7
NECK EXTENSION						
Males lb kg	80.0 36.3	77.5 35.2	75.0 34.0	72.5 32.9	70.0 31.8	60.0 27.2
Females lb kg	52.5 23.8	50.0 22.7	47.5 21.6	45.0 20.4	42.5 19.3	40.0 18.1

Adapted from W. Westcott, 1994, "Strength training for life: Loads: Go figure," *Nautilus Magazine* 3(4): 5–7. By permission of W. Westcott.

the men's 10-repetition maximum loads were approximately 50 percent higher than the women's.

Although men can lift heavier loads than women can, a large-scale study with more than 900 subjects indicated that both sexes are similar in strength when muscle-to-muscle comparisons are made (Westcott 1987). But because men typically have more muscle (43 percent) than women (23 percent), their absolute strength is greater (Baechle and Earle 2006).

Table 7.2 shows that male subjects performed 10 leg extensions with 50 percent more weight than female subjects did, but when the results were adjusted for differences in bodyweight (load divided by bodyweight), males completed 10 leg extensions with 62 percent of their bodyweight and females completed 10 leg extensions with 55 percent of their bodyweight.

When adjusted for differences in lean weight (load divided by estimated lean weight), both males and females completed 10 leg extensions with about 75 percent of their lean weight, suggesting nearly equal quadriceps strength on a muscle-for-muscle basis.

TABLE 7.2

Quadriceps Strength Measured by the 10-Repetition Maximum Load on a Leg Extension Machine (*n* = 907)

	Men	Women
Age	43 yr	42 yr
Bodyweight	191 lb (87 kg)	143 lb (65 kg)
10-rep max	119 lb (54 kg)	79 lb (36 kg)
Strength quotient (bodyweight)	62%	55%
Strength quotient (lean bodyweight)	74%	73%

Adapted, by permission, from W. Westcott, 2003, *Building strength and stamina,* 2nd ed. (Champaign, IL: Human Kinetics), 3.

YMCA Leg Extension Test

The individual training programs presented in chapter 4 frequently referred to the client's present strength fitness level. Our criterion for categorizing a client's strength fitness is the YMCA leg extension test, based on the performance of 907 men and women (Westcott 1987). This easy-to-administer assessment addresses the large and frequently used quadriceps muscles, making it appropriate for older adults. The YMCA leg extension test also evaluates muscle performance relative to bodyweight, making it a fair strength assessment for men and women of various sizes. Because it uses the 10-repetition maximum load, which is well below the clients' maximum capacity, this is a low-risk test. Nonetheless, before using this test, determine whether it may aggravate the knee joint, especially with clients that have arthritic conditions.

The original strength classifications used in the YMCA leg extension test were derived from scores of men and women in their mid-40s. Modified assessment categories have been developed for men and women in their 50s, 60s, and 70s, based on a study of strength changes over six decades of adult life (Westcott 1994).

The YMCA leg extension test procedures are as follows (refer to figure 7.1):

- Select a load on a leg extension machine that is about 25 to 35 percent of the client's bodyweight and encourage her or him to perform 10 repetitions in the following manner:

    1. Lift the roller pad in 2 seconds to full knee extension.

    2. Hold the fully contracted position for 1 second.

    3. Lower the roller pad in 4 seconds until the starting position is reached.

- Take a 2-minute rest, select a load that is about 40 to 50 percent of the client's bodyweight, and encourage the participant to perform 10 repetitions in the prescribed manner.

- Continue testing with progressively greater resistance until you determine the 10-repetition maximum load.

- Divide this load by the client's bodyweight to obtain a strength quotient and then determine the participant's present strength fitness category (see tables 7.3 and 7.4).

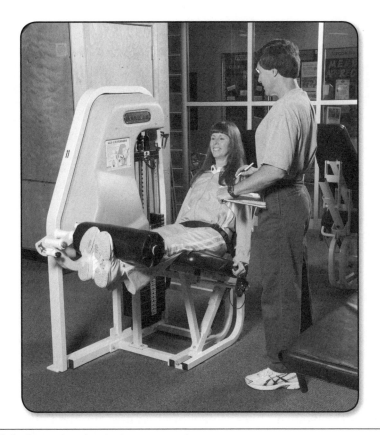

Figure 7.1 Leg extension test.

TABLE 7.3

YMCA Leg Extension Test Score Categories for Men

	Ages 50-59	Ages 60-69	Ages 70-79
Muscle strength	**(% bodyweight)**	**(% bodyweight)**	**(% bodyweight)**
Low	≤44%	≤39%	≤34%
Below average	45-54%	40-49%	35-44%
Average	55-64%	50-59%	45-54%
Above average	65-74%	60-69%	55-64%
High	≥75%	≥70%	≥65%

Example: A 55-year-old male who weighs 180 pounds (82 kg) and completes 10 leg extensions with 120 pounds (54 kg) has a strength quotient of 66% and has an above-average level of strength in his quadriceps muscles.

TABLE 7.4

YMCA Leg Extension Test Score Categories for Women

	Ages 50-59	Ages 60-69	Ages 70-79
Muscle strength	(% bodyweight)	(% bodyweight)	(% bodyweight)
Low	≤34%	≤29%	≤24%
Below average	35-44%	30-39%	25-34%
Average	45-54%	40-49%	35-44%
Above average	55-64%	50-59%	45-54%
High	≥65%	≥60%	≥55%

Example: A 70-year-old female who weighs 120 pounds (54 kg) and completes 10 leg extensions with 40 pounds (18 kg) has a strength quotient of 33% and has a below-average level of strength in her quadriceps muscles.

Bench Press Test for the Upper Body

A 1RM bench press exercise may also be used to assess upper-body strength fitness levels, provided that clients do not have orthopedic conditions at the elbow and shoulder joints that would be aggravated by performing the bench press exercise. Although there are concerns about older adults performing strength assessment tests using 1RM, its use has been found to be safe with older clients and those with some chronic diseases (ACSM 2010). Using data compiled at the Women's Exercise Research Center and the Cooper Institute for Aerobics Research and adapted by Heyward (2010) (see table 7.5), 1RM test results were divided by bodyweight and put into a percentile table for 50 to 59 and 60 and older age groups (and younger age groups). If you elect to include the 1RM bench press for assessing strength fitness levels, refer to the older age group norms and consider categorizing percentile results of your clients in the

TABLE 7.5

Age-Sex Norms for 1RM Bench Press (1-RM/BM)

	AGE	
Percentile rankings for men	50-59	60+
90	0.97	0.89
80	0.90	0.82
70	0.84	0.77
60	0.79	0.72
50	0.75	0.68
40	0.71	0.66
30	0.68	0.63
20	0.63	0.57
10	0.57	0.53

Percentile rankings for women	AGE		
	50-59	60-69	70+
90	0.40	0.41	0.44
80	0.37	0.38	0.39
70	0.35	0.36	0.33
60	0.33	0.32	0.31
50	0.31	0.30	0.27
40	0.28	0.29	0.25
30	0.26	0.28	0.24
20	0.23	0.26	0.21
10	0.19	0.25	0.20

Adapted, by permission, from V. Heyward, 2010, *Advanced fitness assessment and exercise prescription,* 6th ed. (Champaign, IL: Human Kinetics), 136; Data for men from Cooper Institute for Aerobics Research, 2005, *The physical fitness specialist manual* (Dallas, TX: The Cooper Institute). Data for women from Women's Exercise Research Center, 1998 (Washington, DC: The George Washington University Medical Center).

following manner: Low = 30 to 39; below average = 40 to 49; average = 50 to 69; above average = 70 to 79; and high = 80 or above. A table (20-3) of 1RM norms by age groups for the bench press is also provided in ACSM's Resource Manual for Guidelines for Exercise Testing and Prescription (2010).

ASSESSING HIP AND TRUNK FLEXIBILITY

Joint flexibility, which refers to the movement range of a given joint structure, is related to the muscles' capacity to stretch beyond their resting length. Because poor hip–trunk flexibility may be related to low-back problems, this area is the most frequently evaluated in flexibility tests. Clients with acceptable hip–trunk flexibility should be able to touch their toes without bending their knees, but to reduce the possibility of back strain, have your clients perform this assessment in a sitting position rather than a standing position. This assessment is typically referred to as the sit-and-reach test.

Although specially designed testing devices facilitate assessments of hip–trunk flexibility (figure 7.2), a simple testing procedure requires only a measuring stick (figure 7.3). After your client warms up, have her or him sit on the floor with the

Tracking Load Increases Over Time

If appropriate testing equipment is not available, you can periodically evaluate strength by comparing your client's exercise loads over time. As a rule, loads should increase about 45 percent during the first 2 months of training and about 15 percent during the next 2 months. Thereafter, a 5 percent strength gain every 2 months represents a productive training program. For example, if a senior male begins with 100 pounds (45 kg) in the leg press, he may be expected to use about 145 pounds (66 kg), or 145 percent of 100 pounds (45 kg), after 8 weeks of training; about 167 pounds (76 kg), or 115 percent of 145 pounds (66 kg), after 16 weeks; and about 175 pounds (79 kg), or 105 percent of 167 pounds (76 kg), after 24 weeks.

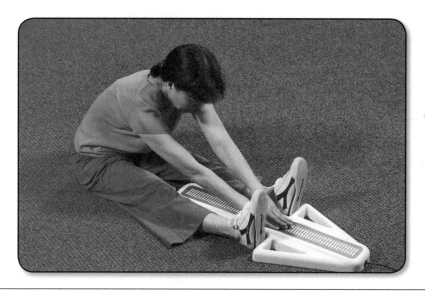

Figure 7.2 Hip-trunk flexibility assessment—electronic measurement.

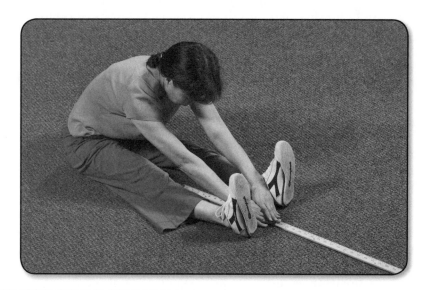

Figure 7.3 Hip-trunk flexibility assessment—yardstick measurement.

measuring stick between the legs and the 15-inch (38 cm) mark even with the heels. Encourage the client to reach forward as far as possible without straining and with the knees straight. Record the farthest reach of three trials and determine flexibility fitness according to table 7.6.

If your clients can reach the 15-inch (38 cm) mark (by the heels), they are reasonably flexible in the hip–trunk area. If they cannot, an increase of 1 inch (2.5 cm) per month represents an excellent rate of improvement in hip–trunk flexibility during the first few months of training.

TABLE 7.6

Hip–Trunk Flexibility Assessments for Men and Women Over Age 45 Based on Sit-and-Reach Test Scores

Assessment	Men	Women
Excellent	19-23 in. (48-58 cm)	21-24 in. (53-61 cm)
Good	16-18 in. (41-46 cm)	19-20 in. (48-51 cm)
Above average	14-15 in. (36-38 cm)	17-18 in. (43-46 cm)
Average	12-13 in. (30-33 cm)	16 in. (41 cm)
Below average	10-11 in. (25-28 cm)	14-15 in. (36-38 cm)
Poor	7-9 in. (18-23 cm)	11-13 in. (28-33 cm)
Very poor	1-6 in. (3-15 cm)	4-10 in. (10-25 cm)

Data from Golding, Myers, and Sinning 1989.

A study by Westcott, Dolan, and Cavicchi (1996) found that combined strength training and flexibility exercises are effective in significantly increasing movement ranges in shoulder abduction, hip flexion, and hip extension. Girouard and Hurley (1995) observed significant improvements in shoulder abduction and shoulder flexion following 10 weeks of combined strength training and flexibility exercises. These results indicate that training programs including both strength training and stretching exercises can increase range of movement in selected joint actions.

BODY COMPOSITION

Body composition is a relative measure of the two basic components of bodyweight—fat weight and lean weight. Fat weight consists solely of fat tissue, whereas lean weight includes muscle, bones, organs, blood, skin, and all other nonfat tissues. The ratio of fat weight to lean weight is usually reported as percent body fat. Ideally, adult males should be about 15 percent fat weight and 85 percent lean weight. That is, a 200-pound (91 kg) male with desirable body composition should have about 30 pounds (14 kg) of fat weight and 170 pounds (77 kg) of lean weight.

Because they have greater fat requirements for reproduction purposes, women should be about 25 percent fat weight and 75 percent lean weight. In other words, a 120-pound (54 kg) female with a desirable body composition should have about 30 pounds (14 kg) of fat weight and 90 pounds (40 kg) of lean weight.

Two of the most accurate ways to assess body composition are underwater weighing and dual-energy X-ray absorptiometry (DEXA). Because the trainee must exhale all air and sit totally submerged in a tank of water, however, underwater weighing is too challenging for most senior men and women, and DEXA machines are typically too expensive. The most frequently used and affordable method for determining percent body fat is skinfold measurement

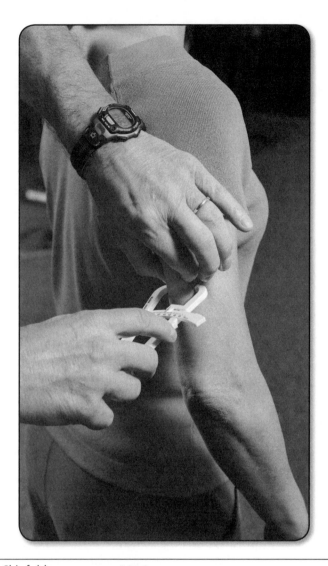

Figure 7.4 Skinfold measurement test.

using calipers—a field technique that trained fitness instructors can administer efficiently and effectively (see figure 7.4). A recent 6-month study with senior women (average age 59 years) showed that approximately 2.5 pounds (1.1 kg) of lean weight gain occurred during the first 3 months, and another 2.5 pounds of lean weight gain occurred during the second 3 months. Their fat loss showed a similar pattern; approximately 4.5 pounds (2.0 kg) of fat loss occurred during the first 3 months, and another 4.5 pounds of fat loss occurred during the second 3 months (Westcott et al. 2008).

Why not simply use body weight alone or the body mass index (BMI)? Body weight and BMI measurements may not be particularly helpful because fat losses in response to training may not be apparent. For example, a senior who adds 4 pounds (1.8 kg) of muscle and loses 4 pounds of fat will weigh the same in spite of an 8-pound (3.6 kg) improvement in body composition. One way to monitor improvements in body composition is to take periodic midsection measurements. Have clients stand tall, and place a measuring tape around the waist just above the belt. A 0.5-inch (1.3 cm) reduction in waist girth every month during the first few months of training indicates an excellent rate of body composition improvement and a successful strength training program.

PERSONAL PERCEPTIONS

Assessing physical improvements in which we can make fairly precise before-and-after measurements—muscle strength, joint flexibility, and body composition—is relatively simple. But in some respects, psychological outcomes may be even more important to seniors than physical progress. Are your clients' personal perceptions more positive because of their strength training programs? Ideally, older adults should not only be stronger but also feel better, have more self-confidence, and function more independently after the exercise program. Numerous research publications by Dr. James Annesi have demonstrated significant improvements in a variety of psychological parameters in older adults following several weeks of regular strength exercise (Annesi et al. 2004; Annesi, Westcott, and Gann 2004; Annesi and Westcott 2004, 2007). Because these personal perceptions appear closely associated with exercise compliance and continuation, you may want to perform some simple psychological assessments with your senior clients.

Although personal perceptions are not easy to quantify, a brief questionnaire may serve this purpose satisfactorily. Consider using the Lifestyle Questionnaire (figure 7.5) developed by Westcott (1995), in which participants rate themselves on several fitness-related parameters by recording their physical and personal perceptions on a 5-point scale: low, below average, average, above average, or high. The questionnaire is administered before and after the training program to identify the participants' perceptual changes.

After an 8-week strength and endurance exercise program, participants in the Westcott (1995) study reported perceived improvements in muscle

Assessing the Functional Status of Older Adults

Although professionals can use the tests described previously to help determine the readiness of their clients to undertake a strength training program and to set an appropriate level of intensity, others may want only to determine their clients' ability to maintain independence in activities of daily living. For that purpose, the article by Varela, Ayan, and Cancela (2008) is especially helpful. Performance assessment criteria developed by American Alliance of Health, Physical Education, Recreation and Dance; the Senior Fitness Association; the National Institute on Aging; and the popular test battery developed by Rikli and Jones (2000) as well as criteria developed by 12 other researchers are carefully reviewed in this article. The strength of the review by Varela, Ayan, and Cancela is that it addresses test selection, administration considerations, and the interpretation of results.

strength, cardiovascular endurance, joint flexibility, overall physical fitness, coordination, energy level, activity level, and self-confidence. These positive perceptions reinforced the beneficial effects of their exercise efforts and encouraged over 90 percent of the participants to continue their fitness programs. If you choose to use the Lifestyle Questionnaire (figure 7.5) with your clients, you may want to copy it at 120 percent to obtain an 8.5-inch-by-11-inch version. For further information on personal perceptions and exercise adherence, we recommend Rod Dishman's excellent *Exercise Adherence* text (Human Kinetics, 1988).

Summary of Progress Assessments

Some seniors are content to evaluate their strength training program by noting load increases in their training log. Others prefer formal assessments of their progress, and some want specific feedback that enables them to compare their fitness level to that of their peers.

- The YMCA leg extension test effectively and safely measures lower-body muscle strength, providing research-based ratings of muscle strength for men and women in their 50s, 60s, and 70s. The test evaluates the large quadriceps muscles, relative to the subject's bodyweight, using the 10-repetition maximum load.

- You can assess joint flexibility with the sit-and-reach test. This evaluation targets the hip and trunk muscles, which are closely related to low-back health. Research indicates that properly performed strength training improves hip and trunk flexibility.

- Body composition, which refers to the ratio of fat weight to lean weight, is usually reported as percent body fat. The most common and practical method for assessing percent body fat is skinfold measurement using calipers. Regular strength training improves body composition by increasing lean weight and decreasing fat weight.

- We suggest administering self-rating questionnaires before and after exercise programs to assess personal perceptions of fitness-related parameters. Preliminary results indicate that strength training improves older adults' perceptions of their fitness and performance levels, as well as their self-confidence.

Recommended Reading

National Institutes of Health Technology Assessment Conference Statement. (1994). Bioelectrical impedance analysis in body composition measurement. (December 12–14). Washington, DC.

Lifestyle Questionnaire

Age _____   Gender _____   Date _____

Please indicate the most accurate response to each of the following questions.
Thank you.

	High	Above average	Average	Below average	Low
1. My overall level of physical fitness is . . .	❏	❏	❏	❏	❏
2. My level of muscular strength is . . .	❏	❏	❏	❏	❏
3. My level of cardiovascular endurance is . . .	❏	❏	❏	❏	❏
4. My level of joint flexibility is . . .	❏	❏	❏	❏	❏
5. My general energy level is . . .	❏	❏	❏	❏	❏
6. My daily activity level is . . .	❏	❏	❏	❏	❏
7. My desire to do physical activities is . . .	❏	❏	❏	❏	❏
8. My ability to walk a mile is . . .	❏	❏	❏	❏	❏
9. My ability to lift and carry large objects (groceries, suitcases, vacuum cleaners, etc.) is . . .	❏	❏	❏	❏	❏
10. My level of self-confidence is . . .	❏	❏	❏	❏	❏
11. My level of personal independence is . . .	❏	❏	❏	❏	❏
12. My level of coordination is . . .	❏	❏	❏	❏	❏

Figure 7.5   Lifestyle Questionnaire.
Data from South Shore YMCA Fitness Research Department.

8

Working With Special Populations

The aging process is associated with a variety of conditions, diseases, and disabilities that make it difficult for some older adults to participate in strength training activities. This chapter discusses some of the more common of these and suggests sensible training modifications that you can employ with senior men and women that will enable them to strength train safely and productively. The conditions and diseases addressed in this chapter include overweight and obesity, diabetes, cardiovascular disease, osteoporosis, low-back pain, arthritis, fibromyalgia, depression, visual and auditory impairments, strokes, and general frailty. Before designing a program for clients with these conditions and diseases, a medical evaluation should be performed that includes a thorough health history and physical examination. Disabilities, limitations, and health problems should be inventoried, and clearance should be acquired from the physician for participation in the resistance training exercises and programs suggested in this chapter.

OBESITY

Over two-thirds of American adults are overweight or obese (National Health and Nutrition Examination Survey, 2004), with many estimates even higher (ACSM 2010). People must be more than 20 percent heavier than the recommended bodyweight for their height to be considered obese, yet bodyweight based on height chart assessments alone does not identify how much extra fat a person is carrying. Another method that does not identify body fat but rather uses bodyweight relative to height (kg/m^2) is the body mass index (BMI). The National Institutes of Health (2007) use BMI values between 25 and 29.9 and those greater than 30 for classifying people who are overweight and obese, respectively. When skinfold measurements, or the more precise method of underwater weighing, are used to determine body-fat percentage, values that exceed the normal range by at least 5 percent are considered obese. In older populations, ACSM (2010) has suggested that satisfactory body-fat values for men and women age 50 to 59 are between 10 and 22 percent and 20 and 32 percent, respectively. Average body-fat values reported by the Cooper Institute for men age 60 to 69 and 70 to 79 are 22.6 and 23.1 percent, respectively, and those for women are 27.9 and 28.6 percent, respectively (ACSM 2010). Although girth measurements may also be used with older adults, they may not be as helpful because there are no well-established values for persons over 56 years of age. Regardless of the method used for assessing body composition, the lifestyles of many Americans clearly contribute to their weighing too much.

It is also easy to understand why many senior men and women are debilitated by obesity—nonexercising adults lose over 5 pounds (2.3 kg) of muscle and add about 15 pounds (6.8 kg) of fat each decade, bringing about an increase in body fat that may be 50 percent greater than the increase in bodyweight (Evans and Rosenberg 1992). Thus, older clients may come to you with simply too much fat and too little muscle, which makes every one of their physical tasks more strenuous, almost as if they are driving a semitrailer truck with a motor scooter engine. Fortunately, sensible strength training can remediate this situation (Campbell et al. 1994; Westcott 2009).

Equipment Considerations

Because of the weight and size of their bodies, obese people have difficulty moving, including getting up, getting down, and engaging in all types of ambulatory activities. In choosing equipment, then, obese adults typically prefer upright or recumbent stationary cycles that support their weight instead of treadmills and stair-climbing machines that do not. Therefore, for your overweight clients, try to include machine exercises that can accommodate their larger frames and that are structurally sturdy enough to support their weight (plus that of the load or weight that they are using). Avoid exercises such as the machine hip/leg press because of the challenges it presents in getting into position to perform the exercise as well as simply getting into and out of the machine.

When working with obese clients, be sure that the equipment can accommodate their weight. Most manufacturers provide a weight limit in the product manual; if they do not, contact them to ascertain the weight limit for each piece of equipment that heavier clients will use. Free-weight exercises that require lifting dumbbells instead barbells from the floor to start an exercise may be easier. The width of the free-weight bar may also be too narrow to allow proper performance of exercises such as the biceps curl and back squat, indicating the need to use an Olympic-size bar, which is longer. Additional consideration should be given to selecting machine equipment that will be easy for overweight clients to get into and out of, and to avoiding some floor exercises (e.g., crunches, modified push-ups, stretching) that require clients to get down and up. If arthritis or joint pain is present, consider alternating the strength training exercises with lower-impact activities such as elliptical machines and stationary cycling activities or swimming. Regardless of the equipment used or the exercises being performed, programs for overweight and obese clients should include exercises that can be performed correctly and that clients feel more comfortable performing.

Calisthenic Limitations

Including calisthenic exercises such as sit-ups, push-ups, and pull-ups is an option, but excess bodyweight significantly limits the number of repetitions that overweight or obese clients can perform. Therefore, these activities may limit improvement and be embarrassing for them to attempt. Designing programs that include the use of machines or free-weight equipment may avoid this problem, because resistance loads can be easily adjusted to match each client's strength level. For example, the free-weight bench press works the same muscles as push-ups do, and the weight-assisted chin and dip machine is nearly identical to pull-ups in its effect on the muscles worked. Although your client may not have the strength to complete push-ups or pull-ups, load assignments in the bench press and weight-assisted chin and dip machine, respectively, can be reduced enough to enable him or her to perform the 8 to 12 reps recommended in chapter 4.

> ### *Cardiovascular Endurance Issues*
>
> Cardiovascular exercise is an important component of well-designed fitness programs and is especially helpful for clients who desire to lose weight. Some obese adults, however, find it hard to complete weight-supported endurance activities such as treadmill or hard-surface jogging. Therefore, supported activities such as swimming, deep-water running, and cycling (stationary usually preferred) are good alternatives for them. Cardiovascular training programs such those described by Vega and Jimenez (in Earle and Baechle 2004) provide excellent guidelines for developing cardiovascular fitness programs for overweight clients.

Training Protocols

Given that many older adults suffer from obesity, you will likely have some of these clients coming to you for help in losing fat and increasing muscle mass and strength. Of course, strength training along with sensible eating can be instrumental in bringing about desired changes in overall body composition. Using the workouts in chapter 4, you can easily adjust training loads or resistances to match current strength levels while selecting exercises that can be performed safely on sturdy and properly sized machine and free-weight equipment.

Although strength training programs have been shown to reduce body weight significantly (and increase muscle mass), convincing overweight clients to eat properly is even more important in helping them lose fat. Consult a registered dietician and use the information in chapter 10 that discusses food selection and substitutions for heart-healthy eating to help your overweight clients attain a more desirable bodyweight. Also, encourage them to drink lots of water before, during, and after workouts, especially in hot and humid weather or in training areas without ideal air circulation. Suggest that they wear loose clothing to decrease chafing and dress in layers so that they can remove articles to avoid overheating (Flood and Constance 2002).

DIABETES

Diabetes mellitus, commonly called diabetes, is a metabolic dysfunction that prevents glucose, the body's primary fuel source, from being efficiently transported and utilized. In type 1 diabetes, the pancreas does not produce insulin, the hormone responsible for getting glucose into the body cells. In type 2 diabetes, the pancreas manufactures sufficient insulin but the body cells become resistant to its effects. According to Dr. David Nathan, director of the diabetes center at Massachusetts General Hospital, diabetes is difficult to treat after it develops, and it is the leading cause of blindness, kidney failure, and limb amputations, as well as a predisposing factor in heart disease and stroke (Foreman 1997). The number of people in the United States diagnosed with diabetes has been estimated to be 17.9 million, and another 5.7 million are unaware that they have the disease (American Diabetes Association 2008).

Genetic factors appear to be involved in some cases of type 2 diabetes, but age, inactivity, impaired glucose tolerance, and obesity are major predisposing factors. Obesity alone appears to be associated with 80 percent of the type 2 diabetes cases reported (National Institute of Diabetes and Digestive and Kidney Diseases 2004). Dr. Nathan's research revealed that this disease is about six times more common in adults over age 45 than in those aged 30 through 44. People with impaired glucose tolerance have about a 50 percent greater chance of developing diabetes than do others, and the risk essentially doubles for those with impaired glucose tolerance who are also obese.

Because all older adults have one risk factor for developing diabetes (age), many have a second (obesity), and some have a third (impaired glucose tolerance), taking preventive measures with all your clients is prudent. Although most diabetes publications rightly recommend endurance exercise, such as walking (Weil 1993), support is now overwhelming for adding strength training to the overall fitness program for those with diabetes (Eriksson 1997). Strength training not only improves insulin sensitivity to about the same extent that aerobic exercise does but also improves blood glucose control by increasing storage of glucose in skeletal muscle in those with type 2 diabetes (Eves and Plotnikoff 2006). Besides increasing glucose utilization, strength training may be the best means for improving body composition, bone mineral density, mobility, and physical self-reliance (Stewart 2004), thus reversing many negative aspects of the aging process (see chapter 1). Strength training, however, may be contraindicated for those with diabetes who have high blood pressure and retinopathy, and those who have had recent laser treatments (ACSM 2010).

Training Protocols

Based on information currently available and support from organizations such as the American Diabetes Association, American Heart Association, and the American College of Sports Medicine, it is clear that a program of strength training is appropriate for people with diabetes, contingent on physician approval. No evidence indicates that strength training will have adverse effects on those with diabetes or that high-intensity exercise is harmful. In fact, studies involving people with diabetes indicate that higher intensity exercises may be better than lower intensity activities for producing desirable metabolic changes (President's Council on Physical Fitness and *Sports Research Digest* 1997; Segal et al. 1991). Clients should be reminded, however, to use proper technique and to minimize the occurrence of sustained grips, static positions, and breath holding when performing exercises, so as to avoid high spikes in blood pressure. We recommend starting with the basic workout program presented in chapter 4 when training older adults with diabetes, with one exception. The initial training loads should be light enough to permit 10 to 15 repetitions (65–75 percent of 1RM). As strength improves, the load should be increased so that 8 to 10 repetitions (75–80 percent of 1RM) will result (Eves and Plotnikoff 2006). As clients attain greater strength, muscle development, and endurance levels, the more advanced training protocols described in chapter 5 may be indicated.

Precautions

The common problem when training insulin-dependent diabetics is that they may experience hypoglycemia (an acute low blood sugar episode) resulting from the combined effects of insulin supplementation and exercise. Always maintain a supply of canned fruit juice or diabetic glucose tablets in your activity area. Be sure that clients have taken the necessary precautions (such as eating the right amount of carbohydrate) before they work out. Snacks containing complex carbohydrates and protein will help provide a more level or continuous energy source, keeping the blood sugar at a more level rate. Instruct any client who shows signs of an adverse insulin reaction (such as dizziness, weakness, sweating, headache, blurred vision, slurred speech, disorientation, or lack of coordination) to sit down immediately and drink 6 to 8 ounces (180 to 240 ml) of fruit juice or consume some other significant source of sugar (Rimmer 1997). Hypoglycemia can occur during exercise and up to 6 hours following an exercise bout. To counteract this response, the client with diabetes may need to reduce his or her insulin dosage or increase carbohydrate intake before exercising, according to his or her physician's recommendations.

You should note the following when working with clients with diabetes:

- Encourage clients to drink a lot of water before, during, and after workouts, especially when training in hot and humid conditions and in facilities that do not have good air circulation.

- Be aware that exercising in excessive heat or humidity may cause problems in those with diabetes, particularly those with peripheral neuropathy. Loose-fitting and layered clothing is also recommended, especially for overweight clients.

- Be aware that the use of beta-blockers (which is common among those with diabetes) and other medications may interfere with the ability to discern hypoglycemic symptoms or angina (and heart rate and blood pressure readings).

- Be sure also to encourage clients with diabetes to practice proper foot hygiene and to wear appropriate footwear.

- Blood glucose levels should be taken and recorded before and after exercise sessions, especially when a client is starting a program.

- If insulin injections are required for diabetes management on training days, clients should be reminded to make injections into a nonactive muscle site.

Blood Sugar Levels and Exercise

Some general recommendations regarding blood sugar levels (American Diabetes Association 2008) follow, but each client's physician should determine specific levels because diabetes is rarely the only serious health risk factor.

- Lower than 100 mg/dL (5.6 mmol/L). Your client's blood sugar may be too low to exercise safely. Clients should be reminded to eat small carbohydrate-containing snacks, such as fruit or crackers, before they begin their workout.

- 100 to 250 mg/dL (5.6 to 13.9 mmol/L). For most people, this is a safe preexercise blood sugar range.

- 250 mg/dL (13.9 mmol/L) or higher. This level is considered a caution zone for clients with type 2 diabetes. Clients should check their urine for ketones. Excess ketones indicate that the body does not have enough insulin to control blood sugar levels. If ketones are present the client should forgo exercise until the blood sugar level returns to a more normal range *and* ketones are no longer present. For those with type 1 diabetes (inadequate insulin production), 250 mg/dL (regardless of ketone levels) is a contraindication to exercise, requiring physician consultation because of the risk of a further increase in blood glucose and production of ketones. But if the high blood sugar level is the result of a dietary indiscretion (rather than forgetting to take insulin), exercise may be carefully undertaken, if blood sugar can be monitored during the exercise bout.

- 300 mg/dL (16.7 mmol/L) or higher. The blood sugar may be too high to exercise safely, putting clients at risk of ketoacidosis. Physician consultation is necessary before training your client. Postpone workouts until the blood sugar level drops to a safe preexercise range. For additional guidelines on diabetes and glucose levels, refer to ACSM's logic model for risk stratification (ACSM 2010).

Your clients with diabetes may also need to adjust their daily carbohydrate intake or insulin. They should consult with their physicians and seek the expertise of a registered dietitian who has experience working with those with diabetes when making the changes needed.

CARDIOVASCULAR DISEASE

Cardiovascular disease, the leading cause of death in the United States, is prevalent among many older adults at varying levels of physical impairment, and it is the leading cause of death in people with diabetes. Sadly, every 25 seconds an American will have a coronary event, and about every minute one will die. Fortunately, about 7.9 million have survived heart attacks (AHA 2007) leaving many in need of an exercise program that can speed their recovery.

Traditionally, postcoronary patients have been advised to begin strength training with about 40 percent of their maximum resistance (40 percent of 1 RM) in each exercise (Drought 1995; Kelemen et al. 1986; Vander et al. 1986). Although using 40 percent of 1RM may not appear heavy enough to stimulate improvement, a review of resistance training studies involving cardiac rehabilitation patients disclosed that similar gains occurred in muscular strength and endurance among those using training loads as low as 30 percent compared with those using training loads as high as 80 percent of 1RM (Wenger 1995).

Percent of 1RM and Heart Rate Considerations

Although it is clearly understood that cardiac patients should not undertake training or use higher 1RM percentage training loads without their physician's permission, loads up to 80 percent of maximum may be safe for many postcoronary participants (Faigenbaum et al. 1990; Ghilarducci, Holly, and Amsterdam 1989). Westcott and O'Grady (1998) studied the relationship between training intensity and heart rate responses in middle-aged males and determined that lighter loads (70 percent of 1RM) offered more control over cardiovascular responses on a repetition-by-repetition basis than did heavier loads (85 percent of 1RM). They concluded that postcoronary exercisers could begin with lighter training loads (40 to 60 percent of 1 RM) and then progress to heavier loads. Thus, cardiac patients probably do not need to train with loads of more than 70 percent of 1RM (Westcott 2009; Westcott and Guy 1996; Westcott, Dolan, and Cavicchi 1996), because lighter loads have been shown to produce significant muscle strength development in low- to moderate-risk postcoronary patients (ACSM 2010; Pierson et al. 2001; Wenger et al. 1995).

Clients who have recently completed a cardiac or pulmonary rehabilitation program should obtain a copy of their exercise program from the hospital or rehabilitation staff and provide this information to you. This information should describe loads and workouts used so that you can safely and effectively direct the client's exercise program. The American Association of Cardiovascular and Pulmonary Rehabilitation (AACVPR) (2006) recommends including 8 to 10 exercises and training loads that the client can comfortably perform for one set of 10 to 15 repetitions (65–75 percent of 1RM). In our opinion, assigning loads even as low as 30 percent or as high as 70 percent of 1RM is appropriate when introducing strength training programs to postcoronary clients, as long as the client's effort level does not exceed a "somewhat hard" perceived exertion rating of 12 to 13 (Borg et al. 1988). After a successful response to the initial strength training program, physicians may approve progressively heavier loads and eliminate the requirement for medically monitored exercise sessions. We recommend that trainers who work with postcoronary patients implement the following exercise guidelines adapted from AACVPR (2006) and American Senior Fitness Association (Clark 1997).

- Instruct clients to warm up and cool down thoroughly before and after each strength training session, for a minimum of 10 minutes at low intensity.

- Monitor and document heart rate and perceived exertion throughout each workout, as well as blood pressure if recommended by the physician.
- Emphasize the importance of breathing continuously during every repetition and never holding the breath.
- Instruct clients to use a relaxed grip, thus avoiding the use of excessive pressure to hold handles, dumbbells, and bars.
- Remind clients to move the resistance continuously (never holding the weight in a static position) and in a slow, controlled manner (2 seconds up, 4 seconds down) throughout the full range of motion of each exercise and during every repetition.
- Increase the training loads gradually, by about 1 pound (0.45 kg) in upper-body exercises and 2.5 pounds (1.1 kg) in lower-body exercises, when clients can comfortably complete more than 15 repetitions in each set with proper form.
- Include exercises for all the major muscle groups unless there are reasons not to do so (e.g., creates discomfort or pain).
- Organize exercises so that they usually follow a general sequence from larger to smaller muscles.
- Keep overhead exercises to a minimum, especially during the early stages of strength training.
- Instruct clients to complete two or three strength workouts per week and allow at least 48 hours between training sessions.
- Emphasize the importance of discontinuing exercise at the first sign of cardiovascular stress, including dizziness, abnormal heart rhythm, unusual shortness of breath, or chest discomfort. Instruct clients to notify you if any of these symptoms occur.
- Obtain a complete list of medications from each physician (some clients have several doctors) and research their exercise indications.

Training Protocols

Cardiac patients or clients with unstable conditions (refer to ACSM Guidelines 2010), as well as those who have not received physician release from a monitored rehabilitation program, should not be trained until medical clearance has been obtained. Cardiac patients who are cleared for medically supervised strength training should exercise in accordance with the information obtained from their symptom-limited stress test. The introductory weeks of the strength training program presented in chapter 4 meet a good number of the aforementioned exercise guidelines and should work well for most clients with cardiovascular disease who have been cleared for resistance training. But additional modifications are indicated. For instance, keep in mind that the suggested starting loads in chapter 4 represent 70 to 80 percent of 1RM and therefore are a little heavier than the previously recommended loads of 65 to 75 percent of 1RM (AACVPR 2006). Ultimately, the loads assigned should be determined by the level of cardiovascular and muscle stress that they impose; you must be sure that the loads do not result in undue exertion or overstress the heart or cardiovascular system. The bottom line is that cardiac patients can safely perform strength training exercises if they adhere to their physician's recommendations, perform exercises correctly (including avoiding the Valsalva maneuver), and follow the training protocol guidelines presented in this chapter.

OSTEOPOROSIS

Osteoporosis is a condition characterized by a deterioration of bone tissue that leads to bone fragility and susceptibility to fracture. According to the National Osteoporosis Foundation (NOF 2009) 10 million Americans probably have osteoporosis, and another 34 million have low bone mass or osteopenia, which places them at increased risk for the disease. Of the 10 million who have osteoporosis, 8 million are women (NOF 2009). Osteoporosis has no obvious symptoms, and unfortunately it is usually determined after an injury. Therefore, you must ask older clients, especially women, if they have had a bone scan, and if they have, you should request a copy of the report.

After acquiring approval from the client's physician, you can generally apply basic strength training guidelines to clients with osteoporosis (Menkes et al. 1993; Hughes et al. 1995; Rhodes et al. 2000; Kerr et al. 2001). Because such clients may have extremely weak bones, you should assign very light resistances or loads at the start. We suggest starting with training loads that are equivalent to 50 to 60 percent of 1RM, as Nelson and colleagues did in their study (1994), and instruct clients to perform only 8 to 12 repetitions. When they can perform 14 or more repetitions with correct technique during two consecutive workouts, cautiously increase the load. Over time, you should increase training loads to 70 to 80 percent of 1RM (and maybe heavier), because heavier loads appear to be more effective in increasing bone mineral density (ACSM 2010; Maddalozzo and Snow 2000) and building muscle mass and strength. Exercises that involve flexing at the waist (e.g., bent-over row) or twisting the spine (e.g., twisting crunch) and high-impact aerobics should not be included (ACSM 2010).

We also recommend following the exercise program described in chapter 4 with a couple of modifications and suggestions. Start with machine or bench exercises that provide hip and back support. Proper body positioning and alignment and range of movement are easier to control using machines. We find that our clients do much better when they start with machines instead of free weights, especially if they are new to strength training. With older clients who demonstrate good muscle coordination, consider introducing free-weight and elastic band exercises, because these activities may assist them in maintaining or increasing their kinesthetic awareness, dynamic movement, and balance. Balance exercises are critically important to helping your clients avoid falls. Regardless of which mode of training you use with your osteoporotic clients, avoid including too many spinal flexion exercises (e.g., crunches, sit-ups) that place stress on the vertebrae, because they may cause fractures (Clark 1997). Thus, the trunk curl exercise should be deleted from the list of exercises in chapter 4, or the range should be reduced considerably. Hip, back, and neck extensor exercises (e.g., hip adductor and abductor, flexion and extension exercises, back and neck extension exercises, respectively) should be emphasized (Bennell et al. 2000). Instruct clients to maintain a straight back position and to flex from the hips, not the spine, during workouts (National Institute on Aging Information Center 2008). Ultimately, exercises that minimize flexion loading on the spine, promote an extended posture, improve chest expansion (e.g., dumbbell chest flies, chest crossover), and strengthen the legs, abdomen, and back are ideal for clients with osteoporosis.

LOW-BACK PAIN

Affecting four out of five adults, low-back pain is a major malady among both older and younger men and women. Researchers at the University of Florida have demonstrated that isolated trunk extension exercise can increase strength and decrease pain in the low-back area (Risch et al. 1993). Resistance exercises that provide full-range trunk extension while minimizing hip extension are most productive for strengthening the low-back muscles (Jones et al. 1988).

Although clients should avoid exercise during periods of discomfort, strength training appears to be an effective means for rehabilitating, as well as preventing, low-back problems. Unfortunately, strength training does not help everyone with low-back discomfort. Therefore, you must determine from the client's physician (with the client's approval) whether resistance training is appropriate, and if so, which exercises are indicated or contraindicated, and what range of motion and spinal loading limitations exist. Also, determine what signs and symptoms should be closely monitored for referral or program modification.

As mentioned previously, we recommend that clients with low-back pain (acute and chronic, and back pain associated with leg pain, or sciatica) first consult their physicians regarding participation in a strength training program.

The exercises selected for clients with low-back problems should strengthen the trunk, low-back extensor, and abdominal muscle areas. By strengthening these and other muscles surrounding the spinal column, clients may decrease the stress on vertebral discs and decrease pain. Therefore, exercises selected for inclusion in workouts should target strengthening the low-back and abdominal muscles, and strengthening and stretching the iliopsoas, hamstrings, piriformis, gluteal complex, quadriceps, and quadratus lumborum.

Start your clients with the basic exercises presented in chapter 4 that target the muscles just discussed and assign lighter training loads that permit 10 to 15 repetitions (65–75 percent of 1RM). For instance, we recommend including the machine low-back exercise (see chapter 4) that targets the trunk extensor muscles and deemphasizes the hip extensor muscles, thereby enhancing essential low-back strength development. The trunk extension is another low-back exercise, and one that is easy to execute. It involves using the low-back muscles to raise the torso from a hip-supported prone position from the floor. By using the arms for assistance, even clients with weak low-back muscles should be able to perform this movement productively. Low-back pain patients at the University of Florida experienced excellent results by performing one set of

8 to 12 machine trunk extensions, 2 or 3 days per week (Risch et al. 1993). We recommend a similar training protocol after several weeks of pretraining using loads of 10 to 15 repetitions. Physicians in the Boston area also believe that the rotary torso machine is an effective exercise for increasing trunk strength and function by complementing the low-back muscles with strong oblique muscles. They recommend, however, that the nonpulling arm (refer to chapter 3, page 74) be elevated slightly to maintain a more erect torso position throughout performance of the exercise. You must closely monitor each client's response to the exercises mentioned here and those listed in chapter 3, and eliminate any that result in low-back discomfort. If a client feels low-back pain, radiating pain, numbness or tingling, or muscular weakness at any time during the exercise session, the exercises should be discontinued and his or her physician should be contacted immediately. If the client has been working with a physical therapist or back specialist, you should also communicate to these professionals the client's response to the program.

Ideally, the aforementioned strength training program will be effective, the low-back discomfort will diminish, and your client will be able to progress to some of the more advanced training protocols presented in chapter 5.

ARTHRITIS

The pain and swelling that accompany arthritic conditions frequently are limiting factors for strength training by older adults. Therefore, addressing questions with the client's physician (with the client's approval), such as what type of arthritis the client has, which joints are involved and are unstable, and what specific exercises should be avoided, will enable you to design a safe and effective program. With rheumatoid arthritis, the amount of exercise and type of exercise that can be tolerated can vary greatly from one day to the next depending on the amount of inflammation that she or he is experiencing. Osteoarthritis, on the other hand, does not vary from day to day, although flare-ups occasionally occur with this type of arthritis too.

According to Clark (1997), president of the American Senior Fitness Association, most strength training exercises can be modified to decrease arthritic discomfort and increase ease of execution, and every reasonable effort should be made to accomplish these outcomes. If an exercise causes joint discomfort that persists for more than 1 hour, it should be replaced. Clark also advised that brief exercise sessions are better tolerated than long workouts. For example, instead of combining strength exercise and aerobic activity into a 1-hour workout on Mondays, Wednesdays, and Fridays, clients with arthritis may respond more favorably to 30 minutes of strength exercise on Mondays, Wednesdays, and Fridays and 30 minutes of aerobic activity on Tuesdays, Thursdays, and Saturdays. Ultimately, the goals for training should be an increase in muscular endurance and strength that improves function but does not cause pain, inflammation, or joint damage.

We suggest starting and ending workouts with an active low- (or no-) impact warm-up (cycling or elliptical or stepping machines, not jogging or walking on pavement) of at least 5 to 15 minutes, followed by flexibility and range-of-motion exercises to help decrease stiffness, increase joint mobility, and prevent soft-tissue contractures. All movements should be pain free. We think that the basic strength training program presented in chapter 4 is a good starting point for clients with arthritis (Nelson 2002). The number of repetitions recommended is from 2 to 3 with a light load (e.g., 40 percent of 1RM) for a beginning client (to determine whether the range of movement causes pain) to 10 to 15 reps (65–75 percent of 1RM) for more advanced clients with arthritis. ACSM (2006) recommends stopping at volitional fatigue, or 2 or 3 repetitions before fatigue occurs.

Starting clients with arthritis with only six exercises as shown in chapter 4 (first 2 weeks) and instructing them to perform only one set of each provides a good foundation for subsequent weeks when the number of exercises increases, requiring a higher level of muscular strength and endurance. Use pain tolerance and improvement as a guide for training progression in each workout and modify ranges of motion during exercises as needed.

Regarding equipment issues, machines are typically preferred (over free weights) when training clients with arthritis because they provide greater support and usually do not require as firm a grip, but free weights, elastic bands, and isometric exercises may also be used effectively. For some with osteoarthritis, isometric exercises may be a more comfortable option.

Consider the following additional recommendations, adapted from those of Janie Clark (1997) and Dorothy Foltz-Gray (1997), when designing and implementing programs for clients with arthritis:

- Monitor pain levels during training sessions and modify loads, exercise group, and range of movement to decrease arthritic discomfort, as needed.
- Decrease loads and reduce the number of repetitions and sets during periods of acute inflammation.
- Brief training sessions are better tolerated than long ones. Begin with only one set of a few exercises.
- Avoid overtraining a specific muscle–joint area.
- Avoid exercises that require a tight grip if it causes discomfort (e.g., lat pull-down).
- Emphasize proper technique and posture.
- Reduce the stress on joints (e.g., by incorporating machine exercises, increasing the diameter of handles or bars with tape, and using wrist straps or gloves).
- If joint pain persists for more than an hour after a training session, replace the exercise associated with the pain.

FIBROMYALGIA

As discussed in chapter 1, fibromyalgia is not a disease but a rheumatologic syndrome characterized by chronic musculoskeletal (muscles, ligaments, and joints) aches, pains, stiffness, fatigue, and muscle spasms as well as heightened tenderness at discrete anatomical points (ACSM 2010). Additionally, many people with fibromyalgia have postural imbalances and poor range of movement. Their loss in function can lead to depression and a variety of other complications.

Be sure to learn the client's experience and history with exercise before being diagnosed with fibromyalgia. Consult with his or her physician to make sure that the client is cleared for participation and that the physician approves of the strength training program that you are considering for the client.

Although published research-based recommendations are lacking regarding the intensity or frequency of training clients with fibromyalgia, training loads of between 50 and 70 percent of 1RM and 2 or 3 days of training per week are generally accepted (ACSM 2010). We recommend starting fibromyalgia clients with very light weights or no weights for one set in the six exercises listed for the first 2 weeks of the basic program in chapter 4.

Experiment with different types of exercises; some may be more uncomfortable to perform than others. Identify where tender points are and modify ranges of movements to increase comfort levels. Although clients with fibromyalgia may need to train through some pain, do not encourage them to train through excessive pain.

Focus your client's attention on proper body alignment. Posture is important, and it should be closely monitored during workouts; make sure to correct rounded shoulders and swayback positions and the tendency for clients to lean forward.

Fatigue is a common side effect of fibromyalgia. Make decisions regarding when to increase training intensity based on whether the client is able to recover fully from previous workouts in 2 to 3 days. If the client cannot recover adequately, back off on the number of exercises, loads used, or the number of reps and sets. Also, allow longer recovery between sets and different exercises (e.g., 3 minutes or longer). Clients should not start a 3-day-a-week program until they have demonstrated the ability to recover completely from 2 days of training per week. Flexibility training is important to the progress of those with fibromyalgia. Include a minimum of 5 to 10 minutes of mild stretching before and after each session, and instruct clients to move slowly into and out of stretched positions.

DEPRESSION AND SELF-CONFIDENCE

Strength training can improve self-concept in children (Faigenbaum et al. 1997) and increase self-confidence (Westcott 1995), self-efficacy (Baker et al. 2001), and emotion and well-being in older adults. In a study conducted at Harvard Medical School (Singh, Clements, and Fiatarone 1997), strength training also resulted in significantly reduced depression levels in people over 60 years of age. Of 16 clinically depressed subjects, 14 no longer met the criteria for depression following 10 weeks of strength training. An important outcome of this study was the finding that participants who trained at higher levels of intensity (more than 80 percent of maximum resistance) made significantly more improvement in their depression scores than those who trained at lower levels (less than 80 percent of 1 RM).

It appears that depressed older adults may participate safely and success-fully in supervised strength training programs. We recommend starting with the basic program presented in chapter 4 and progressing to more advanced programs when appropriate. As discussed previously, higher training intensities may be more effective in reducing depression; therefore, we suggest assigning training loads equal to 75 percent of 1RM (10 reps) for the first 2 weeks and then increasing loads to 80 percent of 1RM (8 reps) when two or more sets can be completed during two consecutive workouts.

VISUAL AND AUDITORY IMPAIRMENTS

Working with clients who have visual and auditory limitations presents addi-tional challenges, but procedures and precautions to enhance their experiences are many and easy to implement. A good starting point is to make sure that the exercise facility has ample lighting and good acoustics. Eliminate barriers that can increase the likelihood of falls or collisions, remove weights and obstacles from walkways and workout areas, and see that doors are not left half open. Place machines with cables and hanging bars, such as lat pull-down machines, into areas separate from where the equipment that they will be using is located. Be sure that areas are uncluttered and that a minimum of 3 feet (1 m) of clear-ance exists around all equipment, in accordance with ACSM guidelines (ACSM 2006). Adequate lighting and nonskid floor surfaces are also a high priority in working with this clientele.

Especially important is to provide visually impaired clients with precise exercise demonstrations and to speak loudly and slowly to those with hearing difficulties. Because many people with impaired hearing read lips, be sure to face your clients as much as possible (Clark 1997).

For the visually impaired, avoid including in their programs exercises that produce unnecessary pressure in the eyes, as well as actions that elevate blood pressure excessively. Make sure that clients do not hold their breath, hold the resistance in a static position, or strain to complete a final repetition. Because both visually and auditorily impaired individuals may have difficulty with balance and postural alignments, we suggest starting with machines or free-weight exercises that clients can perform from supported positions. For example, incline bench dumbbell presses are preferable to standing dumbbell presses.

You should develop and follow a consistent pattern of exercise sequencing, moving from station to station in a routine manner. Introduce additional exer-cises one at a time and take care to establish new movement procedures and pathways around the training facility.

We recommend that older adults with visual or auditory impairment attempt the basic training program presented in chapter 4, assuming that the exercise stations are arranged appropriately and are easy to access. Although you may need to make minor exercise adjustments along the way, the training progres-sions should not be problematic, and improvements in strength should be no different from those of other older adults.

STROKES

When we were asked to assist in the rehabilitation of a former National Football League rushing champion, we did not know how to strengthen the limbs affected by his stroke. How do you apply resistance to a hand that cannot grip and an arm that cannot move? We first learned that a Velcro glove enabled him to hold the handle of the biceps curl machine. We then discovered that, although he could not lift any amount of resistance (concentric muscle action), he could lower a little resistance (eccentric muscle action) after we placed his arm in the fully contracted, flexed-elbow position. By progressively training with the eccentric phase of the muscle action, Jim gradually increased his biceps strength until he was eventually able to lower and lift relatively heavy training loads. Again, stroke clients tend to be unique in their responses to training, so although this approach worked with Jim, it may not be as effective with other clients. You may find, however, that this and similar strength training procedures work well for clients with similar disabilities (Weiss et al. 2000). If so, just be patient with their progress, especially in the early stages of the exercise program.

Special Considerations

Training to improve balance, stability, and neuromuscular coordination is essential to a well-designed program for stroke patients. Incorporate functional balance and stability exercises into as many sessions as possible. Any type of functional exercise training (especially those that involve activities of daily living) is highly beneficial. Because balance is a concern, begin exercises in a stable (e.g., seated) position and watch for the client's response; provide support as needed. Provide hands-on support when clients are attempting standing movements. Also, do not forget that normal feedback systems may be impaired; therefore, it is beneficial to ask clients whether they can feel the difference between correct and incorrect posture.

Because stooped postures when sitting and standing are typical among those who have had strokes, posture retraining exercises are important because they will help restore normal movement patterns. Emphasize extension of the head, neck, hip, and knee, as well as spinal rotation exercises. Also, consider incorporating manual tension exercises. For example, try putting your hand on the back of the client's head and ask him or her to push the head back gently (extending, not rotating, to flatten the cervical spine curve). Give mild resistance to this movement as tactile feedback. Of particular importance is instructing and reminding poststroke clients to avoid holding their breath or holding static positions when working out because these actions may significantly increase blood pressure. Equipment that features independent movement arms, such as chest press, seated row, shoulder press, and arm curl machines, allows the client to exercise one side at a time (left and right). Equipment adaptations such as splints or orthotic devices can help stroke victims control joint positioning and unwanted movements and reduce injuries and pain. Gripping bars and handles can be improved with the use of Velcro gloves and by increasing the thickness of bars and handles.

Training Protocols

We suggest following the basic strength training exercises presented in chapter 4 with the modifications presented here. We also encourage you to consider incorporating the negative (eccentric) training approach, in which you perform the lifting (concentric) phase and the stroke client lowers the weight in the eccentric phase of the exercise. Follow these suggestions, which were adapted from ACE's *Clinical Exercise Specialist Manual* (1999).

Monitor and record blood pressure and heart rates during strength training sessions. Always know what medications the client is taking and what effects they have on blood pressure, heart rate, and balance.

Before designing a strength training program for a client who has had a stroke, try to obtain the following information from her or his physician (with the client's permission):

1. What is the official diagnosis of this client's medical condition and what are her or his limitations and capabilities? Please elaborate.

2. Are cognitive deficits present?

3. What are your specific recommendations for exercise heart rate and maximum blood pressure?

4. What medications have been prescribed, and what are their effects on exercise heart rate and blood pressure? What other side affects should I be aware of?

5. What warning signs, if any, should I watch for while she or he is exercising?

GENERAL FRAILTY

For some older adults, especially those in higher age categories, the major physical problem is general frailty—years of inactivity have resulted in severe muscle atrophy and strength loss. Fortunately, the Tufts University research on nonagenarians discussed in chapter 1 demonstrates that even the oldest and weakest adults respond positively to properly designed strength exercise (Fiatarone and Singh 2002; Fiatarone et al. 1994; Tufts 1994; Fiatarone et al. 1990; Frontera et al. 1988).

We recommend that frail older adults begin by performing single sets of the six exercises presented at the beginning of chapter 4, unless doing so aggravates an existing musculoskeletal or arthritic condition. In that regard, shoulder problems are common among older adults, so caution should be exercised when selecting overhead exercises for them. To err on the side of caution, the American College of Sports Medicine (2010) recommends starting with a 10- to 15-repetition protocol (65–75 percent of 1RM) for older adult exercisers and then increasing loads that will result in a range of 8 to 12 reps (70–80 percent of 1RM) as described in chapter 4. As clients become stronger and are able to train harder and longer, consider assigning them to the more challenging workouts presented later in chapter 4. If necessary, modify the machine and free-weight programs in chapter 4 by deleting some exercises and adding others (combining some machine exercises with free-weight exercises and vice versa) or by also adding some elastic resistance exercises. Encourage older clients to exert an effort similar to that applied by younger clients when training in order to improve their functional performance (Kalapotharakos 2005; Noble et al. 1983).

Summary

The strength training programs that you design for older clients should incorporate the precautions detailed in this chapter and advocated by the various health care organizations (e.g., American Diabetes Association, American Heart Association) and professional organizations (e.g., AACVPR, ACSM). The training principles presented in chapter 2 and the basic exercise programs described in chapter 4 are generally applicable, although the workout intensity recommended in this chapter may be lower and the rate of progression slower.

Sport-Specific Training

Many of your older clients are like us—they still enjoy participating in organized recreational and sport activities and take their performance in them seriously. Although some of your exercisers who are older than 50 continue to participate in team sporting activities such as basketball, softball, and soccer, most choose to participate in individual sports such as running, cycling, swimming, tennis, and golf. This chapter will assist you in developing programs that are based on the training principles presented in chapter 2 and that are designed specifically to enhance your clients' performance in their chosen sports activity. The approach taken here emphasizes the importance of including exercises in clients' programs that create balanced strength and are sport specific; the former will help reduce injuries and the latter will enhance performance.

Our first objective is to help seniors avoid sports-related injuries typically caused by disproportionate strength and muscle imbalance. By helping to develop balanced strength in the muscles most frequently injured in a particular sport, we can accomplish this objective. If the quadriceps muscles of the front of the thigh of runners become disproportionately stronger than the opposing hamstring muscles of the rear thigh, the chances of injury to the hamstrings increase. Conversely, if the hamstring muscles of the rear thigh become disproportionately stronger than the quadriceps muscles of the front thigh, the likelihood that the quadriceps will become injured increases. We therefore recommend that you include a balanced program of hamstring and quadriceps strengthening exercises for your clients who are runners to reduce their risk of injuries to the thigh. This concept of balancing strength and avoiding disproportionate strength levels across joints applies not only to the hip and knee joints and their opposing muscle groups but also to other joints and opposing muscle groups of the body.

Our second objective is to strengthen the muscles that are most prominent (prime movers) in the specific athletic activity to increase performance power, often referred to as sport-specific training. Success in every sport is related to developing strength in sport-specific muscles and ultimately performance power, which is essentially the product of muscle force and movement speed.

$$\text{Performance power} = \text{muscle force} \times \text{movement speed}$$

Increasing movement speed involves complex neuromuscular phenomena and technical training programs that are beyond the scope of this book. Increasing muscle force, on the other hand, is a relatively simple process that is best accomplished by implementing the strength training principles, protocols, and procedures presented in chapters 2 and 3. As your clients increase their muscle strength, they automatically improve their ability to produce performance power.

Consider what you have just read regarding strength training for sports. First, to reduce their injury risk, older adults should strengthen the muscles that are less involved in the athletic activity. Second, we want seniors to strengthen the muscles that are more involved in the athletic activity to increase their power production and improve their performance ability. In other words, we want them to work all of their major muscle groups for best results in both quality and quantity of sport participation.

For example, in our golf studies, our relatively brief but comprehensive approach to overall muscle conditioning produced many positive outcomes, both expected and unexpected. In addition to building muscle, losing fat, improving strength, enhancing performance power, and increasing club head speed, the golfers found that they could play their favorite activity more frequently and for longer durations without fatigue. Best of all, none of the golf conditioning participants (including those who had been injured previously) reported a golf-related injury as long as they continued their strength training program.

In this chapter we present specific strength training programs for the sports of running, cycling, swimming, skiing, tennis, golf, rock climbing, hiking, triathlon, rowing, and softball. Although the exercises and training protocols are different for each activity, each program works the major muscle groups in the most appropriate manner to ensure overall muscle strength, muscle balance, and power enhancement. You will learn how the major muscles are involved in each athletic event and how to train clients properly for integrated strength development and improved sports performance.

RUNNERS

Distance running is a sport enjoyed at a variety of levels by millions of competitive and recreational athletes. Whether clients are jogging a couple of miles through the neighborhood or are training to complete a marathon, distance running is a highly effective and efficient means of aerobic conditioning. Unfortunately, distance running is considerably less beneficial for the musculoskeletal system. Injury rates among runners are extremely high. In fact, at the high school level, cross country runners experience more injuries than athletes in any other sport do, including football and gymnastics.

Why is a noncontact sport like running such a high-risk activity? Actually, running involves an incredible amount of contact, but it is with road surfaces rather than other athletes. Every running stride places about three times the person's bodyweight on the foot, ankle, knee, and hip joints. These landing forces may also transmit excessive stress to lower-back structures.

The repetitive pounding encountered by running long distances produces a degree of microtrauma to the shock-absorbing tissues (especially muscles and tendons). Under ideal conditions, these tissues recover completely within a 24-hour period. But numerous factors may interfere with normal recovery processes, eventually resulting in weakened and injury-prone tissues. These factors include longer running sessions, faster running paces, shorter recovery periods between workouts, more downhill running, more hard-surface running, more racing, more general fatigue, and undesirable changes in eating or sleeping patterns.

Of course, you may encourage distance-running clients to take steps that reduce the amount of tissue trauma and decrease the risk of running-related injuries. Such precautions include making gradual increases in training distances and speeds, taking sufficient recovery periods (particularly between hard training sessions), selecting user-friendly running courses (soft surfaces and level terrain), competing in fewer races, avoiding overfatigue, and paying careful attention to proper nutrition and sleep.

But one of the most effective means for minimizing tissue trauma is to develop stronger muscles, tendons, fascia, ligaments, and bones. Primarily for that reason, every runner should perform strength training exercises on a regular basis. Consider the results of our four-year strength training project with the Notre Dame High School girls' cross country and track teams (see the highlight box).

Although the first six strength training benefits should be self-explanatory, you may be intrigued by improved running economy. In a 1995 study at the University of New Hampshire, the women cross country runners who did strength training experienced a significant improvement in running economy. They required 4 percent less oxygen at submaximal running speeds (7:30, 7:00, and 6:30 mile paces, or 4:40, 4:20, and 4:00 km paces), meaning that they could run more efficiently and race faster than before.

> ### *Notre Dame High School Strength Training Program*
>
> For 4 consecutive years, 30 distance runners from Notre Dame High School participated in a basic and brief strength training program during the summer and winter months between their cross country and track seasons. Every Monday, Wednesday, and Friday, they performed 30 minutes of strength training (12 weight-stack machines) that addressed all of their major muscle groups. In each of those years, the cross country team won both the Massachusetts championship and the New England championship in the sport. More important, during the 4 years that they did strength training, only one girl experienced an injury that resulted in a missed practice session or meet.
>
> The Notre Dame runners realized that a sensible strength training program provides many benefits for runners. These include the following:
>
> - Greater muscle strength
> - Greater muscle endurance
> - Greater joint flexibility
> - Better body composition
> - Reduced injury risk
> - Improved self-confidence
> - Improved running economy

Concerns

With the many advantages offered by strength training, why do so few runners regularly do it? Consider four concerns that keep many runners from strength training and the facts that dispel these misconceptions.

- *Increased bodyweight*. In fact, few people who perform strength training exercises have the genetic potential to develop large muscles, especially distance runners, who typically have ectomorphic (thin) physiques. Strength training increases muscle strength and endurance but rarely results in significant weight gain.

- *Decreased movement speed*. With respect to running speed, our studies and many others have shown that greater strength results in faster movement speeds. We need only look at sprinters and middle-distance runners to realize that strength training has a positive effect on running speed, because essentially all these athletes perform regular, high-level strength training.

- *Less fluid running form*. Running involves coordinated actions of the legs and arms, and one set cannot function without the other. Your right arm moves in mirror image with your left leg, and your left arm counterbalances your right leg in perfect opposition. It is almost impossible to run fast and move your arms slow or to move your arms fast and run slow. Strengthening the upper-body muscles makes it possible to share the running effort between the arms and legs more effectively, resulting in a more fluid running form.

- *Fatigued muscles*. A strenuous strength training session can certainly cause a considerable amount of muscle fatigue that could adversely affect the quality and quantity of a client's running program. For that reason we recommend brief strength workouts that do not leave exercisers feeling enervated or exhausted. Remember that your clients are strength training to enhance their running performance, not to become competitive weightlifters. Our recommended program of strength training for runners requires just one set of exercise for each major muscle group, which does not take much time and does not produce much lasting fatigue. You may also choose to strength train clients only 1 or 2 days per week, which should make interfering muscle fatigue even less likely.

Runners' Strength Training Program

The strength training protocol followed by the Notre Dame athletes, and all of our runners, is a comprehensive conditioning program that addresses all the major muscle groups in the body. We do not attempt to imitate specific running movements or emphasize specific running muscles because this approach typically results in an overtrained, imbalanced, and injury-prone musculoskeletal system.

For example, the calf (gastrocnemius and soleus) muscles are used extensively in running. Because of their involvement in every running stride, many people think that runners should strengthen their calf muscles. Indeed they should, but even more important is strengthening their weaker counterpart, the shin (anterior tibial) muscles. If clients strengthen only the larger and stronger calf muscles, they will eventually overpower the smaller and weaker shin muscles, which may lead to shin splints, stress fractures, Achilles tendon problems, and other lower-leg difficulties. With this in mind, our runners always conclude their strength workouts with a set of weighted toe raises to strengthen the shin muscles and maintain balance within the lower-leg musculature.

Some people believe that runners should complete numerous sets and many repetitions with light resistance to enhance their endurance capacity. But this is not our purpose in performing strength training. Remember that running is the best way to improve cardiovascular endurance and that strength training is the best way to increase musculoskeletal strength.

Most athletes best develop muscle strength by training with moderate loads (about 75 percent of 1RM) for 8 to 12 repetitions per set. Distance runners, however, typically possess a higher percentage of slow-twitch muscle fibers and therefore attain better results by training with about 12 to 16 repetitions per set. You should add 1 to 5 pounds (0.45 to 2.3 kg) more resistance when your client can complete 16 repetitions in good form. One set of each exercise is sufficient for strength development.

Training with fast movement speeds is unnecessary because training fast will not necessarily make clients faster runners and training slow will not cause them to run slower. Exercising with controlled movement speeds maximizes muscle tension and minimizes momentum for a better training effect. We recommend 6-second repetitions, taking 2 seconds for each lifting movement and 4 seconds for each lowering movement. Your clients can develop muscle strength with a variety of exercises using free weights or machines. The following section presents recommended strength exercises for the major muscle groups.

Leg Muscles

Although barbell squats are the traditional leg exercise, most runners may do better to avoid placing a heavy barbell across their shoulders. Dumbbell squats are an acceptable alternative, but many clients may have difficulty holding enough weight to apply appropriate stress to the large leg muscles.

Our recommendation is leg presses on a well-designed machine that offers a full movement range and good back support. It may be advisable to precede leg presses with leg extensions that target the quadriceps and leg curls that target the hamstrings. One set of each exercise is sufficient, but clients may perform additional sets if you desire.

Upper-Body Muscles

The standard exercises for the upper body are bench presses for the chest muscles, bent rows for the middle- and upper-back muscles, and overhead presses for the shoulder muscles. These are acceptable exercises, but they are much safer when performed with dumbbells rather than barbells. For example, because there is no back support in a barbell bent row, the stress to the low-back area is 10 times the weight of the barbell. By using one dumbbell, clients may place the other hand on a bench for back support and therefore perform this exercise more safely and effectively.

If your clients have access to machines, we recommend chest crosses for the chest muscles, pullovers for the middle- and upper-back muscles, and lateral raises for the shoulder muscles. These machines require rotary movements that isolate the target muscle groups better. If you prefer linear movements that involve more muscle groups, well-designed chest press, seated row, and shoulder press machines provide combined training for essentially all the upper body and arm muscles.

Arm Muscles

The basic exercise for the biceps muscles is the arm curl, performed with barbells, dumbbells, or machines. Training the triceps involves some form of arm extension, with either free weights or machines.

A good means for working the biceps and upper-back muscles together is chin-ups with bodyweight or on a weight-assisted chin and dip machine. A good means for working the triceps and chest muscles together is bar dips with bodyweight or on a weight-assisted chin and dip machine.

Midsection Muscles

Machines provide the best means for safely and progressively conditioning the muscles of the midsection. In our opinion, the abdominal machine and low-back machine provide key exercises for developing a strong and injury resistant midsection. We also recommend the rotary torso machine for strengthening the oblique muscles surrounding the midsection.

If appropriate machines are not available, the basic trunk curl may be the best alternative for abdominal conditioning. The recommended counterpart for the low-back muscles is a front-lying (face-down) back extension. Although both of these exercises are performed with bodyweight resistance, they are reasonably effective for strengthening the midsection muscles.

Neck Muscles

The neck muscles maintain head position throughout each run. Because the head weighs up to 15 pounds (6.8 kg), this is an important function. In fact, the first place where many runners fatigue and tighten up is the neck and shoulder area. We therefore recommend the four-way neck machine to strengthen these muscles. If your clients do not have access to this machine, the best alternatives are shoulder shrugs (dumbbell or barbell) and manual resistance. To perform manual resistance for the neck muscles, place your hands in front of your client's forehead to resist slow neck flexion movements, and place your hands behind your client's head to resist slow neck extension movements.

Table 9.1 presents the recommended strength training exercises for an overall conditioning program that should be beneficial for runners. After your clients have mastered the basic exercise program, you may want to add some of the exercises presented in table 9.2.

TABLE 9.1

Recommended Strength Training Program
for Runners: Basic Exercises

Major muscle groups	Machine exercises	Free-weight exercises
Quadriceps	Leg extension	Dumbbell squat
Hamstrings	Leg curl	Dumbbell squat
Chest	Chest crossover	Dumbbell bench press
Upper back	Pullover	Dumbbell one-arm row

Major muscle groups	Machine exercises	Free-weight exercises
Shoulders	Lateral raise	Dumbbell overhead press
Biceps	Biceps curl	Dumbbell standing curl
Triceps	Triceps extension	Dumbbell lying triceps extension
Low back	Low-back extension	Trunk extension
Abdominal	Abdominal flexion	Trunk curl

TABLE 9.2

Recommended Strength Training Program for Runners: Additional Exercises

Muscle groups	Machine exercises	Free-weight exercises
Quadriceps and hamstrings	Leg press	Dumbbell lunge
Chest and triceps	Weight-assisted bar dip	Bar dip
Upper back and biceps	Weight-assisted pull-up	Pull-up
Internal and external obliques	Rotary torso	Twisting trunk curl
Neck flexors and extensors	Neck extension and flexion	Manual resistance neck flexion and extension
Calves	Heel raise	Dumbbell heel raise
Shins	—	Weight plate toe raise

Summary of Strength Training for Runners

When developing a sensible strength training program for runners we recommend that you carefully consider the following exercise guidelines:

Exercise selection: Include exercises in table 9.1, and consider additional exercises in table 9.2, making sure to include at least one exercise for each major muscle group

Exercise sets: One set of each exercise

Exercise resistance: Approximately 60 to 70 percent of 1RM

Exercise repetitions: Between 12 and 16 controlled repetitions

Exercise progression: A resistance increase of 5 percent when 16 repetitions can be completed (typically 1 to 5 pounds or 0.45 to 2.3 kg)

Exercise speed: Moderate, typically 2 seconds of lifting and 4 seconds of lowering

Exercise range: Full-range movements but avoid the lockout position on the leg press exercise

Exercise frequency: Train 1 or 2 nonconsecutive days per week

Time required: 20 to 30 minutes per session

CYCLISTS

The bicycle is an extremely energy-efficient machine, and cycling is an excellent exercise for enhancing cardiovascular endurance. As in running, power is generated by the leg muscles. Unlike running, cycling produces no landing forces to the feet, legs, and back, which reduces the risk of impact injuries. Nonetheless, like any repetitive movement activity, cycling stresses some muscles more than others, which may lead to overuse injuries.

Let's examine the major muscle involvement in cycling. The power stroke in cycling is produced primarily by contraction of the quadriceps muscles (knee extension) and the hamstring muscles (hip extension). Although the gluteal muscles are also involved in hip extension, the biomechanics of cycling emphasizes the knee extensors (quadriceps).

Lower-leg contributions to cycling include the calf muscles for ankle extension and the anterior tibial (shin) muscles for ankle flexion. Although the calf muscles are involved in every pedal push, the anterior tibial muscles are limited to upward pulling movements against the toe clips or pedals.

The cycle racing position places considerable stress on the upper-body muscles, including the triceps, shoulders, lower back, upper back, chest, forearms, and neck extensors. Properly positioned handlebars more evenly distribute the upper-body muscle involvement, but longer rides may fatigue some muscles more than others. For example, the neck extensor muscles work continuously to hold the head up and are likely to tire before the other upper-body muscles do.

The triceps muscles, front shoulders, and lower back are primarily responsible for maintaining the torso position. The upper-back and chest muscles provide stability for the upper arms, and the forearm muscles enable the hands to maintain a firm grip on the handlebars.

Like all athletes, cyclists should strengthen all their major muscle groups through a comprehensive program of resistance exercise. That is, they should train both the prime mover muscle groups and the antagonist muscle groups to develop balanced muscle strength and ensure joint integrity. Training only the prime mover muscles typically leads to overuse injuries because one side of a joint becomes much stronger than the other, and the weaker structure is eventually overpowered and damaged.

This caution does not imply that opposing muscle groups should be trained to equal strength. For example, the neck extensor muscles are inherently larger and stronger than the neck flexor muscles. But both of these muscle groups should be addressed in a sensible strength training program.

Concerns

Perhaps the greatest concerns for older cyclists (other than accidents) are pain in the posterior muscle groups (lower back, upper back, neck) and injury to the knee joints. We believe that the best approach for preventing these problems is an overall strength training program that features resistance exercises for the lumbar spine, shoulder retraction, and neck extension muscles, as well as for the knee extension and knee flexion muscles. Developing a strong and balanced musculature is definitely an injury deterrent and a performance enhancer. Generally, most older cyclists should limit their training rides to 60 to 90 minutes of continuous cycling.

Cyclists' Strength Training Program

It is usually advisable to work the larger muscle groups of the legs before the smaller muscle groups of the torso, arms, and neck. Within each muscle group, however, it may be preferable to perform rotary exercises before linear exercises. In this manner, single-joint exercises performed with less resistance precede multijoint exercises performed with more resistance. This exercise sequence is sometimes called prefatigue training, because the rotary exercise fatigues a specific muscle and the linear exercise further fatigues the same muscle with assistance from another muscle. For example, the lateral raise exercise fatigues the deltoid muscles, and the succeeding shoulder press exercise further fatigues the deltoid muscles with help from the fresh triceps muscles. Training in this manner is tough, but it is highly effective and time efficient because the successive rotary and linear exercises are performed with minimal rest (10 to 20 seconds).

Training Frequency

During a strength training session, the exerciser fatigues the exercised muscles. The exercise stimulates strength development if the exerciser allows sufficient recovery and building time between workouts. Research shows that two or three properly spaced training sessions per week are effective for improving muscle strength. Cycling clients who are scheduled for two strength workouts per week invest only 1 hour of their time for excellent improvement in muscle strength. Research with older people reveals that they attain approximately 50 percent more muscle strength after 2 months of twice-a-week resistance training.

Number of Sets

Research indicates that one set of properly performed strength training exercises is sufficient for stimulating gains in muscle strength. We therefore suggest that your cycling clients start with one good set of each exercise. Each exercise set should be completed during a period of approximately 60 to 90 seconds. At about 90 seconds per exercise and 30 seconds between stations, our recommended circuit training program should require just over 30 minutes per session.

Training Resistance

Of course, the exercise resistance should be sufficient to fatigue the target muscles within the anaerobic energy system. For most practical purposes, this goal requires using a resistance of about 75 percent of 1RM, because empirical evidence indicates this load level provides a safe and productive training stimulus.

Number of Repetitions

Research demonstrates that most people can complete between 8 and 12 repetitions with about 75 percent of 1RM. Persons with low-endurance muscles (sprinters), however, typically perform fewer than 8 repetitions, and those with high-endurance muscles (marathoners) typically perform more than 12 repetitions. Because cycling is essentially an endurance activity, most cyclists should attain excellent strength gains training with approximately 12 to 16 repetitions per set.

Note that for maximum benefit, each set of strength training exercises must be performed to muscle fatigue. To reach this state, referred to as temporary muscle failure, your clients must continue exercising until their muscles can no longer lift the resistance. For best results, the training intensity should be high and the exercise progression should be consistent.

Exercise Selection

Table 9.3 presents recommended exercises for the major muscle groups in appropriate order of performance.

Cyclists require considerable time and energy to perform their daily training distance. Therefore, cyclists should not spend unnecessary time and energy in the strength training facility. Fortunately, endurance building and strength building are complementary activities. Whereas building endurance requires exercise of lower intensity and long duration, building strength requires exercise of higher intensity and short duration.

Training Progression

We prefer a double progressive system of strength development. Begin with a resistance that your clients can perform 12 times. Have them continue training

TABLE 9.3

Recommended Strength Training Program for Cyclists

Major muscle groups	Machine exercises	Free-weight exercises
Quadriceps	Leg extension	Dumbbell squat
Hamstrings	Leg curl	Dumbbell squat
Quadriceps, hamstrings, and gluteals	Leg press	Barbell squat
Pectoralis major	Chest crossover	Dumbbell chest fly
Pectoralis major and triceps	Chest press	Barbell bench press
Latissimus dorsi	Super pullover	Dumbbell pullover
Latissimus dorsi and biceps	Seated row	Dumbbell one-arm row
Deltoids	Lateral raise	Dumbbell lateral raise
Deltoids and triceps	Shoulder press	Dumbbell bench press
Biceps	Biceps curl	Barbell curl
Triceps	Triceps extension	Dumbbell kickback
Erector spinae	Low-back extension	Trunk extension
Abdominals	Abdominal flexion	Trunk curl
Upper trapezius, levator scapulae, and sternocleidomastoids	Neck extension and flexion	Dumbbell shrug

with this load until they can complete 16 repetitions in two consecutive workouts. When they can complete 16 properly performed repetitions, increase the resistance by about 5 percent. Stay with this resistance until your clients can again complete 16 repetitions and then increase the load again by about 5 percent.

Speed

There is a myth that strength training at fast speeds develops fast muscles, whereas strength training at slow speeds develops slow muscles. This notion is categorically untrue. Muscles respond to sensible strength training by becoming stronger. Speed is developed by practicing an athletic event with emphasis on increased movement velocity and proper technical execution.

From a practical perspective, clients are unlikely to be able to perform strength training exercises involving the legs faster than they can pedal a bicycle, because they would have to perform about 90 repetitions per minute. The recommended approach, therefore, is to train in a controlled manner to maximize strength development and minimize injury risk. Research has demonstrated that excellent strength gains occur from exercising with moderate movement speeds. Because muscles are stronger in negative movements than in positive movements, we recommend lifting the weight in about 2 seconds and lowering the weight in about 4 seconds. This 6-second training protocol requires about 70 to 95 seconds of continuous muscle effort to complete an exercise set of 12 to 16 repetitions.

Range of Motion

Although cycling involves midrange movements of the leg muscles and static contractions of the upper-body muscles, performing full-range strength training exercises is beneficial. For performance purposes, doing part-range movements may be acceptable, but for safety purposes, performing full-range movements is advisable. Weakness in the ends of the movement range may reduce joint integrity and increase injury risk.

Cyclists should perform rotary exercises, such as leg extensions, from the fully stretched position to the fully contracted position. Pressing movements, however, such as leg presses, should end just short of the lockout position. Locking out the knee joint against heavy resistance increases the potential for injury, so exercisers should avoid doing so.

Summary of Strength Training for Cyclists

In our experience with cyclists and triathletes, stronger muscles lead to better cycling performance. Because every pedal revolution requires a certain percentage of maximum leg strength, more strength is of considerable advantage. After strength training, many of our cyclists are able to use higher gears at the same pedal frequency, thereby increasing their road speed.

(continued)

Summary *(continued)*

When developing a sensible strength training program for cyclists we recommend that you carefully consider the following exercise guidelines:

Exercise selection: Include exercises in table 9.3, and make sure that you have at least one exercise for each major muscle group

Exercise sets: One set of each exercise

Exercise resistance: Approximately 60 to 70 percent of 1RM

Exercise repetitions: Between 12 and 16 controlled repetitions

Exercise progression: A resistance increase of 5 percent when 16 repetitions can be completed (typically 1 to 5 pounds or 0.45 to 2.3 kg)

Exercise speed: Moderate, typically 2 seconds of lifting and 4 seconds of lowering

Exercise range: Full-range movements but avoid the lockout position on the leg press exercise

Exercise frequency: 2 or 3 exercise sessions per week

Time required: Approximately 30 minutes

SWIMMERS

Swimming has often been called the perfect physical activity, because it appears to address all of the major muscle groups of the body. Indeed, swimming does involve both the upper body and the lower body through pulling movements of the arms and kicking actions of the legs. Nonetheless, some of the major muscle groups are used much more than others, thereby increasing the risk for overuse and imbalance injuries. For example, the upper-body muscles that pull the arms through the water work considerably harder than the opposing muscles that recover the arms through the air. In addition, the leg muscles, which are continuously active when swimming, move through a relatively short and repetitive range of motion, which can also lead to muscle imbalance problems. Because swimming is largely an aerobic activity, it provides little muscle-strengthening benefit, and because the water-supported body encounters no impact forces (unlike jogging), it does not promote bone development. Let's examine each of these areas more closely by looking at how strength training can enhance your clients' swimming performance and reduce their risk of injury.

Concerns

Although swimmers can experience a variety of overuse injuries, the most common are those involving the shoulder joints. This common problem is at least partly because the relatively large pectoralis major and latissimus dorsi muscles pull the arms through the greater water resistance, whereas the relatively small deltoid muscles recover the arms through the lesser air resistance. Older swimmers must therefore strengthen their deltoid muscles and upper trapezius muscles. Older adults should also schedule swimming sessions of reasonable duration (30 to 60 minutes) to reduce the risk of overtraining injuries.

Muscle Balance

To produce the requisite propulsive actions, most standard swimming strokes emphasize the muscle groups presented in table 9.4

Although strengthening these prime mover muscles is certainly important for improved swimming performance, strengthening the opposing muscles is just as necessary for maintaining muscle balance and joint integrity to reduce injury risk in the shoulder structures. These muscles include the deltoids, biceps, and upper trapezius. Therefore, the exercises in table 9.5 are recommended to develop overall musculoskeletal strength in the upper body.

Although we could add biceps curls and triceps extensions to the exercise protocol, we want to avoid overtraining, and these arm muscles are already addressed in the five basic upper-body exercises. With respect to muscle balance, we also want to train the leg muscles through a full range of joint motion. So let's add these exercises to the training program (see table 9.6).

The eight exercises recommended (leg extension, leg curl, leg press, chest press, lat pull-down, shoulder press, seated row, and incline press) make up a reasonably comprehensive strength training program for swimmers. But if time permits, senior swimmers should also work the midsection muscles that

TABLE 9.4

Major Muscles Involved in Swimming Propulsion

Muscle groups	Propulsive action
Pectoralis major	Pull arm back through water
Latissimus dorsi	Pull arm back through water
Triceps	Extend elbow at end of arm stroke

TABLE 9.5

Recommended Upper-Body Exercises for Swimmers

Muscle groups	Machine exercises	Free-weight exercises
Pectoralis major and triceps	Chest press	Barbell bench press
Latissimus dorsi and biceps	Lat pull-down	Dumbbell pullover
Deltoids, triceps, and upper trapezius	Shoulder press	Dumbbell bench press
Latissimus dorsi, biceps, rear deltoids, rhomboids, and trapezius	Seated row	Dumbbell one-arm row
Pectoralis major, triceps, and front deltoids	Incline press	Dumbbell incline press

TABLE 9.6

Recommended Leg Exercises for Swimmers

Muscle groups	Machine exercises	Free-weight exercises
Quadriceps	Leg extension	Dumbbell step-up
Hamstrings	Leg curl	Dumbbell step-up
Quadriceps, hamstrings, and gluteals	Leg press	Barbell squat

TABLE 9.7

Recommended Midsection and Neck Exercises for Swimmers

Muscle groups	Machine exercises	Free-weight exercises
Internal and external obliques, low back, and abdominal muscles	Rotary torso	Twisting trunk curl
Neck flexors	Neck flexion	Dumbbell shrug
Neck extensors	Neck extension	Dumbbell shrug

connect the upper and lower body, as well as the neck muscles. The midsection and neck muscles are responsible for the torso- and head-positioning movements that accompany every swimming stroke. Consider adding the strength training exercises in table 9.7 for these stroke-sustaining muscle groups.

We now have 11 strength training exercises that address essentially all the major muscle groups. Your older swimming clients should strength train 2 or 3 nonconsecutive days per week. They should begin with the larger muscle groups of the legs, work through the upper-body muscles, and finish with the muscles of the midsection and neck. The suggested strength training program for swimmers should require approximately 20 minutes for completion (one set of 11 exercises with about 1 minute between exercises). Although strength training should not interfere with your clients' swimming practice, workouts should probably be scheduled on nonswimming days if possible. Be sure that clients eat enough calories to fuel their combined physical activities by consuming a little more carbohydrate and protein and lots of water. Finally, encourage senior swimmers to obtain at least 8 hours of sleep nightly so that they enter every exercise session with energy and enthusiasm. This balanced strength training program will enhance their swimming performance and lessen the likelihood of overuse and imbalance injuries.

Movement Range and Speed

Although standard swimming strokes work the upper-body muscles through a fairly full range of motion, the kicking action of the legs uses only midrange movements. To compensate for this potentially harmful limitation, every strength training exercise should be performed through a full movement range. Instruct clients to attain full joint flexion and full joint extension on every repetition but never to move into uncomfortable positions. Strength training through the full movement range is safe and effective only when the exercise repetitions are performed with controlled movement speed. Ballistic and momentum-assisted movements may place excessive stress on joint structures, so exercisers should avoid doing them. Besides being safe, moderate movement speeds provide greater strength-building stimulus. Generally, 6-second repetitions are recommended for prudent and productive strength training—2 seconds for each lifting movement and 4 seconds for each lowering movement. Proper posture requires trainees to sit or stand tall throughout each exercise.

Muscle and Bone Strengthening

As good as swimming is for improving cardiovascular endurance and general fitness, it does not provide sufficient stimulus to build stronger muscles or bones. To strengthen the musculoskeletal system, your clients must progressively stress their muscles with enough resistance to cause fatigue in less than 90 seconds. For that reason, strength training is the perfect complementary activity to swimming. Strength training is a high-intensity and short-duration anaerobic activity, whereas swimming (depending on the distance involved in the event) may be a low-intensity and long-duration aerobic activity. Although landing forces can stimulate bone remodeling, swimming does not offer this option, making strength training exercises especially important for swimmers.

Summary of Strength Training for Swimmers

To ensure sufficient resistance for strength, muscle, and bone development without overstressing body structures, we recommend that you carefully consider the following exercise guidelines:

Exercise selection: Select exercises from table 9.5, 9.6 and 9.7, making sure that there is at least one exercise for each major muscle group

Exercise sets: One set of each exercise

Exercise resistance: Approximately 70 to 80 percent of 1RM

Exercise repetitions: Between 8 and 12 controlled repetitions

Exercise progression: A resistance increase of 5 percent when 12 repetitions can be completed (typically 1 to 5 pounds or 0.45 to 2.3 kg)

Exercise speed: Moderate, typically 2 seconds of lifting and 4 seconds of lowering

Exercise range: Full-range movements but avoid the lockout position on the leg press exercise

Exercise frequency: 2 or 3 exercise sessions per week on non-swimming days

Time required: Approximately 20 minutes

SKIERS

In spite of the fact that chairlifts take people up the mountain, downhill skiing is a physically demanding activity. The body positions that provide the best combination of balance, stability, control, and speed are those that require relatively high levels of muscle strength. Besides enhancing skiing performance, a strong musculoskeletal system is the best protection against acute and overuse injuries that are all too common in this sport.

Although no one would argue the value of cardiovascular conditioning, aerobic fitness is clearly not the limiting factor in downhill skiing. And although lack of joint flexibility may lead to performance limitations, excessive joint mobility is typically more harmful than helpful. The key to better skiing is greater muscle strength, pure and simple. For overall health and fitness, clients should do their favorite endurance activities and stretching exercises. But for confidence and competence on the black diamond trails, they should perform sensible strength training.

Downhill skiing is essentially a power activity that emphasizes the anaerobic energy system. Forceful contractions of the quadriceps and hamstring muscles provide the body positioning that can use the snow and gravity to best advantage. Be thankful for turns, because no one can hold the power position for long without experiencing formidable muscle fatigue. Turns offer both challenge and change of position. The brief unloading phase provides momentary release and relief for the hard-working quadriceps and hamstrings. The turning action also activates the rotational muscles of the midsection and the lateral movement muscles of the thighs. More specifically, smooth turns are closely related to strong external and internal oblique muscles that control midsection rotation, and to strong hip abductor and adductor muscles that shift the hips from side to side.

Although not as important for power production, the muscles of the shoulders, torso, and arms are responsible for effective pole plants and for safely absorbing impact forces in the event of a fall. Other muscles that serve an essential function in terms of postural support and injury prevention are the low-back and neck muscles.

Finally, the anterior tibial muscles of the shin surround and largely control the ankle joint with respect to skiing movements. Although modern ski boots reduce ankle injuries, strong anterior tibial muscles certainly enhance foot action and functional ability for downhill skiing.

Concerns

Regardless of skill, senior skiers must be careful on the slopes and conscientious in the weight room. Weak leg muscles lead to premature fatigue, and fatigue is frequently a forerunner of injury. Weak low-back muscles are at greater risk for injury during skiing and can result in discomfort after skiing. Clients should therefore strengthen these and all other major muscle groups before the ski season. We recommend the following ski conditioning resistance exercises and training protocols.

Skiers' Strength Training Program

Because strength development is more closely related to training intensity than to training duration, excellent results may be attained with a relatively brief time commitment.

Training Frequency

Research reveals that two training sessions per week produce about the same strength development as three training sessions per week. Training 2 days per week may therefore be preferable to ensure plenty of recovery time for muscle remodeling.

Number of Sets

Many studies show similar strength-building benefits for single-set and multiple-set training. The number of sets that your clients perform is largely a matter of personal preference and time availability. Our ski conditioning program participants have experienced excellent results by doing a warm-up set with a training load of 50 percent of 1RM, resting for 60 seconds, and then performing one set to momentary muscle fatigue with their training load. You may want to experiment with this effective yet time-efficient training protocol.

Training Resistance and Number of Repetitions

Muscle strength is best developed by fatiguing the target muscle within the anaerobic energy system, which for most practical purposes is between 30 and 90 seconds. At a controlled movement speed of 6 seconds per repetition, a set of 8 to 12 repetitions should fatigue the exerciser in the middle of the anaerobic energy system (50 to 70 seconds). Most people can perform 8 to 12 repetitions with about 70-80 percent of 1RM, which is a safe and productive exercise workload. Although you may periodically want to train your client with more or fewer repetitions, 8 to 12 repetitions per set is our recommended repetition range.

Exercise Selection

Based on our downhill skiing needs analyses, the following machine and free-weight exercises are recommended. To ensure muscle balance and lessen injury potential, training opposing muscle groups is advisable. For example, skiers should work both the anterior tibial muscles and the calf muscles for balanced muscle development in the lower leg. Generally, it is best to begin with exercises for the larger muscle groups of the legs and proceed to the smaller muscle groups of the torso, arms, midsection, and neck. Table 9.8 presents a comprehensive selection of strength exercises for skiers.

Although this program represents a comprehensive selection of strength training exercises, some skiers may not have time to do this workout before and particularly during the ski season. In this case, we recommend the "big six" ski strengthening exercises that address most of the major muscle groups in a short training season (see table 9.9).

TABLE 9.8

Recommended Strengthening Exercises for Skiers (Comprehensive Program)

Muscle group	Ski function	Machine exercise	Free-weight exercise
Quadriceps	Power position	Leg extension	Barbell squat
Hamstrings	Power position	Leg curl	Barbell squat
Hip adductors	Turns	Hip adduction	Dumbbell step-up
Hip abductors	Turns	Hip abduction	Dumbbell step-up
Pectoralis major	Pole action	Chest crossover	Dumbbell bench press
Latissimus dorsi	Pole action	Pullover	Dumbbell one-arm row
Deltoids	Pole action	Lateral raise	Dumbbell bench press
Biceps	Pole action	Biceps curl	Dumbbell standing curl
Triceps	Pole action	Triceps extension	Dumbbell kickback
Spinal erectors	Posture support	Low-back extension	Trunk extension
Rectus abdominis	Posture support	Abdominal flexion	Trunk curl
Internal and external obliques	Turns and posture support	Rotary torso	Twisting trunk curl
Neck flexors and neck extensors	Posture support	Neck extension and flexion	Dumbbell shrug
Anterior tibials	Ankle function		Weight plate toe raise
Calves	Ankle function	Heel raise	Dumbbell heel raise

TABLE 9.9

"Big Six" Ski Strengthening Exercises

Major muscle groups	Machine exercises	Free-weight exercises
Quadriceps, hamstrings, gluteals, and calves	Leg press	Dumbbell squat
Hip adductors	Hip adduction	Dumbbell step-up
Hip abductors	Hip abduction	Dumbbell step-up
Pectoralis major, deltoids, and triceps	Chest press	Dumbbell bench press
Latissimus dorsi, biceps, rear deltoids, rhomboids, and trapezius	Seated row	Dumbbell one-arm row
Internal and external obliques, low back, and abdominal	Rotary torso	Twisting trunk curl

Training Progression

If your clients use the recommended 8 to 12 repetitions per set, then they need a sensible progression policy. Because muscle strength develops gradually, they should not increase the resistance more than 5 percent between successive training sessions. Older exercisers should stay with a given load until they can complete 12 repetitions in good form.

They should then add 5 percent more resistance (usually 1 to 5 pounds, or 0.45 to 2.3 kg) to their next workout. This double progressive system, first adding more repetitions and then adding more resistance, is a safe method for stimulating consistent strength gains.

Exercise Technique

Strength training should occur in a safe, effective, and efficient manner. In terms of training technique, this means using full movement range and moderate movement speed on every repetition.

- *Full movement range*. Strength is best developed in the movement range that is exercised against the resistance. To develop strength throughout the entire joint action, training through the full movement range is necessary. That is, the target muscle should be worked from the fully stretched position to the fully contracted position.

- *Moderate movement speed*. Slower strength training movements are more productive than explosive strength training movements. Slower movement speeds produce more muscle force and more muscle tension than faster movement speeds do. Slower movement speeds also place less emphasis on momentum and more emphasis on the target muscles. Because downhill skiing involves mostly eccentric muscle contractions, it may be advisable to emphasize the negative (lowering) phase of each repetition. Our recommendation is 6-second repetitions using approximately 2 seconds for each lifting movement and 4 seconds for each lowering movement.

- *Breathing*. Your clients must breathe on every repetition, because breath holding can lead to undesirable increases in blood pressure as well as restricted blood flow. The recommended breathing pattern is to exhale during each lifting movement and to inhale throughout each lowering movement.

Summary of Strength Training for Skiers

When developing a sensible strength training program for skiers we recommend that you carefully consider the following exercise guidelines:

Exercise selection: Include exercises in table 9.8, or consider the "Big Six" program in table 9.9, making sure to include at least one exercise for each major muscle group

Exercise sets: One set of each exercise

(continued)

Summary *(continued)*

Exercise resistance: Approximately 70 to 80 percent of 1RM

Exercise repetitions: Between 8 and 12 controlled repetitions

Exercise progression: A resistance increase of 5 percent when 12 repetitions can be completed (typically 1 to 5 pounds or 0.45 to 2.3 kg)

Exercise speed: Moderate, typically 2 seconds of lifting and 4 seconds of lowering

Exercise range: Full-range movements but avoid the lockout position on the leg press exercise

Exercise frequency: Train 2 or 3 nonconsecutive days per week and 1 to 2 days during the season

Time required: 30 minutes per session; 12 minutes for the Big Six

TENNIS PLAYERS

Tennis is a superb sport. It requires excellent eye–hand coordination, good agility, and keen spatial awareness. Besides the physical and mental challenge, a good singles match provides both anaerobic and aerobic conditioning. Although skill is essential for top-level tennis, technique development is easier for players who are fit—which is also the critical factor for staying power during the second and third sets.

Fitness comes in many forms, and conditioning is specific to the training program. For example, joint flexibility is enhanced through stretching exercises, cardiovascular endurance is improved through aerobic activity, and muscular strength is increased through resistance training. Certainly, all these fitness components may contribute to better tennis performance. If you were to focus on one area of physical conditioning for senior tennis players, however, it should undoubtedly be strength training.

Concerns

Singles tennis is one of the sports that can be played at relatively high levels of skill and performance well into the senior years, and doubles tennis can be played competitively even longer. The major areas of concern for older tennis players are the stop-and-go, forward-and-backward, and side-to-side movements, which place considerable stress on the legs, as well as the shoulder, elbow, and wrist joints of the racket arm, which are subject to overuse injuries. Proper strength training can reduce the risk of these typical tennis injuries and enhance performance power in the process.

Basic Strength Training Exercises

Tennis play involves a lot of musculoskeletal activity, including all kinds of movements in the legs, midsection, upper body, and arms. Tennis players should

TABLE 9.10

Recommended Basic Exercises for Tennis Players

Target muscles	Machine exercises	Free-weight exercises
Quadriceps	Leg extension	Dumbbell step-up
Hamstrings	Leg curl	Dumbbell squat
Pectoralis major	Chest crossover	Dumbbell chest fly
Latissimus dorsi	Pullover	Dumbbell pullover
Deltoids	Lateral raise	Dumbbell lateral raise
Biceps	Biceps curl	Dumbbell standing curl
Triceps	Triceps extension	Dumbbell kickback
Spinal erectors	Low-back extension	Trunk extension
Rectus abdominis	Abdominal flexion	Trunk curl
Neck flexors and extensors	Neck extension and flexion	Dumbbell shrug

therefore train all their major muscle groups. This approach ensures overall strength and balanced muscle development to enhance performance power and reduce the risk of injuries. The machine and free-weight exercises presented in table 9.10 provide a solid base of conditioning from which to progress into more advanced training when clients are ready to do so.

The exercises are presented from the larger muscles of the legs to the smaller muscles of the neck, which is the recommended order of performance. One set of each exercise is sufficient, as long as clients train with good form to the point of muscle fatigue. Because intensity is the key to strength development, they should use enough resistance to fatigue the target muscle groups within about 50 to 70 seconds. In general, this level of resistance corresponds to the heaviest weight load that they can lift for 8 to 12 controlled repetitions.

Each repetition should be completed in approximately 6 seconds—2 seconds for the lifting movement and 4 seconds for the lowering movement. The slower lowering phase emphasizes the stronger negative muscle contraction, which should make each exercise set more productive. Clients should perform each repetition through a full range of movement to enhance both joint integrity and joint flexibility.

As muscles become stronger, progressively increasing the work effort is essential. This objective is best accomplished by gradually increasing the exercise resistance. When your clients can complete 12 repetitions in two consecutive workouts, the weight load is no longer heavy enough to produce maximum strength benefits. By increasing the resistance by about 5 percent (typically 1 to 5 pounds, or 0.45 to 2.3 kg), they can continue to stimulate strength development.

Depending on a tennis player's activity schedule, strength training should be performed 1 or 2 days per week. Research shows that two sessions per week are more effective than one session, but one weekly workout should be sufficient during the competitive season as long as the recommended strength training guidelines are followed.

Advanced Strength Training Exercises

After 2 months of basic training, your client may be ready for advanced strength training exercises. Some of these will replace the introductory exercises, and others will provide supplementary training relevant to tennis performance.

Leg Muscles

Let's begin with the powerful leg muscles that generate the force for hard-hitting ground strokes as well as fast movements across the court. Instead of training the quadriceps and hamstrings separately, replace the leg extension and leg curl with the leg press that works both of these muscle groups and the gluteals concurrently. The leg press permits heavier loads and is the best exercise for developing functional leg strength. Like the quadriceps and hamstrings, the hip adductors and abductors play a major role in weight shifts and lateral movements. These opposing muscle groups on the inner and outer thighs are best trained with the hip adductor and hip abductor machines, which should be added to your clients' strength training program.

Because of the stop-and-go movements that require almost continuous force production and shock absorption in the lower-leg muscles, performing some calf strengthening exercises is prudent. Calf presses or standing calf raises are highly effective for targeting the gastrocnemius and soleus muscles of the lower leg, and they serve as an excellent supplement to the upper-leg exercises.

Midsection Muscles

The power generated by the large leg muscles is transferred to the upper body through the muscles of the midsection. Swinging movements (ground strokes and serves) involve the internal and external oblique muscles on both sides of the midsection. These important muscles may be effectively strengthened on the dual-action rotary torso machine, which works the right internal and left external obliques on clockwise movements and the left internal and right external obliques on counterclockwise movements. Add the rotary torso exercise to the low-back and abdominal machine exercises for comprehensive midsection conditioning.

Upper-Body Muscles

The major upper-body muscles involved in swinging a tennis racket are the pectoralis major, latissimus dorsi, and deltoids of the torso and the biceps and triceps of the arms. Although the basic strength training program addresses these muscles individually, it may be advantageous to work some of the groups together. This goal is best accomplished by doing pushing and pulling exercises such as bench presses, seated rows, overhead presses, and pull-downs.

The chest press and bench press are popular pushing exercises that strengthen the pectoralis major and triceps muscles at the same time. Conversely, the seated row and bent row are effective pulling exercises that work the opposing latissimus dorsi and biceps muscles simultaneously.

One of the best means of training the shoulder and triceps muscles together is the overhead press. The counterpart to this exercise is the pull-down, which involves both the latissimus dorsi and the biceps muscles.

TABLE 9.11

Recommended Advanced Exercises for Tennis Players

Target muscles	Machine exercises	Free-weight exercises
Quadriceps, hamstrings, and gluteals	Leg press	Barbell squat
Hip adductors	Hip adduction	Dumbbell step-up
Hip abductors	Hip abduction	Dumbbell step-up
Gastrocnemius and soleus	Heel raise	Barbell heel raise
Pectoralis major and triceps	Chest press	Barbell bench press
Latissimus dorsi, biceps, rear deltoids, rhomboids, and trapezius	Seated row	Dumbbell one-arm row
Deltoids and triceps	Shoulder press	Dumbbell bench press
Latissimus dorsi and biceps	Lat pull-down	Pulley pull-down
Spinal erectors	Low-back extension	Trunk extension
Rectus abdominis	Abdominal flexion	Trunk curl
External and internal obliques	Rotary torso	Twisting trunk curl
Neck flexors and extensors	Neck extension and flexion	Dumbbell shrug

Table 9.11 presents an advanced tennis strength training program. These exercises should be performed in the same manner as the basic program exercises, namely, one set of 8 to 12 well-controlled repetitions.

Arm Muscles

Although both the basic and advanced strength training programs should provide excellent tennis conditioning and reasonable injury protection, one more step should be taken to address particularly vulnerable muscle groups that undergo significant stress during tennis play.

The first of these smaller and frequently injured muscle groups is the rotator cuff complex that surrounds and stabilizes the shoulder joint.

The shoulder rotator muscles, which lie beneath the large deltoid muscles, enable us to turn the arm in various positions. Rotating the arm backward, called external rotation, uses the teres minor and infraspinatus muscles. Rotating the arm forward, called internal rotation, involves the subscapularis muscles. Keeping the arm within the shoulder joint structure is the primary function of the supraspinatus muscle. Together, these four muscle groups surround the shoulder joint, providing both structural stability and the ability to produce forehand, backhand, and serving movements.

The good news is that these four relatively small muscle groups respond well to proper strength training. The bad news is that most people do not perform any specific exercises for their rotator cuff. This circumstance is unfortunate because rotator cuff injuries occur frequently in tennis players and typically require a long recovery period.

Although the standard strength exercises offer some rotator cuff conditioning benefit, your clients should definitely do at least one workout per week specifically for the shoulder rotator muscles.

The best means for specifically training the rotator cuff muscles is the rotary shoulder machine, a dual-action exercise that provides full-range rotational resistance for both the external and internal shoulder rotator muscles.

If this machine is not available, clients can strengthen these important muscles with resistance bands. After attaching the band to a door at waist level, have your client stand with the right side toward the door, keep the right elbow against the right side, and pull the band across the midsection using the right hand. This exercise works the right internal shoulder rotator muscles. Next, have your client keep the left elbow against the left side and pull the band away from the midsection using the left hand to work the left external shoulder rotator muscles. Have your client repeat these two exercises standing with the right side toward the door and using the opposite hands. See figure 9.1. Rotator cuff exercises can also be performed using a dumbbell as shown in figure 9.2. After completing the external and internal rotator cuff exercises on the right side, have your client repeat these two exercises with a dumbbell in the left hand.

Because of the extensive wrist action required in tennis play, the forearm muscles can easily be overstressed, leading to injuries at the elbow or wrist joints. The forearm machine provides five separate wrist movements to condition all the forearm muscles. Few exercises are better suited to tennis players, especially for increasing grip strength and reducing injury potential.

If this training device is not available, an excellent alternative exercise is the wrist roller. Simply attach a 5-pound (2.3 kg) weight plate to a 2-foot (60 cm) rope and tie the other end to a round wooden dowel. Have your client hold the dowel in both hands and alternately turn the wrists clockwise to wind the rope around the dowel and lift the weight. This action addresses the forearm flexor muscles. When the weight touches the dowel, have your client alternately turn the wrists counterclockwise to unwind the rope and lower the weight. This action works the forearm extensor muscles. See figure 9.3.

If your clients play tennis 3 or 4 days per week, then doing strength training on 2 nontennis days is probably best. That schedule permits plenty of recovery time after each activity. If they practice tennis every day, strength training should probably be performed about 4 hours after tennis training for best overall results. For example, if they play tennis every morning from 9 to 11, you may schedule their strength training program around 3 p.m. For most purposes, 1 or 2 equally spaced strength training days are recommended.

Remember that skill training is the most important factor for improving a player's tennis game. Physical conditioning, however, can enhance tennis-playing efforts and outcomes. The cornerstone of physical conditioning is muscular strength, and a stronger tennis player should always be a better tennis player.

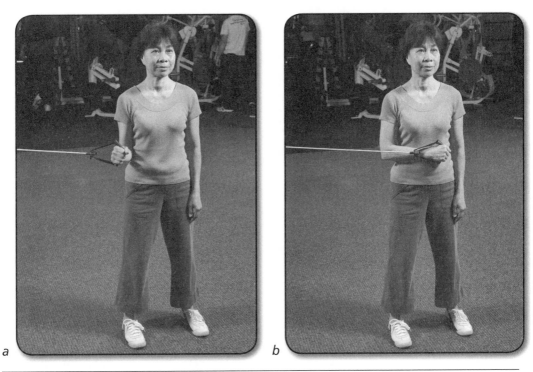

Figure 9.1 Elastic resistance band internal rotator cuff exercise *(a)* start and *(b)* finish positions.

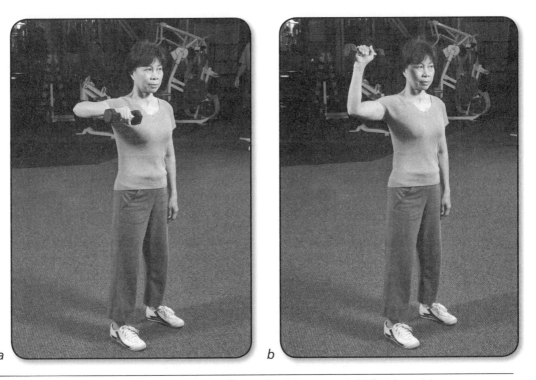

Figure 9.2 Dumbbell external rotator cuff exercise *(a)* start and *(b)* finish positions.

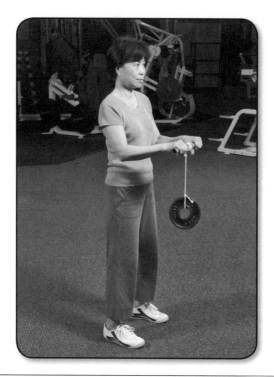

Figure 9.3 Wrist roller.

Summary of Strength Training for Tennis Players

When developing a sensible strength training program for tennis players we recommend that you carefully consider the following exercise guidelines:

Exercise selection: Select from the basic exercises in table 9.10 and/or the advanced exercises in table 9.11, making sure that you include at least one exercise for each major muscle group

Exercise sets: One set of each exercise

Exercise resistance: Approximately 70 to 80 percent of 1RM

Exercise repetitions: Between 8 and 12 controlled repetitions

Exercise progression: A resistance increase of 5 percent when 12 repetitions can be completed (typically 1 to 5 pounds or 0.45 to 2.3 kg)

Exercise speed: Moderate, typically 2 seconds of lifting and 4 seconds of lowering

Exercise range: Full-range movements but avoid the lockout position on the leg press exercise

Exercise frequency: Train 2 times a week on nonconsecutive days and on the days that the client does not play tennis, or twice a week on the same day, but at least 4 hours afterward

Time required: Approximately 25 minutes

GOLFERS

More than 50 million Americans enjoy playing the great game of golf. If your clients are like most golfers, they want to play more golf, at a higher level, without sustaining injuries. They want to play stronger and drive longer, both of which they can accomplish through a well-designed senior golfer strength training program.

Our recommended approach to golf conditioning involves two brief exercise sessions per week, leaving plenty of time for your clients to practice and play their favorite sport. Each workout includes strength training, stretching exercise, and optional aerobic activity. Golfers have traditionally avoided strength training for fear of adding bodyweight, developing large muscles, feeling tight, losing speed, compromising coordination, experiencing errant drives, and posting higher scores. But our research has shown that golfers who perform regular strength training achieve significant benefits (Westcott, Dolan, and Cavicchi 1996). As you can see in table 9.12, the 77 adult golfers who completed just 2 months of our strength training program made impressive improvements in their health, fitness, and driving power. Consider that they reduced their mean resting blood pressures by almost 5 mmHg, increased their muscle strength by more than 50 percent, added 4 pounds (1.8 kg) of muscle, lost 4 pounds of fat, and increased their club head speed (driving power) by 6 percent.

KEY POINTS FROM THIS STUDY INCLUDE THE FOLLOWING:

• *Flexibility exercise.* Our golf conditioning participants attained greater increases in club head speed when they combined stretching exercise with the strength training program. They performed six basic stretches for the major muscle groups, including the thighs, hips, lower back, upper back, chest, and shoulders. Each flexibility exercise was performed slowly, with a 20-second stationary hold in the fully stretched position.

• *Endurance exercise.* Although we did not include cardiovascular conditioning in our golf research studies, we recommend regular aerobic activity in conjunction with the golf power training program. On an effort scale of 1 to 10, the warm-up and cool-down segments should be performed at low intensity (levels 3 to 4) and the conditioning segment should be performed at moderate intensity

TABLE 9.12

Results of 77 Men and Women Who Completed 8 Weeks of the Golf Strength Training Program

Mean resting blood pressure	Decreased	–4.5 mmHg
Muscle strength	Increased	+56.0%
Bodyweight	Decreased	–0.2 lb (–0.1 kg)
Percent fat	Decreased	–2.0%
Muscle weight	Increased	+3.9 lb (+1.8 kg)
Fat weight	Decreased	–4.1 lb (–1.9 kg)
Club head speed	Increased	+6.1%

Performance Power

In simplest terms, performance power is muscle force multiplied by movement distance divided by movement time. That is, driving power can be improved by increasing muscle force, increasing swing distance, or decreasing swing time. Strength training is the best means for increasing muscle force, and stretching exercise is the best means for increasing swing distance. Decreasing swing time is a more complex task that involves practice and coordination, but it is certainly facilitated by stronger muscles and more flexible joints.

Performance power =
muscle force × movement distance ÷ movement time

(levels 6 to 8). Have your clients choose their favorite endurance exercise (e.g., walking, jogging, cycling, stepping) or combine activities for a cross-training effect. Although improved cardiovascular fitness has little direct effect on golf driving power, it may enable clients to play stronger and longer by increasing their resistance to fatigue. Therefore, if time is available, we advise 20 to 30 minutes of aerobic activity on 3 nonconsecutive days per week.

Concerns

Older golfers often experience injuries to their backs, shoulders, elbows, and wrists, as well as their hips. Although some of these injuries may be attributed to overuse, the more probable cause is the powerful ballistic swinging action involved in golf drives. Senior golfers must therefore do sufficient strength training to condition the muscles and joint structures that both produce and receive these high force levels.

Golfers' Strength Training Program

Our senior golfers have experienced excellent results with a progressive program of 12 basic strength training exercises. All the strength training exercises are performed for one set of 8 to 12 repetitions using moderate movement speed (2 seconds of lifting and 4 seconds of lowering), full movement range, and gradual progression (a load increase of 1 to 5 pounds, or 0.45 to 2.3 kg, on completing 12 repetitions). Two strength training sessions per week are preferable, but if your clients have time limitations, one weekly workout is sufficient.

The following sections present our recommended exercises, training principles, and workout progressions for improving overall muscle strength. Let's begin with the muscles of the trunk, which are important for two reasons. First, many golfers experience low-back problems that are largely due to weak trunk muscles, particularly the erector spinae muscles in the low-back area. Second, the trunk muscles (abdominal muscles and obliques) play the key role in transferring the power produced by the large hip and thigh muscles to the club-swinging muscles of the upper body and arms. As shown in table 9.13, these muscles may be conditioned with machine (low-back, abdominal, rotary torso) or bodyweight exercises (trunk extension, trunk curl, twisting trunk curl).

The second group of muscles that golfers should strengthen are the power-producing groups of the thighs and hips. The front thigh muscles (quadriceps)

TABLE 9.13

Recommended Strength Training Exercises for Golfers: Muscles of the Trunk

Muscle groups	Machine exercises	Bodyweight exercises
Low back	Low-back extension	Trunk extension
Abdominal muscles	Abdominal flexion	Trunk curl
External and internal obliques	Rotary torso	Twisting trunk curl

and rear thigh muscles (hamstrings) are major force generators, especially in conjunction with the gluteus maximus muscles of the hips. The leg press and squat exercises are ideal for strengthening these large muscle groups. Because weight transfer and hip thrust are critical components of powerful golf drives, we also recommend specific strength training exercises for the inner-thigh muscles (hip adductors) and outer-thigh muscles (hip abductors). The recommended exercises for the power production muscles of the legs are presented in table 9.14.

The third group of muscles that should be addressed for improved golf driving power are those of the torso. These include the chest muscles (pectoralis major), upper-back muscles (latissimus dorsi), and shoulder muscles (deltoids). These muscles not only produce the swinging action of the arms but also control the shoulder joint movements. The pectoralis major, latissimus dorsi, and deltoid muscles must therefore be strengthened in a balanced manner. Our recommended training exercises for the torso muscles (machine chest press, pull-down, lateral raise or dumbbell bench press, one-arm row or lateral raise) are presented in table 9.15.

TABLE 9.14

Recommended Strength Training Exercises for Golfers: Muscles of the Thighs and Hips

Muscle groups	Machine exercises	Free-weight exercises
Quadriceps, hamstrings, and gluteals	Leg press	Dumbbell squat
Hip adductors	Hip adduction	Dumbbell step-up
Hip abductors	Hip abduction	Dumbbell step-up

TABLE 9.15

Recommended Strength Training Exercises for Golfers: Muscles of the Torso

Muscle groups	Machine exercises	Free-weight exercises
Pectoralis major and triceps	Chest press	Dumbbell bench press
Latissimus dorsi and biceps	Lat pull-down	Dumbbell one-arm row
Deltoids	Lateral raise	Dumbbell lateral raise

Finally, if time permits, we suggest that senior golfers perform specific strength training exercises for the muscles of the arms and neck. The muscles of the front arm (biceps) and rear arm (triceps) are involved in club control, which is a key component of consistent swinging actions. Although the triceps are worked in chest presses and bench presses, we recommend an additional exercise that better isolates this muscle group. Likewise, although the biceps are worked in pull-downs and bent rows, we advise performing a more exclusive biceps exercise. These arm exercises (triceps machine and biceps machine or dumbbell triceps extension and dumbbell curl) are presented in table 9.16.

Head stability is an essential condition for successfully performing sports skills that require hand–eye coordination. We therefore consider neck strengthening exercises to be an important part of our golf conditioning program. Our recommended resistance exercises for the neck muscles (neck machine or dumbbell shrug) are presented in table 9.16.

We suggest that older golfers perform all the exercises during each workout, in the order presented in table 9.17. Clients should use a moderate movement speed, taking about 2 seconds to lift the resistance and about 4 seconds to lower

TABLE 9.16

Recommended Strength Training Exercises for Golfers: Muscles of the Arms and Neck

Muscle groups	Machine exercises	Free-weight exercises
Triceps	Triceps extension	Dumbbell lying triceps extension
Biceps	Biceps curl	Dumbbell standing curl
Neck flexors and extensors	Neck extension and flexion	Dumbbell shrug

TABLE 9.17

Recommended Order of Golf Conditioning Exercises

Machine exercises	Free-weight exercises
Leg press	Dumbbell squat
Hip adduction	Dumbbell step-up
Hip abduction	Dumbbell step-up
Chest press	Dumbbell bench press
Lat pull-down	Dumbbell one-arm row
Lateral raise	Dumbbell lateral raise
Triceps extension	Dumbbell lying triceps extension
Biceps curl	Dumbbell standing curl
Low-back extension	Trunk extension
Abdominal flexion	Trunk curl
Rotary torso	Twisting trunk curl
Neck extension and flexion	Dumbbell shrug

the resistance. They should perform each repetition through a full range of joint movement as long as they can do so without discomfort.

Senior golfers should train with an exercise resistance that enables them to complete between 8 and 12 repetitions to the point of momentary muscle fatigue. When they can do 12 repetitions with correct technique in two consecutive workouts, increase the load by approximately 5 percent (typically 1 to 5 pounds, or 0.45 to 2.3 kg). Although one good weekly workout is sufficient, clients will improve muscular fitness and increase driving power at a faster rate by training on 2 nonconsecutive days each week. Keep accurate records of your clients' workouts and watch how their driving power correlates with their strength gains.

Summary of Strength Training for Golfers

When developing a sensible strength training program for golfers we recommend that you carefully consider the following exercise guidelines:

Exercise selection: Select from the trunk, thigh, hip, torso, arms and neck exercises in tables 9.13 to 9.16, making sure that there is at least one exercise for each major muscle group

Exercise sets: One set of each exercise

Exercise resistance: Approximately 70 to 80 percent of 1RM

Exercise repetitions: Between 8 and 12 controlled repetitions

Exercise progression: A resistance increase of 5 percent when 12 repetitions can be completed (typically 1 to 5 pounds or 0.45 to 2.3 kg)

Exercise speed: Moderate, typically 2 seconds of lifting and 4 seconds of lowering

Exercise range: Full-range movements but avoid the lockout position on the leg press exercise

Exercise frequency: Train 2 times a week on nonconsecutive days

Time required: Approximately 25 minutes

ROCK CLIMBERS AND HIKERS

Rock climbing and hiking are becoming popular recreational activities among older adults. These challenging activities require relatively high levels of muscular conditioning.

A few years ago we conducted some studies on the physiological benefits of rock climbing, using a mechanical rock climbing apparatus that allowed us to collect data on each exercise session (Westcott 1992). We trained 30 men and women for 20 minutes a day, 2 days per week, for a period of 8 weeks on a Treadwall revolving rock climbing machine. Even this rather limited amount of simulated rock climbing produced significant improvements in body composition, muscle strength, joint flexibility, and cardiovascular endurance. To say the least, we were highly impressed with the physical adaptations associated with regular rock climbing activity.

Of course, there is another side to the rock climbing coin. Because of the intense nature of this muscle-challenging activity, prior physical conditioning is highly recommended, especially a well-rounded program of strength training exercises.

Concerns

Rock climbing uses most of the major muscle groups, but, as with almost all physical activities, some muscles are more involved than others. Holding onto rocks places a lot of stress on the muscles of the arms and forearms, increasing the likelihood of elbow and wrist injuries. Rock climbing also requires sustained tension in the hip, thigh, and calf muscles, as well as a considerable degree of core stability.

Rock Climbers and Hikers' Strength Training Program

Because rock climbing involves almost all the major muscles, we suggest a comprehensive program of strength training. A well-designed strength training program should address the muscles of the legs, torso, midsection, arms, neck, and forearms. Although the forearms are not normally considered a major muscle group, gripping ability is particularly important for successful rock climbing experiences. Table 9.18 presents our recommended single-joint exercises that effectively isolate the target muscles relevant to rock climbing. These are the leg extension, leg curl, hip adduction, hip abduction, chest cross, pullover, lateral raise, biceps curl, triceps extension, low-back extension, abdominal curl, neck extension, neck flexion, forearm extension, and forearm flexion, typically performed on weight-stack machines.

An alternative training approach is presented in table 9.19. This equally productive program uses multiple-joint exercises that work several muscle groups at the same time. The machine exercises are the leg press, chest press, seated row, incline press, pull-down, shoulder press, assisted chin-up, assisted bar dip, rotary torso, forearm extension, and forearm flexion. The free-weight exercises are the squat, bench press, bent row, incline press, pull-down, overhead press, chin-up, bar dip, twisting trunk curl, and wrist roller.

Training Frequency

The general recommendation for strength training frequency is three workouts per week, and recent research reveals that this approach produces excellent results in new exercisers. But these same studies have shown essentially as much muscular development from two training sessions per week. Your clients should attain similar strength gains by training either 2 or 3 days per week. Just be sure that they allow at least 48 hours between successive exercise sessions, because muscle development occurs during the recovery and building periods between workouts.

TABLE 9.18

Recommended Single-Joint Strength Exercises
That Target Muscles Used in Rock Climbing and Hiking

Exercises	Muscle groups
Leg extension	Quadriceps
Leg curl	Hamstrings
Hip adduction	Hip adductors
Hip abduction	Hip abductors
Chest crossover	Pectoralis major
Pullover	Latissimus dorsi
Lateral raise	Deltoids
Biceps curl	Biceps
Triceps extension	Triceps
Low-back extension	Erector spinae
Abdominal flexion	Rectus abdominis
Neck extension	Neck extensors
Neck flexion	Neck flexors
Forearm extension	Forearm extensors
Forearm flexion	Forearm flexors

TABLE 9.19

Recommended Multiple-Joint Strength Exercises
That Work The Muscles Used in Rock Climbing and Hiking

Machine exercises	Free-weight exercises	Muscle groups
Leg press	Squat	Quadriceps, hamstrings, and gluteals
Chest press	Bench press	Pectoralis major, anterior deltoids, and triceps
Seated row	Dumbbell one-arm row	Latissimus dorsi, posterior deltoids, and biceps
Incline press	Incline press	Anterior deltoids, pectoralis major, and triceps
Lat pull-down	Pull-down	Latissimus dorsi, posterior deltoids, and biceps
Shoulder press	Overhead press	Deltoids, triceps, and upper trapezius
Weight-assisted pull-up	Pull-up	Latissimus dorsi, posterior deltoids, and biceps
Weight-assisted bar dip	Bar dip	Pectoralis major, anterior deltoids, and triceps
Rotary torso	Twisting trunk curl	External and internal obliques
Forearm extension	Wrist roller	Forearm extensors
Forearm flexion	Wrist roller	Forearm flexors

Number of Sets

Research has clearly demonstrated that single-set strength training is highly productive for stimulating muscle development. Although exercisers may certainly complete more sets if they so desire, excellent results can be attained by performing one good set of each exercise. If a person does one set of the 15 exercises presented in table 9.18, the entire strength training session should take approximately 30 minutes, assuming about 1 minute per set and about 1 minute between exercises.

Training Resistance and Repetitions

We recommend training with a resistance that permits at least 8 but not more than 12 repetitions per exercise set. If your client cannot perform 8 repetitions the resistance should be reduced, and if the client can perform 13 or more repetitions the resistance should be increased by approximately 5 percent. Most older adults can perform 8 repetitions with about 80 percent of maximum resistance and 12 repetitions with about 70 percent of maximum resistance, which represents a highly effective training range for muscle strength development.

Number of Repetitions

Obviously, muscle endurance plays a major role in rock climbing excursions, so it may be tempting to advocate a strength training program that emphasizes high repetitions with low resistance. Although this approach is certainly acceptable, our studies have revealed excellent improvements in both muscle strength and endurance from the standard training program of 8 to 12 repetitions per set. In fact, we have found no significant differences in strength development when using a low (5 to 10) or high (15 to 20) number of repetitions per set, indicating that a variety of repetition protocols are effective when training is continued to the point of muscle fatigue (Faigenbaum et al. 2005). To increase both muscle strength and endurance in an efficient manner, we recommend the standard protocol of 8 to 12 repetitions.

Exercise Selection

If your client trains on machines, you may consider the following single-joint exercises that tend to isolate specific muscle groups. As presented in table 9.18, these include the leg extension, leg curl, hip adduction, hip abduction, chest cross, pullover, lateral raise, biceps curl, triceps extension, low-back extension, abdominal curl, neck extension, neck flexion, forearm extension, and forearm flexion. If you prefer to train your client with multijoint exercises on either machines or free weights, we recommend machine leg presses, chest presses and seated rows or dumbbell squats, bench presses, and bent rows (see table 9.19), along with standard bodyweight midsection exercises (trunk extensions and twisting trunk curls).

Training Progression

Our recommended training progression is to increase the exercise resistance by approximately 5 percent when clients can complete 12 repetitions in proper form in two consecutive workouts. This approach represents a double progressive training protocol, first adding exercise repetitions and then adding exercise resistance.

Exercise Speed

Because of the tensive nature of rock climbing, we recommend moderate-speed lifting and lowering movements, which work the muscles more effectively. Rather than using fast, momentum-assisted repetitions, the exerciser should maintain constant tension on the target muscle groups with controlled training speeds. Although the standard 6-second speed (2 seconds lifting and 4 seconds lowering) should be sufficient, older rock climbers may experience greater benefits by performing even slower repetitions.

Exercise Range

Contrary to popular understanding, properly performed strength training exercises enhance joint flexibility. Improved joint flexibility, however, is clearly related to full-range exercise movements. In other words, your clients should make every effort to train the target muscles through as full a movement range as possible on every repetition.

Hiking Application

Although strength training is clearly advantageous for rock climbing activity, its benefits for hiking performance are less obvious. Generally, hikers should have a strong and balanced muscular system for all kinds of ambulatory actions up and down trails and mountainsides. The basic strength training program is therefore similar to that for rock climbing, and it should include exercises for the quadriceps, hamstrings, hip adductors, hip abductors, pectoralis major, latissimus dorsi, deltoids, biceps, triceps, low back, abdominals muscles, and neck muscles. With this in mind, both the single-joint strength training program presented in table 9.18 and the multiple-joint program presented in table 9.19 are appropriate for hikers, although the forearm exercises are less relevant to this activity.

Body Weight

Of course, rock climbers do not desire any extra body weight that they must pull up the side of a cliff. Strength training will add a few pounds of muscle, which is analogous to going from a six-cylinder engine to an eight-cylinder engine. Besides increasing muscle power, strength training typically leads to an equivalent (or greater) loss of fat weight. Research with hundreds of participants has shown that 10 weeks of strength training adds 3 pounds (1.4 kg) of muscle and takes away 4 pounds (1.8 kg) of fat (Westcott 2009). In other words, strength training can improve your clients' body composition (more muscle and less fat) without increasing their body weight, which definitely improves athletic ability and climbing performance.

Because of the nature of most hiking outings, strength training technique is extremely important. For example, hiking up a mountain is hard work that places considerable stress on the thigh muscles. But hiking down a mountain can be even harder because it places more stress on the thigh muscles. Downhill hiking emphasizes eccentric muscle contractions that attenuate the force of gravity and prevent the hiker from tumbling head over heels down the mountain. Eccentric muscle contractions cause considerably more microtrauma to the tissues and often lead to muscle soreness on the day following the activity.

With this understanding, it would appear useful for hikers to emphasize eccentric muscle contractions in their strength training programs. We are not in favor of senior exercisers performing eccentric-only workouts with heavier than normal loads, because excessive muscle overload can cause serious tissue damage. But we do recommend performing carefully controlled lowering movements to accentuate the eccentric phase of every repetition. For example, if the exerciser lifts the load in 2 seconds and lowers the load in 4 to 6 seconds, the eccentric muscle contraction receives ample attention. This technique should enhance the overall training effect and translate into better muscle response to both uphill and downhill hiking.

Because hikers frequently carry packs on their backs, they need to develop strong midsection and lower- and upper-body muscles as well as strong leg muscles. The recommended training program should be sufficient in this regard, as long as clients train with reasonable intensity. One set of each exercise is highly effective when the resistance is sufficient to fatigue the target muscle group within 8 to 12 controlled repetitions. Two or three 20- to 30-minute training sessions per week should produce excellent strength gains, and this plan represents an important investment for better activity performance as well as improved physical fitness.

Summary
of Strength Training for Rock Climbers and Hikers

When developing a sensible strength training program for hikers and rock climbers we recommend that you carefully consider the following exercise guidelines:

Exercise selection: Select single and multijoint exercises presented in tables 9.18 and 9.19, respectively, making sure that there is at least one exercise for each major muscle group

Exercise sets: One set of each exercise

Exercise resistance: Approximately 70 to 80 percent of 1RM

Exercise repetitions: Between 8 and 12 controlled repetitions

Exercise progression: A resistance increase of 5 percent when 12 repetitions can be completed (typically 1 to 5 pounds or 0.45 to 2.3 kg)

Exercise speed: Moderate, typically 2 seconds of lifting and 4 seconds of lowering

Exercise range: Full-range movements but avoid the lockout position on the leg press exercise

Exercise frequency: Train 2 or 3 times a week on nonconsecutive days

Time required: Approximately 30 minutes

TRIATHLETES

There is a saying that a stronger athlete is a better athlete. When applied to sports such as football, basketball, and baseball, most people would agree that strength training is highly beneficial. But in the context of endurance activities such as swimming, cycling, and running, opinions vary. In fact, some argue that aerobic athletes need to be as lean as possible and that strength training makes them bigger rather than better.

Although few successful triathletes weigh over 200 pounds (90 kg), the fear of becoming too large and strong is essentially unfounded. To begin, top triathletes typically have an ectomorphic body type. That is, they have a linear physique with firm but trim features. On a comparative basis they are relatively low on fat and muscle. Because ectomorphs have fewer fat cells they do not add fat easily, and because they have fewer muscle cells they do not build muscle easily. In other words, ectomorphic people do not have the genetic potential to develop large, muscular physiques.

But they certainly can become leaner and stronger through a sensible program of strength training. For example, let's say that Tom weighs 150 pounds (68 kg) and is 10 percent fat. He therefore has 15 pounds (7 kg) of fat weight and 135 pounds (61 kg) of lean (muscle) weight. After 10 weeks of regular strength training Tom still weighs 150 pounds. But he has added 2 pounds (1 kg) of muscle for 137 pounds (62 kg) of lean weight, and lost 2 pounds of fat for 13 pounds (6 kg) of fat weight. He is now 8.7 percent fat and is leaner than before even though his bodyweight is still the same.

As an analogy, Tom has changed from a six-cylinder engine to an eight-cylinder engine. Although his bodyweight is the same, he has increased his horsepower and should experience a higher level of athletic performance. Power is essential for endurance events as well as for sprint events. Because power equals work divided by time, the person who completes the triathlon (work) in the least time is the most powerful athlete, and the winner.

Our muscles are the engines of our bodies. But unlike automobile engines, our muscles use energy when we are both moving and resting (for maintenance and repair functions). Regular strength training increases resting metabolic rate by about 7 percent, which is typically more than 100 additional calories burned every day at rest. Other things being equal, that difference amounts to almost 1 pound (0.45 kg) of fat loss per month just to sustain normal metabolic function.

Clearly, triathletes have nothing to lose and much to gain by developing muscles that are more functional. Although not as obvious, the greatest benefit of a well-designed strength training program may be the experiences that triathletes avoid. We are referring to the various overuse injuries that plague many triathletes. Because swimming, cycling, and running all emphasize some muscles more than others, joint structures in the feet, knees, hips, back, shoulders, and neck may become vulnerable to musculoskeletal problems. By performing a comprehensive program of strength training exercises, many potential muscle overuse and imbalance injuries may be prevented.

For example, swimming emphasizes shoulder extension and adduction movements (pulling the arms through the water) more than shoulder flexion and abduction movements (recovering the arms through the air). Consequently, the stronger pectoralis major and latissimus dorsi muscles tend to overpower the weaker deltoid muscles, which frequently leads to shoulder injuries, especially in the vulnerable rotator cuff area.

On the other side of the coin, some muscles require significant strengthening to enhance athletic performance. Consider the discomfort that many cyclists experience in their neck muscles during long rides. Stronger neck muscles may be extremely beneficial in this activity, as well as during the swimming event. Keep in mind that every physical activity uses a certain percentage of maximum muscle strength. As your clients' maximum muscle strength increases, so does their capacity to perform sustained work at any submaximal effort, including swimming, cycling, and running.

Concerns

Does a strength training program have any drawbacks for competitive triathletes? Yes, namely training time and recovery ability. Because triathletes are already spending a lot of time and expending a lot of energy performing three demanding aerobic activities, little may be left for strength training. A traditional 1-hour-per-day, split-routine strength training program would be counterproductive for most triathletes.

Triathletes must take a sensible approach to strength training. Rather than find out how much strength training your client's body can withstand before it breaks down, you should determine how little strength training your client needs to achieve a gradual strengthening of the musculoskeletal system and improve competitive performance.

Triathletes' Strength Training Program

Triathletes should pursue a strength training program that is safe and time efficient, as well as effective. That is, triathletes should not perform high-risk exercises or high-speed exercises, because these activities typically reduce training safety. They should consider a single-set exercise program, because training in this manner requires less time and energy. Studies show that single-set training is effective for strength development and is less time consuming than multiple-set strength training.

Most people assume that endurance athletes should train with more repetitions than strength athletes do, and this idea is correct within certain parameters. Endurance athletes typically have a relatively high percentage of slow-twitch muscle fibers, which fatigue slowly and respond well to slightly higher repetition schemes. We therefore recommend that endurance athletes train with about 12 to 16 repetitions per exercise set.

Of course, a person's training speed determines the time required to perform 12 to 16 repetitions. Research shows that 6-second repetitions are both safe and productive for increasing muscle strength. At 6 seconds per repetition, a set of 12 to 16 repetitions requires about 70 to 95 seconds of continuous muscle effort. Because muscles can produce more force in eccentric contractions (lowering movements) than in concentric contractions (lifting movements), we suggest

TABLE 9.20

Major Muscle Groups Used in Triathlon Events

Major muscle groups	Machine exercises	Free-weight or bodyweight exercises
Quadriceps	Leg extension	Squat
Hamstrings	Leg curl	Squat
Low back	Low-back extension	Trunk extension
Abdominal	Abdominal flexion	Trunk curl
Chest	Chest press	Bench press
Upper back	Seated row	Dumbbell one-arm row
Shoulders	Lateral raise	Overhead press
Biceps	Biceps curl	Dumbbell standing curl
Triceps	Triceps extension	Dumbbell lying triceps extension

2 seconds for each lifting movement and 4 seconds for each lowering movement.

To ensure balanced muscular development, all the major muscle groups must be trained. Therefore, a basic triathlon strength training program for your senior clients may include the machine or free-weight exercises presented in table 9.20.

We recommend that older athletes perform the triathlete strength workout twice a week because studies on strength training frequency show that two sessions per week are essentially as effective as three sessions per week (Westcott et al. 2009).

After your clients have mastered the basic workout, you may add a few specialized strength training exercises that can further improve their triathlon performance. For example, we advise triathletes to perform the four-way neck machine to strengthen one of the most important and vulnerable muscle groups in the body. A stronger neck should help both swimming and cycling performance, and may enhance running ability as well.

The oblique muscles on each side of the midsection are another conditioning consideration. These muscles are used extensively in the turning action of the freestyle stroke. Our choice for strengthening the internal and external oblique muscles is the rotary torso machine or twisting trunk curls.

Because the triceps are used dynamically in swimming and statically in cycling, giving these muscles a little extra attention may be advisable. Bar dips target the triceps muscles and allow clients to master a bodyweight exercise. As they become stronger they can add external resistance for additional strengthening. Just be sure not to let them dip too deeply, because doing so may unduly stress the shoulder joints. We suggest stopping the downward movement when the elbows reach a right angle.

Finally, because the legs are heavily involved in all three events, safely increasing their functional strength is important. Our preference for working the quadriceps, hamstrings, and gluteal muscles together is a well-designed leg press machine, which may be substituted for leg extensions and leg curls. Like squats, properly performed leg presses provide an excellent strength stimulus for all the major leg muscles.

Summary of Strength Training for Triathletes

When developing a sensible strength training program for triathletes we recommend that you carefully consider the following exercise guidelines:

Exercise selection: Include the exercises presented in table 9.20, making sure that there is at least one exercise for each major muscle group

Exercise sets: One set of each exercise

Exercise resistance: Approximately 60 to 70 percent of 1RM

Exercise repetitions: Between 12 and 16 controlled repetitions

Exercise progression: A resistance increase of 5 percent when 16 repetitions can be completed (typically 1 to 5 pounds or 0.45 to 2.3 kg)

Exercise speed: Moderate, typically 2 seconds of lifting and 4 seconds of lowering

Exercise range: Full-range movements but avoid the lockout position on the leg press exercise

Exercise frequency: Train 2 or 3 times a week on nonconsecutive days

Time required: Approximately 30 minutes

ROWERS

If your clients enjoy rowing, canoeing, or kayaking, then the information in this section should be helpful for improving their rowing or paddling performance and reducing their risk of muscle overuse and imbalance injuries. Of course, one objective is to strengthen the muscles used in these activities for more powerful rowing or paddling actions. To do this, we will concentrate on exercises that specifically address the rowing muscles. An equally important objective, however, is to strengthen the muscles not used in these activities, especially the opposing muscle groups that must balance the prime mover muscles and maintain joint integrity throughout thousands of repetitive rowing movements. That is, rowers need a sound and sensible strength training program for comprehensive musculoskeletal conditioning. This guidance becomes obvious when we realize how much musculature is actually involved in rowing and paddling activities.

Let's begin with a basic analysis of the rowing action as produced by the contributing muscle groups and the recommended resistance exercises for effectively strengthening the musculoskeletal system. The first movement in sliding seat rowing is extension of the legs, starting with the muscles that straighten the knees. These are the quadriceps muscles of the front thighs, the largest and strongest muscles in the body. The second and almost simultaneous movement is extension of the hip joint, which is accomplished by the opposing hamstring muscles of the rear thighs and gluteus maximus muscles of the hips. The single best strength training exercise for the quadriceps muscles is the leg extension, and the single best exercise for the hamstring muscles is the leg curl (either seated or prone). The exercise that most effectively works the quadriceps, hamstrings, and gluteus maximus muscles at the same time is the leg press (machine) or the squat (free weights). As shown in table 9.21, these leg exercises should be performed first in the strength training program, because they are responsible for the initial power production of every rowing action.

The next phase of the rowing movement is extension of the trunk, which is produced by contraction of the lower-back muscles. Although the erector spinae muscles can become extremely strong, the lower back is a vulnerable area of the body for many people. Older adults must therefore train these important muscles in a careful and progressive manner to reduce the risk of injury during the strengthening process. Without question, the best exercise for safely developing stronger lower-back muscles is the low-back machine. To ensure comprehensive midsection conditioning, however, you should combine the low-back exercise with the abdominal machine and the rotary torso machine. These three exercises address the erector spinae muscles of the rear midsection, the rectus abdominis muscles of the front midsection, and the oblique muscles (internal and external) on both sides of the midsection, respectively. If these machines are not available, the trunk extension, trunk curl, and twisting trunk curl provide excellent alternatives for midsection conditioning. All these midsection muscles are involved in efficient force transfer from the lower body to the upper body, and exercises that address them should be included in each strength training session. Because they stabilize essentially every strength training exercise, we recommend placing the midsection exercises at the end of each workout (see table 9.21).

The next aspect of the rowing sequence is the arm pulling action that moves the oars through the water to propel the boat forward. Although always challenging, the arm pull is much easier when it is appropriately timed so that it immediately follows the trunk extension movement. The prime mover muscles for the arm pull are the latissimus dorsi and teres major muscles of the upper back, the rear deltoid muscles of the shoulders, and the biceps muscles of the arms. The large shoulder retractor muscles (upper trapezius, middle trapezius, and rhomboids) provide assistance. The super pullover machine is most productive for isolating the latissimus dorsi and teres major muscles, and it should be followed by the compound row machine, which addresses these muscles as well as the posterior deltoids, biceps, upper trapezius, middle trapezius, and rhomboids. Additional biceps conditioning can be obtained by using the biceps machine. These exercises should be performed in the order presented in table 9.21. To ensure muscle balance and joint integrity in the upper body, older rowers should also do exercises for the opposing muscle groups, namely the pectoralis major, anterior and middle deltoids, and triceps. As shown in table 9.21, the chest press, shoulder press, and triceps extension exercises achieve this purpose and should be included in the rowers' strength training program where indicated. If free-weight exercises are preferred, we recommend the pull-down, bent row, and dumbbell curl for the upper-body

TABLE 9.21

Recommended Strength Training Exercises and Training Order for Increasing Rowing or Paddling Power

Machine exercises	Free-weight exercises	Muscle group	Rowing relevance
Leg extension	Dumbbell step-up	Quadriceps	Power production
Leg curl	Dumbbell step-up	Hamstrings	Power production
Leg press	Squat	Quadriceps, hamstrings, and gluteals	Power production
Super pullover, seated row	Pull-down, dumbbell one-arm row	Latissimus dorsi and teres major	Arm pull
Biceps curl	Dumbbell standing curl	Biceps	Arm pull
Chest press	Barbell bench press	Pectoralis major, anterior deltoids, and triceps	Joint integrity
Shoulder press	Dumbbell bench press	Anterior deltoids, middle deltoids, and triceps	Joint integrity
Triceps extension	Dumbbell lying triceps extension	Triceps	Joint integrity
Rotary torso	Twisting trunk curl	Internal and external obliques	Force transfer
Abdominal flexion	Trunk curl	Rectus abdominis	Force transfer
Low-back extension	Trunk extension	Erector spinae	Force transfer

pulling muscles and the bench press, dumbbell press, and triceps extension for the opposing muscles.

All the strength training exercises should be performed on 2 or 3 days per week, typically in a total-body workout that can be completed in less than 25 minutes. One properly performed set of each exercise should be sufficient. Approximately 1 minute of recovery time should be allowed between successive exercises. Proper exercise performance is characterized by full movement range and slow movement speed on every repetition. We suggest taking about 6 seconds for each repetition, allowing 2 seconds for the lifting movement and 4 seconds for the lowering movement. The exerciser should use enough resistance to fatigue the target muscles within the anaerobic energy system, generally during a range of 50 to 70 seconds. At 6 seconds per repetition, this duration corresponds to about 8 to 12 repetitions per exercise set. When the client can complete 12 repetitions in proper form in two consecutive workouts, the load should be increased by approximately 5 percent (or less). For most exercises, this increase requires adding 2 to 10 pounds (0.9 to 4.5 kg), which of course will reduce the number of repetitions that can be performed. The client should train with the higher resistance until he or she can again complete 12 repetitions. An appropriate amount of weight can then be added to the next workout. Keep careful records of all your clients' training sessions for purposes of progression and motivation.

Summary of Strength Training for Rowers

When developing a sensible strength training program for rowers we recommend that you carefully consider the following exercise guidelines:

Exercise selection: Include the exercises presented in table 9.21, making sure that there is at least one exercise for each major muscle group

Exercise sets: One set of each exercise

Exercise resistance: Approximately 70 to 80 percent of 1RM

Exercise repetitions: Between 8 and 12 controlled repetitions

Exercise progression: A resistance increase of 5 percent when 12 repetitions can be completed (typically 1 to 5 pounds or 0.45 to 2.3 kg)

Exercise speed: Moderate, typically 2 seconds of lifting and 4 seconds of lowering

Exercise range: Full-range movements but avoid the lockout position on the leg press exercise

Exercise frequency: Train 2 or 3 times a week on nonconsecutive days

Time required: Approximately 25 minutes

SOFTBALL PLAYERS

Softball is an increasingly popular senior team sport that involves throwing, catching, batting, and sprinting. Successful players must have excellent eye–hand coordination and high levels of performance power. Although softball does not require cardiovascular endurance, muscular strength is a key factor for improved throwing, batting and sprinting. Let's look at the major muscle groups used in these actions and the strength training exercises best suited for their development.

Throwing

Throwing is generally considered an arm action, and good throwers are said to have strong arms. Although the triceps muscles that extend the elbow are certainly involved in delivering the ball, the shoulder joint muscles generate most of the throwing movement, particularly the pectoralis major and deltoids, with assistance from the latissimus dorsi. The propulsive force applied by the arm and upper body represents the final phase of a three-part total-body movement sequence.

The first phase is primary power production by the leg muscles as the person steps forward and shifts the hips in the direction of the throw. This action incorporates the large quadriceps, hamstrings, adductor, abductor, and gluteal muscles of the hips and thighs.

The second phase is the smooth and efficient transfer of force from the lower body to the upper body. This task is accomplished by the muscles of the midsection, namely, the internal obliques, external obliques, rectus abdominis, and erector spinae groups. Working together, these muscles rotate the torso forward with high torque that initiates the whiplike action of the throwing arm. Table 9.22 presents the muscles, actions, and recommended exercises related to throwing a softball.

Batting

Swinging a bat is actually an action similar to throwing a ball; the bat is an extension of the arms. Like throwing, batting is a three-phase sequence of coordinated body movements starting with the step, followed by the turn, and completed with the swing. The forward step and torso rotation use the same muscles and movement pattern used in throwing.

The swing is a horizontal action that involves both arms and essentially all the upper-body muscles. For a right-handed batter, the left arm supplies most of the hitting force by powerful contraction of the rear deltoid, latissimus dorsi, and triceps muscles. The right arm assists by means of the pectoralis major, front deltoid, and triceps muscles.

To address these muscles, you should add two multimuscle exercises to your clients' softball strength training program (see table 9.22). The compound row exercise targets the rear deltoid, latissimus dorsi, and biceps muscles, and it should be performed after the super pullover, which preexhausts the latissimus dorsi muscles, to obtain the most benefit.

The chest press exercise addresses the pectoralis major, front deltoid, and triceps muscles. Have clients perform the chest press after the chest cross to maximize the preexhaustion effect of the pectoralis major muscles.

Sprinting

Although sprinting speed is largely an inherent neuromuscular ability, strength training can definitely enhance movement power. The same leg exercises used for improved throwing and batting will increase baserunning speed and fielding quickness. To place greater emphasis on the hip flexor muscles used in sprinting, be sure to have clients lock their feet behind the ankle anchor pads when doing the abdominal machine exercise.

Softball Players' Strength Training Program

Two strength training sessions per week, performed on nonconsecutive days, are recommended during the off-season, and one or two workouts per week should be sufficient during the season. Clients should require less than 30 minutes to complete the 15 strength training exercises in each training session.

Clients should perform one set of each exercise in good form, emphasizing moderate movement speed and full movement range. We suggest 6-second repetitions consisting of 2 seconds for each lifting action and 4 seconds for each lowering action. Clients should attempt to achieve positions of full joint flexion and full joint extension on every repetition, as long as they do not experience discomfort in the end ranges.

TABLE 9.22

Muscles, Actions, and Recommended Exercises Related to Throwing a Ball

Muscles	Actions	Exercises, machines
Quadriceps	Power production	Leg extension
Hamstrings	Power production	Leg curl
Hip adductors	Power production	Hip adduction
Hip abductors	Power production	Hip abduction
Gluteals	Power production	Leg press
Internal and external obliques	Force transfer	Rotary torso
Rectus abdominis	Force transfer	Abdominal flexion
Erector spinae	Force transfer	Low-back extension
Deltoids	Arm action	Lateral raise
Pectoralis major	Arm action	Chest crossover, chest press
Latissimus dorsi	Arm action	Super pullover, seated row
Triceps	Arm extension	Triceps extension
Biceps	Muscle balance	Biceps curl

Senior softball payers should train with a load that enables them to complete between 8 and 12 repetitions. This resistance typically requires clients to train with about 70 to 80 percent of 1RM, which represents a safe and productive training load. When clients can complete 12 repetitions in good form in two consecutive workouts, about 5 percent more resistance should be added for gradual progression and continued improvement.

A comprehensive strength training program results in stronger muscles that enhance power production for throwing, batting, and baserunning. Just as important, a stronger musculoskeletal system reduces the risk of softball-related injuries. We therefore encourage senior softball players to start strength training at least 2 months before their competitive season.

Summary of Strength Training for Softball Players

When developing a sensible strength training program for softball players, carefully consider the following exercise guidelines:

Exercise selection: Include the exercises and preexhaustion approach previously discussed, and make sure that there is at least one exercise for each major muscle group

Exercise sets: One set of each exercise

Exercise resistance: Approximately 70 to 80 percent of 1RM

Exercise repetitions: Between 8 and 12 controlled repetitions

(continued)

Summary *(continued)*

Exercise progression: A resistance increase of 5 percent when 12 repetitions can be completed (typically 1 to 5 pounds or 0.45 to 2.3 kg)

Exercise speed: Moderate, typically 2 seconds of lifting and 4 seconds of lowering

Exercise range: Full-range movements but avoid the lockout position on the leg press exercise

Exercise frequency: Train 2 or 3 times a week on nonconsecutive days

Time required: Approximately 30 minutes

CHAPTER

10

Nutrition
for Senior Clients

Dietary habits significantly affect your clients' bodyweight, body composition, and physical health. Because most Americans consume too many calories for their level of activity, about two out of three American adults are overweight or obese according to a 2003–2004 National Health and Nutrition Examination Survey (National Institutes of Health 2004), predisposing them to various diseases and degenerative problems. Moreover, being overweight is only the tip of the iceberg. Bodyweight underestimates body fat during the aging process because adults lose 5 to 7 pounds (2.3 to 3.2 kg) of muscle every decade of life unless they perform regular strength exercise. Therefore, a woman who gains 40 pounds (18 kg) of bodyweight between ages 20 and 60 has added 60 pounds (27 kg) of fat because she has lost 20 pounds (9 kg) of muscle. This loss of muscle represents a much more serious situation than the weight gain indicated by the bathroom scale. Your clients should be aware that excessive body fat increases the risk of heart disease, stroke, joint problems, diabetes, low-back pain, and many types of cancer.

Understanding the health risks associated with being overweight is an important step in motivating your clients to make lifestyle changes that can lead to a more desirable bodyweight. Describing the physical improvements that will result from strength training, such as enhanced body composition and personal appearance, will also serve to motivate some seniors to modify their eating habits. Others may need specific nutrition programs that present daily menus and dietary information. Excellent resources in this area are those from the American Dietetic Association (www.eatright.org), the United States Department of Agriculture MyPyramid Web site (www.mypyramid.gov), the U.S. Food and Drug Administration of the Department of Health and Human Services (www.aoa.gov), and textbooks by Drs. Nancy Clark (*Sports Nutrition Guidebook*, Human Kinetics Publishers) and James Rippe (*Exercise Exchange Program*, Simon and Schuster Publishers).

Although most of the interest in diet seems to be about losing bodyweight through low-fat or low-carbohydrate diet plans, we advise against any low-calorie diet program. Low-calorie diet plans almost always fail to result in permanent weight loss. According to the authors (Mann et al. 2007) of a thorough review of the weight-loss research published by the American Psychological Association, essentially everyone who loses weight through dieting regains it.

To emphasize the challenges of dieting, the authors go on to state, "It appears that dieters who manage to sustain a weight loss are the rare exception rather than the rule."

Perhaps the main reason that diets do not work over the long term is that up to 25 percent of the weight lost on low-calorie diets is muscle tissue (Ballor and Poehlman 1994). Of course, muscle loss leads to a reduction in resting metabolic rate, which greatly increases the difficulty of maintaining the weight loss. Because of their lower bodyweight, reduced muscle mass, and slower metabolic rate, dieters who return to their normal eating patterns find that the daily calorie intake that had previously maintained their bodyweight is now excessive.

We take a different nutritional approach to help seniors improve their body composition as well as attain a desirable bodyweight. In fact, our first recommendation is to eat more rather than less, at least when it comes to protein. As you are aware, seniors need to replace the muscle that atrophies through the sedentary aging process. Of course, muscle development depends on strength training stimuli, but it also requires protein building blocks. Although most American adults eat sufficient protein in their daily meals, many seniors do not. Part of the reason may be that seniors need a higher protein intake than the recommended dietary allowance, or RDA (Gersovitz et al. 1982; Fukagawa and Young 1987; Campbell et al. 2001). Also important to know when training older adults is that even higher protein intake is warranted for those who strength train. According to Wayne Campbell, a highly respected nutrition researcher, "Our studies showed that people from their 50s into their 80s who were exercising their muscles needed at least 25 percent more protein than the RDA level just to maintain their muscle mass . . . and to gain muscle tissue, they needed to consume 50 percent more protein than the RDA level" (Schardt 2007). Further emphasizing a need for higher protein intake, evidence indicates that older adults do not process protein as well as younger adults do (Morais et al. 2006).

This being the case, we suggest that seniors consume more protein on a daily basis so that the amount of amino acids actually utilized equals the amount needed for optimal function. As presented in table 10.1, we propose that people in their 50s consume 50 percent more protein, people in their 60s consume 60

TABLE 10.1

Adjusted Minimum Daily Protein Recommendations

Age ranges in years	Recommended daily protein intake	Percent increase for strength trainers	Adjusted daily protein intake for strength trainers
50-59	Men: 56 g	Men: 50%	Men: 85 g
	Women: 46 g	Women: 50%	Women: 70 g
60-69	Men: 56 g	Men: 60%	Men: 90 g
	Women: 46 g	Women: 60%	Women: 75 g
70-79	Men: 56 g	Men: 70%	Men: 95 g
	Women: 46 g	Women: 70%	Women: 80 g

percent more protein, and people in their 70s consume 70 percent more protein than the standard daily recommendations.

The general recommendation for protein consumption is approximately 1 gram of protein for every 2 pounds (0.9 kg) of bodyweight, but a more appropriate guideline for older adults may be approximately 2 grams of protein for every 3 pounds (1.4 kg) of bodyweight. For example, based on the old standard, a 120-pound (54 kg) older woman should consume about 60 grams of protein daily. Our guideline, however, would be for her to take in about 80 grams of protein daily. Rather than take large portions of protein at one meal, it is advisable to take smaller amounts of protein at each meal and in snacks.

To enhance the muscle-building process further, we advise older adults to eat some additional protein at the time of their strength training session. Several studies have demonstrated greater strength and muscle gains when extra protein is consumed just before or just after the weight workout (Esmarck et al. 2001; Anderson et al. 2005; Cribb and Hayes 2006). In one well-designed study (Cribb and Hayes 2006), the subjects who took supplemental protein at the time of the strength training session added almost twice as much lean (muscle) weight as those who consumed the same amount of supplemental protein several hours before or after the weight workout.

We recently completed a 6-month study with women who averaged just less than 60 years of age (Westcott et al. 2008). All the subjects performed one set (8–12 repetitions) of 12 strength exercises and did 20 minutes of endurance activity (cycle or treadmill) on a Tuesday–Thursday schedule or a Monday–Wednesday–Friday schedule. Half of the participants drank a protein–carbohydrate shake (25 grams of protein, 37 grams of carbohydrate, 250 total calories) immediately following their strength training session, and half did not. Those who consumed the protein–carbohydrate shake added 5.5 pounds (2.5 kg) of lean (muscle) weight and lost 9.0 pounds (4.1 kg) of fat weight. Those who did not drink the shake added 3.9 pounds (1.7 kg) of lean (muscle) weight and lost 4.9 pounds (2.2 kg) of fat weight. Based on our results, consuming supplemental protein and carbohydrate right after their weight workouts may benefit senior strength trainers by enhancing both their muscle gain and their fat loss.

Although subjects in this study drank a specific protein and carbohydrate supplement, consuming a particular product is not necessary. Simply drinking a large glass of milk or a yogurt smoothie, or eating protein-rich foods such as cottage cheese, yogurt, or tuna fish may produce similar results. Although consuming excessive protein may place extra stress on the kidneys, this result would occur only with much more daily protein intake than the amounts suggested here.

Besides knowing how to count calories and determine the fat content of various foods, older adults should be aware that eating too little protein, calcium, or vitamin D can lead to a weak musculoskeletal system and even osteoporosis. Insufficient iron in the diet may cause anemia, and excessive sodium intake may contribute to hypertension.

Eating foods high in fiber, low in fat, and rich in vitamins and minerals is essential for optimal health as well as for disease prevention. For example, potassium, which is abundant in bananas and cantaloupe, is involved in every muscle contraction. Vitamins A and C, found in many fruits and vegetables, are important antioxidants (nutritional bodyguards) that protect the body cells from potentially harmful chemical reactions.

Although nutritional supplements can supply vitamins and minerals, dieticians warn that such supplements are not a substitute for a well-balanced diet that includes a variety of vegetables, fruits, and whole grains, as well as lean meats and low-fat dairy products. Human nutrient requirements are too complex (and too little understood) to be adequately supported by pills, and only a varied and well-rounded diet can provide the proper foundation for optimal nutrition. Your clients should be familiar with the food categories and daily servings recommended by the United States Department of Agriculture in MyPyramid. They should also understand that a well-balanced diet is not the same as a low-calorie diet designed for losing weight. Be sure that your client's physician or a registered dietician approves any reduced-calorie diet.

THE BASIC NUTRIENTS

The USDA MyPyramid (figure 10.1) is high in carbohydrate, moderate in protein, and low in fat. The carbohydrate choices are divided into grains, vegetables, and fruits. The suggested protein sources are low-fat milk products and lean meats (including beans, nuts, and tofu), and the recommended fat-rich foods

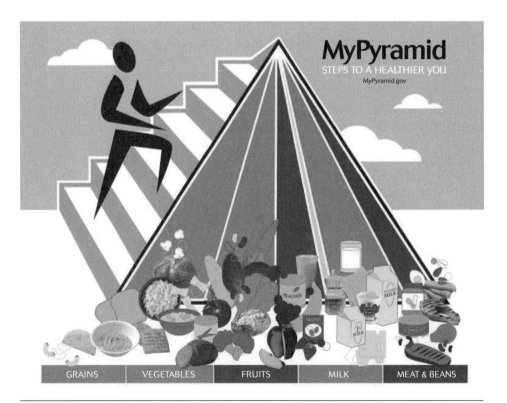

Figure 10.1 United States Department of Agriculture MyPyramid.

U. S. Department of Agriculture and the U.S. Department of Health and Human Services.

are vegetable oils (used sparingly). The Modified MyPyramid for Older Adults presents the same food categories and adds water, calcium, vitamin D, and vitamin B_{12}. The following sections address the basic food categories from a practical perspective. We believe that sharing this essential nutrition information with older adult exercisers is useful.

Grains

Grains include all kinds of foods made from wheat, oats, corn, rice, and the like. Examples of grain foods are cereals, breads, pasta, pancakes, rice cakes, tortillas, bagels, muffins, cornbread, rice pudding, and chocolate cake. Obviously, some grain-based foods such as cakes, cookies, and pastries contain a lot of fat and should be eaten in moderation.

All grains are high in carbohydrate; some grains, or parts of grains, such as wheat germ, are also good sources of protein. Whole grains are typically rich in B vitamins and fiber. Grains are plentiful and inexpensive and should be part of every meal. A serving is equivalent to a slice of bread or 1/2 cup of pasta, so achieving the 6 to 11 servings should not be too difficult for most clients. Refer to page 299 for sample exchange units for popular food choices within the grains category.

◆ GUIDELINES ◆

Grains: MyPyramid recommends 6 to 11 servings of grains every day.

Vegetables

Like grains, vegetables are excellent sources of carbohydrates, vitamins, and fiber. Vegetables come in all sizes, shapes, colors, and nutritional characteristics and are relatively low in calories.

- Orange vegetables (e.g., carrots, sweet potatoes, and winter squash) are typically good sources of vitamin A and beta-carotene.
- Green vegetables are characteristically high in vitamins B_2 and folic acid. Some of the many green vegetables are peas, beans, broccoli, asparagus, spinach, and lettuce.
- Red vegetables generally provide ample amounts of vitamin C. The best-known vegetables in this category are tomatoes and red peppers.
- Other vegetables are essentially white, at least under the skin. These include cauliflower, summer squash, potatoes, and radishes, many of which are good sources of vitamin C.

MyPyramid recommends three to five daily servings of vegetables. One serving is 1/2 cup of any raw vegetable, except for lettuce and sprouts, which require 1 cup per serving. Because heating reduces water content, cooked vegetables require less space than uncooked vegetables do and serving sizes may be smaller. Likewise, vegetable juices are more concentrated and require only 1/2 cup (120 ml) per serving.

The best way to retain nutrients is to eat vegetables raw or to steam or microwave them. Also, fresh and frozen vegetables have more nutritional value and are lower in sodium than canned vegetables.

◆ GUIDELINES ◆

Vegetables: MyPyramid recommends three to five daily servings of vegetables.

Fruit

Fruits are also relatively low in calories and offer just as much variety and nutritional value as vegetables do. Essentially all fruit choices are high in carbohydrates and vitamins, and many provide excellent sources of fiber.

- Citrus fruits, such as oranges, grapefruit, and lemons, are loaded with vitamin C.
- Like orange-colored vegetables, orange fruits—including cantaloupe, apricots, and papaya—are rich in vitamin A and beta-carotene.
- Green fruits, such as honeydew melon and kiwi, and red fruits, such as strawberries and cherries, are also high in vitamin C.
- Yellow fruits—including peaches, mangos, and pineapples—are usually good sources of vitamin C.
- Fruits that are white, at least on the inside—including apples, pears, and bananas—are high in potassium.
- Dried fruit is particularly nutrient dense, and the natural sweetness makes it a healthy substitute for high-fat snacks such as candy bars. Raisins, dates, figs, and prunes are all superb energy sources, and prunes are the single best source of dietary fiber.

MyPyramid recommends two to four servings of fruit every day. Table 10.2 presents sample exchange quantities for a variety of fruits. You will notice that one serving varies considerably depending on the type of fruit eaten. For example, it takes one-quarter of a melon or one-half of a grapefruit to equal three dates or 2 tablespoons of raisins. The difference is water content. Fresh fruit contains lots of water, whereas dried fruit is essentially a high-density carbohydrate. For people who prefer their fruit in liquid form, 1/2 cup (120 ml) of fruit juice equals one serving but has less fiber than whole fruit does.

◆ GUIDELINES ◆

Fruit: MyPyramid recommends two to four servings of fruit every day.

TABLE 10.2

Sample Exchange Units Equivalent to One Serving

ONE GRAIN SERVING			
Cereals	**Grains**	**Breads**	**Snacks**
1/4 cup nugget cereals (Grape Nuts)	1/4 cup wheat germ	1/2 bagel or English muffin	0.75 oz (22 g) pretzels
1/3 cup concentrated bran cereals	1/3 cup brown or white rice	1 slice bread	0.75 oz (22 g) rice cakes
1/2 cup cooked hot cereal (oatmeal or Cream of Wheat)	1/2 cup pasta, macaroni, or noodles	1 piece pita bread	4 crackers (1 oz, or 30 g)
3/4 cup flaked cereals	1/2 cup hominy, barley, or grits	1 tortilla	3 cups air-popped popcorn
1 1/2 cups puffed cereals			
ONE FRUIT SERVING			
2 tbsp raisins	3/4 cup pineapple	3/4 cup berries	1/4 papaya
3 dates	2 kiwi	1 apple	1/4 melon
3 prunes	1/2 pomegranate	1 banana	1/2 mango
1/2 cup grapes	1/4 cantaloupe	1 peach	5 kumquats
1 pear	1 cup honeydew	1/2 grapefruit	1 1/4 cups watermelon
3 apricots	1 1/4 cups strawberries		
ONE DAIRY SERVING			
1 oz (30 g) low-fat cheese	1/2 cup evaporated skim milk	1/4 cup part-skim ricotta cheese	1 cup low-fat or nonfat yogurt
1/4 cup low-fat or nonfat cottage cheese	1 cup nonfat or 1% milk	1/4 cup parmesan cheese	1 cup low-fat buttermilk
ONE MEAT SERVING			
3 oz (90 g) fish	1 tbsp peanut butter	3 oz (90 g) meat (beef, poultry, lamb, and so on)	1/4 cup tuna
3 oz (90 g) poultry	1/4 cup cooked dry beans	1 egg or 2 egg whites	1/4 cup tofu
ONE FAT SERVING			
1 tsp butter	2 tbsp diet salad dressing	1 tbsp diet mayonnaise	2 tbsp sour cream
1 tbsp diet margarine	1 tbsp cream cheese	1 tsp oil	4 tbsp light sour cream
1 tsp mayonnaise	2 tbsp light cream cheese	1 tbsp salad dressing	2 tbsp coffee creamer (liquid)

Milk Products

MyPyramid recommends two to three daily servings of low-fat dairy products, including milk, yogurt, and cheese. These foods are excellent sources of protein and calcium. Because whole-milk products are high in fat, clients should be selective at the dairy counter. For example, skim milk, 1 percent milk, low-fat yogurt, and nonfat cottage cheese offer heart-healthy alternatives to higher-fat dairy selections.

Refer to table 10.2 for exchange units equivalent to one dairy serving. Notice that 1/4 cup of low-fat cheese has similar nutritional value to 1 cup (240 ml) of 1 percent milk. Although there are many sources of dietary protein, seniors may have difficulty obtaining sufficient calcium unless they regularly consume milk products. If clients have problems digesting milk (lactose intolerance), they should be sure to eat other foods that are high in calcium such as tofu, leafy greens, beans, broccoli, and sesame seeds.

◆ GUIDELINES ◆

Milk products: MyPyramid recommends two to three daily servings of low-fat dairy products.

Meats

This category includes meat, poultry, fish, eggs, nuts, and dry beans. All are good sources of protein, although some also contain significant amounts of fat. Table 10.3 presents sample foods in the meat category according to their fat content.

TABLE 10.3

Meat Group Foods Categorized by Fat Content

Low fat	Medium fat	High fat
All fish	Chicken with skin	Beef ribs
Egg whites	Turkey with skin	Pork ribs
Chicken without skin	Roast beef	Corned beef
Turkey without skin	Roast pork	Sausage
Venison	Roast lamb	Lunch meat
Rabbit	Veal cutlet	Ground pork
Top round	Ground beef	Hot dogs
Eye of round	Steaks	Fried chicken
Sirloin tenderloin	Canned salmon	Fried fish
Flank steak	Oil-packed tuna	Nuts
Veal	Whole eggs	Peanuts
Dry beans	Pork chops	Peanut butter

Note that how meat is prepared has a lot to do with how much fat it provides. This nutritional aspect will be presented in more detail in the food preparation section.

Although fat content varies among the foods in the meat category, protein exchange units are quite consistent. As you can see from table 10.2, 3 ounces (90 g) of meat, poultry, and fish (about the size of a deck of cards) have equal exchange value, as do 1/4 cup of dry beans and 1/4 cup of tuna. Encourage your clients to consume two to three servings, for a total of 6 to 9 ounces (175 to 275 g), from the meat group on a daily basis.

◆ GUIDELINES ◆

Meats: MyPyramid recommends two to three daily servings of meat, for a total of 6 to 9 ounces (175 to 275 g).

Fat

The smallest section of MyPyramid is the fat group, which should be consumed sparingly. Although all fat contains over 9 calories per gram, some fats are more desirable than others from a health perspective. For example, consuming saturated fat (such as that found in mayonnaise, butter, and sour cream) presents a higher risk for developing heart disease than consuming polyunsaturated fat (such as that found in margarine and corn oil). Some evidence shows that monounsaturated fat (such as that in olive oil and canola oil) is even more desirable than polyunsaturated fat with respect to coronary health. See table 10.2 to determine serving equivalents for foods in the fat group.

As you are undoubtedly aware, fat consumption has become a major issue in mainstream America. Authorities recommend different amounts of dietary fat intake. Whereas Dr. Dean Ornish (1993) advised that the heart patient eat only 10 percent of daily calories from fat, the American Heart Association (1989) and the American Dietetic Association allow up to 30 percent fat calories in the daily diet. According to the American Council on Exercise's *Personal Trainer Manual* (1996), most athletic people should consume between 20 and 30 percent of their calories from fat. We agree with this recommendation, but prefer diets closer to 20 percent fat calories. Excellent diet plan suggestions for senior strength trainers can be found in Dr. James Rippe's *Exercise Exchange Program* (Simon and Schuster Publishers), which provides about 23 percent fat, 23 percent protein, and 54 percent carbohydrate calories on a daily basis.

◆ GUIDELINES ◆

Fat: We recommend that 20 to 30 percent of calories come from fat, preferably 20 percent (refer to table 10.2 to determine serving equivalents for foods in the fat group).

Water

Water is not included in MyPyramid because it contains no calories and is not technically a food. Yet it is by far the most important human nutrient. The human body is mostly water (muscles are 80 percent water) and can survive only a few days without adequate hydration.

The Modified MyPyramid for Older Adults recommends that seniors consume eight 8-ounce (240 ml) glasses of water daily. Older adults who perform vigorous exercise may need to drink considerably more water on a daily basis. Unfortunately, the natural thirst mechanism declines with age, so have your clients monitor their water consumption to make sure that they are well hydrated. They should drink an extra glass or two on exercise days.

Because coffee, tea, diet drinks, and alcoholic beverages act as diuretics (which have a dehydrating effect), your clients should not count these in their daily water supply; but they may substitute beverages such as seltzer and fruit juices for water. Apple juice is an excellent source of potassium, and orange juice is high in vitamin C. Cranberry juice is close to orange juice in vitamin C content and may help prevent bladder infections. Carrot juice is high in vitamin A, vitamin C, potassium, and fiber.

◆ GUIDELINES ◆

Water: The Modified MyPyramid for Older Adults recommends eight 8-ounce (240 ml) glasses of water daily. We recommend one or two more on workout days.

THREE STEPS TO BETTER NUTRITION

An eating program that provides all the essential nutrients but limits fat consumption requires careful food selection, substitution, and preparation. The following suggestions should be useful to clients who want to implement more healthful eating habits.

Food Selection

If your clients follow the MyPyramid recommendations, emphasizing grains, vegetables, and fruit, along with moderate amounts of milk and meat products, their diets generally will be high in nutrition and low in fat. They should, however, be selective in the fat category. Because saturated fat such as that found in butter, cream, egg yolks, palm oil, and coconut oil raises blood cholesterol levels, your clients should consume these food items sparingly. Instead, have them select monounsaturated fat (such as olive, canola, and peanut oils) or polyunsaturated fat (such as safflower, sunflower, and corn oils). Although both mono- and polyunsaturated oils tend to lower blood cholesterol levels, monounsaturated oils may be preferred for reducing the risk of heart disease.

The following foods contain less saturated fat than other choices in their category and are preferred selections: fish; poultry without skin; low-fat milk, yogurt, and cottage cheese; and olive, peanut, sunflower, safflower, corn, and canola oils.

Your clients should generally avoid prepared foods that contain saturated fat, such as palm and coconut oils, as well as hydrogenated products. These types of fats appear to be most detrimental in raising cholesterol levels, thereby increasing the risk of cardiovascular disease. The container label will indicate whether a food is high in saturated fat or has been hydrogenated.

Food Substitution

Most people have favorite foods that they do not want to give up in spite of the fat content. The good news is that simple substitutions can reduce fat content without detracting from taste. For example, using evaporated skim milk in place of cream cuts fat and cholesterol content by more than 65 percent, and using plain nonfat yogurt or nonfat sour cream in place of sour cream on baked potatoes reduces cholesterol content by 90 percent—and supplies the body with twice as much beneficial calcium.

Other useful substitutes are two egg whites in place of a whole egg, herbs rather than table salt, low-fat frozen yogurt instead of ice cream, cocoa powder in place of chocolate squares in baked goods, and lemon juice or vinegar instead of high-fat salad dressings.

For clients who enjoy sweets, suggest dried fruit (raisins, dates, figs, prunes, dried apricots) in place of candy, cookies, and fat-rich baked goods. People who prefer crunchy snacks like potato chips may appreciate alternatives lower in fat such as pretzels, baked chips, or carrot sticks.

Food Preparation

How food is prepared may increase or decrease the fat content. Frying can double or triple the calories in some foods. Using nonfat vegetable spray or a nonstick skillet can eliminate the fat and oils typically used for frying. It is also better to cook vegetables separate from meat, so that the vegetables will not absorb fat from the meat. Baked or broiled meats and steamed or microwaved vegetables retain the greatest amount of nutrients. Discourage seniors from adding butter and salt to vegetables during cooking; less salt and fat is needed to make food taste good after cooking than during cooking.

ENERGY FOR EXERCISE AND PROTEIN FOR MUSCLE BUILDING

Your clients may be concerned about obtaining enough energy for their workouts and sufficient nutrients for building muscle. Although those who follow the MyPyramid recommendations should be well served in both areas, this section presents specific information about the calorie and protein needs of senior strength trainers.

Strength training generally requires about 8 calories per minute during exercise performance (Wilmore et al. 1978). A client who completes a 25-minute circuit of resistance machines with little rest between successive exercises would therefore burn approximately 200 additional calories (Paffenbarger and Olsen 1996).

Because of its vigorous nature and anaerobic energy requirements, strength training leads to considerable postexercise calorie utilization. Research shows that during the hour following a challenging circuit training session, participants may use up to 25 percent as many additional calories as they burned during the actual workout (Haltom 1999). Using the previous example, the client's additional energy use resulting from a 25-minute circuit strength training workout may total 250 calories.

Besides these direct energy requirements, strength training produces both more muscle and more active muscle—which consumes calories all day long. Seniors who perform 3 to 4 months of standard strength training add 3 to 4 pounds (1.4 to 1.8 kg) of muscle, condition the exercised muscle, and increase their resting metabolic rate by 7 to 8 percent (Campbell et al. 1994; Pratley et al. 1994). Assuming that most seniors have a resting metabolic rate of about 1,300 calories a day, such an increase would result in 100 additional calories per day being used to meet resting energy requirements.

Strength training may therefore be responsible for a total additional energy requirement of approximately 350 calories on exercise days (200 additional calories during the workout, 50 additional calories during the postexercise period, and 100 additional calories during the day because of higher resting metabolism). This number is consistent with the large increase in daily energy utilization experienced by the senior strength trainers in the landmark study at Tufts University discussed in earlier chapters (Campbell et al. 1994).

Based on these numbers, older adults who regularly strength train may eventually need to eat about 350 additional calories on exercise days and about 100 extra calories on nonexercise days to maintain their bodyweight. Although they can accomplish this increase by consuming high-energy drinks, sports bars, or other food supplements, they will do best by having additional servings from MyPyramid. An extra serving each from the grains, fruits, vegetables, and milk groups should total about 350 calories and provide a variety of important nutrients. Of course, clients who want to lose bodyweight may maintain their usual food intake or even reduce their calories slightly.

Strength training enthusiasts should also make a concerted effort to consume a sufficient amount of fluids, especially water, to build more muscle tissue. Because muscle is approximately 75 percent water, maintaining a high level of hydration is important. Clients should drink approximately eight glasses of water every day. Physically active people should drink additional water on days when they exercise.

EATING, EXERCISE, AND ENCOURAGEMENT

Healthy eating is not the same as dieting. Dieting implies reducing calories significantly to lose weight, usually in a short time. Most weight-loss diets involve unnatural eating patterns and the consumption of too few nutrients for optimal physical function. Because most dieters consume reduced levels of important nutrients, they cannot maintain their eating plans for long, and they typically regain the weight that they have lost soon after they discontinue their diets. This outcome occurs because of the reduction in muscle tissue and the slowing of the resting metabolic rate that result from most diet programs. With this in mind, perhaps the most important thing you can do for overweight older clients is to provide sound strength training programs and sincere encouragement for desirable eating behavior. Help your clients set realistic short-term exercise and nutrition goals, and give plenty of positive reinforcement as they make progress in achieving them. Additional recommendations for guiding and motivating clients can be found in chapter 2, "Training Principles and Teaching Strategies."

Emphasize changes in body composition measurements rather than bodyweight, because strength trainers normally lose fat and add muscle at the same time. For example, a male client may add 4 pounds (1.8 kg) of lean weight and lose 8 pounds (3.6 kg) of fat weight during a 10-week training period. Although the bathroom scale shows only a 4-pound weight loss, this client may have made a 12-pound (5.4 kg) change in body composition, which should be obvious by how the person looks and feels in his or her clothes.

On the other side of the coin, essentially all older adults can benefit from higher protein intake than that proposed in the recommended dietary allowance (RDA). More specifically, greater muscle development is attained when supplemental protein and carbohydrate are consumed at the time of the strength training session or shortly afterward.

Summary of Nutrition for Senior Strength Trainers

Nutrition for senior strength trainers is largely the same as nutrition for all older adults who desire good health and body composition. But research indicates that all older adults, especially those who perform muscle-building activity, benefit by ingesting more protein than the present recommended dietary allowance. Clients should find that a sound eating program provides plenty of energy for their strength training workouts and that some supplemental protein at the time of their workouts enhances their muscle development. We generally recommend the food categories and portions presented in the United States Department of Agriculture MyPyramid: 6 ounces (180 g) daily of grains, 2 1/2 cups daily of vegetables, 2 cups daily of fruit, 3 cups (720 ml) daily of milk products, 7 ounces (210 g) daily of meats and beans, and small quantities of fat such as nuts and monounsaturated oils. But because senior strength trainers may use 350 extra calories on exercise days and 100 more calories on nonexercise days, they may want to add a serving from each food category to maintain their bodyweight. Seniors who undertake strength training should also drink plenty of water or fruit juice, especially on their training days.

Senior exercise clients who want to lose bodyweight should experience gradual but consistent fat loss if they maintain their previous level of food consumption during their strength training. You may provide additional motivation by setting short-term goals and giving positive reinforcement as they improve their body composition and progress towards a desirable bodyweight.

Recommended Reading

Rippe, J. (1992). *Exercise Exchange Program.* New York: Simon and Schuster.

Appendix

Training Log

Order	Exercise	Sets	Reps	Day 1 Set 1	Day 1 Set 2	Day 1 Set 3	Day 2 Set 1	Day 2 Set 2	Day 2 Set 3	Day 3 Set 1	Day 3 Set 2	Day 3 Set 3
Name				**Week #**								
1			Weight									
			Reps									
2			Weight									
			Reps									
3			Weight									
			Reps									
4			Weight									
			Reps									
5			Weight									
			Reps									
6			Weight									
			Reps									
7			Weight									
			Reps									
8			Weight									
			Reps									
9			Weight									
			Reps									
10			Weight									
			Reps									
11			Weight									
			Reps									
12			Weight									
			Reps									
13			Weight									
			Reps									
14			Weight									
			Reps									
Bodyweight												
Date												
Comments												

From T. Baechle and W. Westcott, 2010, *Fitness Professional's Guide to Strength Training Older Adults,* Second Edition (Champaign, IL: Human Kinetics).

References

INTRODUCTION

American College of Sports Medicine. 2010. *Guidelines for exercise testing and prescription*, 8th ed. Philadelphia: Lippincott, Williams and Wilkins.

Baker, K., Nelson, M., Felson, D., Layne, J., Sarno, R., and Roubenoff, R. 2001. The efficacy of home based progressive strength training in older adults with knee osteoarthritis: A randomized controlled trial. Journal of Rheumatology 28:155–1665.

Bayramoglu, M., Akman, M., Cetin, N., Yauz, N and R. Ozker. (2001). Isokinetic measurement of trunk muscle strength in women with low back pain. Physical Medicine and Rehabilitation 80 (9), Sept. 650-655.

Campbell, C., Robertson, M., Gardner, R., Norton, R. and D. Buckner (1999) Falls prevention over 2 years: A randomized controlled trial in women 80 years and older. Ageing 28:515-528

Campbell, W., Crim, M., Young, V., and Evans, W. 1994. Increased energy requirements and changes in body composition with resistance training in older adults. *American Journal of Clinical Nutrition* 60:167–175.

Evans, W., and Rosenberg, I. 1992. *Biomarkers*. New York: Simon and Schuster.

Fiatarone, M., Marks, E., Ryan, N., et al. 1990. High-intensity strength training in nonagenarians. *Journal of the American Medical Association* 263 (22): 3029–3034.

Forbes, G. 1976. The adult decline in lean body mass. *Human Biology* 48:161–173.

Frontera, W., Meredith, C., O'Reilly, K., et al. 1988. Strength conditioning in older men: Skeletal muscle hypertrophy and improved function. *Journal of Applied Physiology* 64 (3): 1038–1044.

Hakkinen, A. (2004) Effectiveness and safety of strength training in rheumatoid arthritis. Arthritis and Rheumatism 16 (2) March 132-137.

Harris, K., and Holy, R. 1987. Physiological response to circuit weight training in borderline hypertensive subjects. *Medicine and Science in Sports and Exercise* 10: 246–252.

Haskell, W., Lee, I-Min, Pate, R., et al. 2007. Physical activity and public health: Updated recommendation for adults from the American College of Sports Medicine and the American Heart Association. *Medicine and Science in Sports and Exercise* 39:1423–1434.

Hedley, A., Ogden, C., Johnson, C., et al. 2004. Prevalence of overweight and obesity among US children, adolescents, and adults, 1999–2002. *Journal of the American Medical Association* 291:2847–2850.

Hurley, B. 1994. Does strength training improve health status? *Strength and Conditioning Journal* 16:7–13.

Kell, RT., and GJG Asmundson (2009). A comparison of two forms of periodized exercise rehabilitation programs in the management of chronic nonspecific low back pain. Journal of Strength and Conditioning Resrach 23 (2): 513 – 523.

Kesaniemi, Y., Danforth, E., Jensen, M., et al. 2001. Dose-response issues concerning physical activity and health: An evidence-based symposium. *Medicine and Science in Sports and Exercise* 33 (6 supplement): S531–S538.

Koffler, K., Menkes, A., Redmond, A., et al. 1992. Strength training accelerates gastro-intestinal transit in middle-aged and older men. *Medicine and Science in Sports and Exercise* 24:415–419.

Layne, J. and Nelson, M. 1999. The effects of progressive resistance training on bone density: A review. *Medicine and Science in Sports and Exercise* 31: 25-30.

Nelson, M., Fiatarone, M., Morganti, C., et al. 1994. Effects of high-intensity strength training on multiple risk factors for osteoporotic fractures. *Journal of the American Medical Association* 272 (24): 1909–1914.

Pratley, R., Nicklas, M., Rubin, J., et al. 1994. Strength training increases resting metabolic rate and norepinephrine levels in healthy 50- to 65-year-old men. *Journal of Applied Physiology* 76:133–137.

Risch, S., Nowell, N., Pollock, M., et al. 1993. Lumber strengthening in chronic low back pain patients. *Spine* 18: 232–238.

Rooks, C., Silverman, C., and C. Kantrowitz (2002). The effects of progressive strength training and aerobic exercise on muscle strength and cardiovascular fitness in women with fibromyalgia: A pilot study. Arthritis Care and Research 47 (1) p 22-28.,

Singh, N., Clements, K., and Fiatarone, M. 1997. A randomized controlled trial of progressive resistance training in depressed elders. *Journal of Gerontology* 52A (1): M27–M35.

Westcott, W. 2009. ACSM strength training guidelines. *ACSM's Health & Fitness Journal* 13 (4): 14-22.

Westcott, W., Martin, W., LaRosa Loud, R., and Stoddard, S. 2008. Protein supplementation and body composition changes. *Fitness Management* 24(5): 50-53.

Westcott, W., Richards, M., Reinl, G., and Califano, D. 2000. Strength training elderly nursing home patients. *Senior Fitness Association*. www.seniorfitness.net: 1–8.

Westcott, W., and Guy, J. 1996. A physical evolution: Sedentary adults see marked improvements in as little as two days a week. *IDEA Today* 14 (9): 58–65.

CHAPTER 1

Ades, P., Savage, P., Brochu, M., et al. 2005. Resistance training increases daily energy expenditure in disabled older women with coronary heart disease. *Journal of Applied Physiology* 98:1280–1285.

Ades, P., Ballor, D., Ashikaga, T., et al. 1996. Weight training improves walking endurance in healthy elderly persons. *Annuals of Internal Medicine* 124:658–572.

Alexander, H. 2002. Efficacy of a resting metabolic rate based energy balance prescription in a weight management program. Presentation at Nutrition Week Obesity Research Conference.

American Association of Cardiovascular and Pulmonary Rehabilitation. 1995. *Guidelines for cardiac rehabilitation programs*, 2d ed. Champaign, IL: Human Kinetics.

American College of Sports Medicine. 2010. *Guidelines for exercise testing and prescription, 8th ed.* Philadelphia: Lippincott, Williams and Wilkins.

American Heart Association and American College of Sports Medicine. 2007. Physical activity and health: Updated recommendations for adults from the American College of Sports Medicine and the American Heart Association. *Circulation* 116:1081–1093.

Arthritis Foundation. Arthritis Facts (2009). http://www.arthritis.org/facts.php.

Baechle, T., and Earle, R. 2006. *Weight training: Steps to success*, 3rd ed. Champaign, IL: Human Kinetics.

Baker, K., Nelson, M., Felson, D., Layne, J., Sarno, R., and Roubenoff, R. 2001. The efficacy of home based progressive strength training in older adults with knee osteoarthritis: A randomized controlled trial. *Journal of Rheumatology* 28:155–1665.

Balducci, SF, Leonetti. UD, Mario and F. Fallucca (2004) Is a long term aerobic plus weight training program feasible for and effective on metabolic profiles in type 2 diabetics? *Diabetes Care* 27:841-842.

Ballor, D., Katch, V., Becque, M., and Marks, C. 1988. Resistance weight training during caloric restriction enhances lean body weight maintenance. *American Journal of Clinical Nutrition* 47:19–25.

Ballor, D., and Poehlman, E. 1994. Exercise training enhances fat-free mass preservation during diet-induced weight loss: A meta analytic finding. *International Journal of Obesity* 18:35–40.

Bayramoglu, M., Akman, M., Cetin, N., Yauz, N and R. Ozker. (2001). Isokinetic measurement of trunk muscle strength in women with low back pain. Physical Medicine and Rehabilitation 80 (9), Sept. 650-655.

Bell, N., Godsen, R., and Henry, D. 1988. The effects of muscle-building exercise on vitamin D and mineral metabolism. *Journal of Bone Mineral Research* 3:369–373.

Blessing, D., Stone, M., and Byrd, R. 1987. Blood lipid and hormonal changes from jogging and weight training of middle-aged men. *Journal of Applied Sports Science Research* 1:25–29.

Borst, S. 2004. Interventions for sarcopenia and muscle weakness in older people. *Age and Ageing* 33(6):548–555.

Boyden, T., Pamenter, R., Going, S., Lohman, T., Hall, M., Houtkooper, L., Bunt, J., Ritenbaugh, C., and Aickin, M. 1993. Resistance exercise training is associated with decreases in serum low-density lipoprotein cholesterol levels in premenopausal women. *Archives of Internal Medicine* 153:97–100.

Brehm, B., and Keller, B. 1990. Diet and exercise factors that influence weight and fat loss. *IDEA Today* 8:33–46.

Butler, R., Beierwaltes, W., and Rogers, F. 1987. The cardiovascular response to circuit weight training in patients with cardiac disease. *Journal of Cardiopulmonary Rehabilitation* 7:402–409.

Butts, N., and Price, S. 1994. Effects of a 12-week weight training program on the body composition of women over 30 years of age. *Journal of Strength and Conditioning Research* 8 (4): 265–269.

Campbell, C., Robertson, M., Gardner, R., Norton, R. and D. Buckner (1999) Falls prevention over 2 years: A randomized controlled trial in women 80 years and older. *Ageing* 28:515-528

Campbell, A., Robertson, M., Gardener, M., et al. 1997. Randomised control trial of a general practice programme of home based exercise to prevent falls in elderly women. *British Medical Journal* 315:1065–1069.

Campbell, W., Crim, M., Young, V., and Evans, W. 1994. Increased energy requirements and changes in body composition with resistance training in older adults. *American Journal of Clinical Nutrition* 60:167–175.

Carpenter, D. and Nelson, B. 1999. Low back strengthening for the prevention and treatment of low back pain. *Medicine and Science in Sports and Exercise* 31(1):18-24.

Castaneda, C., Layne, J, Munoz-Orians, L., et al. 2002. A randomized controlled trial of resistance exercise training to improve glycemic control in older adults with type 2 diabetes. *Diabetes Care* 25(12): 2335-2341.

Charette, S., McEvoy, L., Pyka, G., et al. 1991. Muscle hypertrophy response to resistance training in women. *Journal of Applied Physiology* 70:1912–1917.

Chomiak, JA, Abadie, BR, Koh, YS and DR Chilek (2003). Resistance training exercises acutely reduce intraocular presuure in physically active men and women. *J. Strength Cond Res* Nov 17 (4):715-20.

Colletti, L., Edwards, J., Gordon, L., Shary, J., and Bell, N. 1989. The effects of muscle-building exercise on bone mineral density of the radius, spine and hip in young men. *Calcified Tissue International* 45:12–14.

Conte, M, Scarpi, MJ, Rossin, RA, Beteli, HR, Lopes, RG and HL Marcos (2009). Intra-occular pressure variation after submaximal strength test in resistance training. *Arq Bras Oftalmol* May0June 72 (3): 351-4

Cordain, L., Latin, R., and Behnke, J. 1986. The effects of an aerobic running program on bowel transit time. *Journal of Sports Medicine* 26:101–104.

Council on Exercise of the American Diabetes Association (1990). Technical review: Exercise and NIDDM. *Diabetes Care* 13:785-789.

Craig, B., Everhart, J., and Brown, R. 1989. The influence of high-resistance training on glucose tolerance in young and elderly subjects. *Mechanisms of Ageing and Development* 49:147–157.

DeGroot, DW, Quinn, TJ, Kertzer, NB, and WB Olney (1998). Circuit weight training in cardiac patients: determining optimal workloads for safety and energy expenditure. *Cardiopulmonary Rehabilitation* 18 (2): 145-152.

Draovitch, P., and Westcott, W. 1999. *Complete conditioning for golf*. Champaign, IL: Human Kinetics.

Dudley, A. 2001. The unceasing process of sarcopenia. www.sarcopenia.com/.

Durak, E. 1989. Exercise for specific populations: Diabetes mellitus. *Sports Training, Medicine and Rehabilitation* 1:175–180.

Durak, E., Jovanovis-Peterson, L., and Peterson, C. 1990. Randomized crossover study of effect of resistance training on glycemic control, muscular strength, and cholesterol in type I diabetic men. *Diabetes Care* 13:1039–1042.

Eriksson, J., Taimela, S., Eriksson, K., Parviainen, S., Peltonen, J., and Kujala, U. 1997. Resistance training in the treatment of non-insulin dependent diabetes mellitus. *International Journal of Sports Medicine* 18(4):242–246.

Evans, W., and Rosenberg, I. 1992. *Biomarkers*. New York: Simon and Schuster.

Faigenbaum, A., Skrinar, W., Cesare, W., Kraemer, W., and Thomas, H. 1990. Physiologic and symptomatic responses of cardiac patients to resistance exercise. *Archives of Physical Medicine and Rehabilitation* 70:395–398.

Fiatarone, M., O'Neil, E., and Ryan, N. 1994. Exercise training and supplementation for physical fraility in very elderly people. *New England Journal of Medicine* 330:1769–1765.

Fiatarone, M., Marks, E., Ryan, N., Meredith, C. Lipsitz, L., and Evans, W. 1990. High-intensity strength training in nonagenarians. *Journal of the American Medical Association* 263 (22): 3029–3034.

Fiatarone, M.A., and Singh, M. 2002. Exercise comes of age: Rationale and recommendations for a geriatric exercise prescription. *Journal of Gerontology Series A: Biological Sciences and Medical Sciences* 57 (A): M262–28

Frontera, W., Meredith, C., O'Reilly, K., Knuttgen, H., and Evans, W. 1988. Strength conditioning in older men: Skeletal muscle hypertrophy and improved function. *Journal of Applied Physiology* 64 (3): 1038–1044.

Ghilarducci, L., Holly, R., and Amsterdam, E. 1989. Effects of high resistance training in coronary heart disease. *American Journal of Cardiology* 64:866–870.

Gillette, C., Bullough, R., and Melby, C. 1994. Postexercise energy expenditure in response to acute aerobic or resistive exercise. *International Journal of Sport Nutrition* 4:347–360.

Goldberg, L., Elliot, L., Schultz, R., and Kloste, F. 1984. Changes in lipid and lipoprotein levels after weight training. *Journal of the American Medical Association* 252:504–506.

Grimby, G., Aniansson, A., Hedberg, M., Henning, G., Granguard, U., and Kvist, H. 1992. Training can improve muscle strength and endurance in 78 to 84 year old men. *Journal of Applied Physiology* 73:2517–2523.

Haennel, R., Quinney, H., and Kappagoda, C. 1991. Effects of hydraulic circuit training following coronary artery bypass surgery. *Medicine and Science in Sports and Exercise* 23:158–165.

Hakkinen, A. (2001) Effectiveness and safety of strength training in rheumatoid arthritis. Arthritis and Rheumatism 16 (2) March 132-137.

Haltom, R., Kraemer, R., Sloan, R., Herbert, E., Frank, K., and Tryniecki, J. 1999. Circuit weight training and its effect on post-exercise oxygen consumption. *Medicine and Science Sports Exercise* 31 (11): 1613–1618.

Harris, K., and Holly, R. 1987. Physiological response to circuit weight training in borderline hypertensive subjects. *Medicine and Science in Sports and Exercise* 10:246–252.

Haslam, D., McCartney, S., McKelvie, R, et al. 1988. Direct Measurements of arterial blood pressure during formal weight lifting in cardiac patients. *Journal of Cardiopulmonary Rehabilitation* 8: 213–225.

Hempel, L., and Wells, C. 1985. Cardiorespiratory cost of the Nautilus express circuit. *The Physician and Sports Medicine* 13: 82–97.

Hughes, V., Frontera, W., Dallal, G., Lutz, K., Fisher, E., and W. Evans (1995). Muscle strength and body composition: Associations with bone density in older subjects. *Medicine and Science in Sports and Exercise* 7(27):967-974.

Hunter, G., Wetzstein, C., Fields, D., Brown, A., and Bamman, M. 2000. Resistance training increases total energy expenditure and free-living physical activity in older adults. *Journal of Applied Physiology* 89: 977–984.

Hurley, B. 1994. Does strength training improve health status? *Strength and Conditioning Journal* 16:7–13.

Hurley, B., Hagberg, J., Goldberg, A., Seals, D., Ehsani, A., Brennan, R., and Holloszy, J. 1988. Resistive training can reduce coronary risk factors without altering $\dot{V}O_2$max or percent body fat. *Medicine and Science in Sports and Exercise* 20:150–154.

Ibanez, J, Izuierdo, M, Inaki, A, Forga, L, Larrion, JL, Garcia-Unciti, M, Idoate, F, and EN Gorostiaga (2005) Twice weekly progressive resistance training decreases abdominal fat and improves insulin sensitivity in older men with type 2 diabetes. *Diabetes Care* 28:662-667.

Johnson, C., Stone, M., Lopez, S., Hebert, J., Kilgoe, L., and Byrd, R. 1982. Diet and exercise in middle-aged men. *Journal of the Dietetic Association* 81:695–701.

Jones, A., Pollock, M., Graves, J., Fulton, M., Jones, W., MacMillan, M., Baldwin, D., and Cirulli, J. 1988. *Safe, specific testing and rehabilitative exercise for muscles of the lumbar spine.* Santa Barbara, CA: Sequoia Communications.

Katz, J., and Wilson, B. 1992. The effects of a six-week, low-intensity Nautilus circuit training program on resting blood pressure in females. *Journal of Sports Medicine and Physical Fitness* 32:299–302.

Kelley, G. 1997. Dynamic resistance exercise and resting blood pressure in healthy adults: A meta-analysis. *Journal of Applied Physiology* 82:1559–1565.

Kelley, G., and Kelley, K. 2009. Impact of progressive resistance training on lipids and lipoproteins in adults: A meta-analysis of randomized controlled trials. *Preventive Medicine* 48 (1): 9–19.

Kerr, D.T., Ackland, T. Masland, B., Morton, A., and Rice, R. (2001) Resistance training Over 2 Years Increases Bone Mass in Calcium Replete Postmenopausal Women. *Journal of Bone and Mineral Research* (16: 175-81).

Koffler, K., Menkes, A., Redmond, A., Whitehead, W., Pratley, R., and Hurley, B. 1992. Strength training accelerates gastrointestinal transit in middle-aged and older men. *Medicine and Science in Sports and Exercise* 24: 415–419.

Kokkinos, P., Hurley, B., Vaccaro, P., Patterson, J., Gardner, L., Ostrove, S., and Goldberg, A. 1988. Effects of low- and high-repetition resistive training on lipoprotein-lipid profiles. *Medicine and Science in Sports and Exercise* 20:50–54.

Kokkinos, P., Hurley, B., Smutok, M., Farmer, C., Reece, C., Shulman, R., Charabogos, C., Patterson, J., Will, S., DeVane-Bell, J., and Goldberg, A. 1991. Strength training does not improve lipoprotein lipid profiles in men at risk for CHD. *Medicine and Science in Sports and Exercise* 23:1134–1139.

Larsson, L. 1983. Histochemical characteristics of human skeletal muscle during aging. *Acta Physiological Scandinavia* 117:469–471.

Limke, JC., Rainville, J., Pena, E., and L. Childs (2008) Randomized trial comparing the effects of one vs two sets of resistance exercises for outpatients with chronic low back pain and leg pain. *Eur J Phys Rehabil Med.* Dec; 44 (4):399-405

Lohmann, D., and Liebold, F. 1978. Diminished insulin responses in highly trained athletes. *Metabolism* 27 (5): 521–523.

Mann, T., Tomiyama, J., Westling, E., Lew, A., Samuels, B., and Chatman, J. 2007. Medicare's search for effective obesity treatments: Diets are not the answer. *American Psychologist* 62 (3): 220–232.

Marks, R. 1993. The effect of isometric quadriceps strength training in mid-range for osteoarthritis of the knee. *Arthritis Care Research* 6:52–56.

McCartney, N., Hicks, A., Martin, J., and Webber, C. 1996. A longitudinal trial of weight training in the elderly continued improvements in year two. *Journals of Gerontology Series A—Biological Sciences and Medical Sciences* 51(6): B425–B433.

Melby, C., Scholl, C., Edwards, G., and Bullough, R. 1993. Effect of acute resistance exercise on postexercise energy expenditure and resting metabolic rate. *Journal of Applied Physiology* 75 (4):1847–1853.

Menkes, A., Mazel, S., Redmond, R., Koffler, K., Libanati, C., Gundberg, C., Zizic, T., Hagberg, J., Pratley, R., and Hurley, B. 1993. Strength training increases regional bone mineral density and bone remodeling in middle-aged and older men. *Journal of Applied Physiology* 74:2478–2484.

Messier, S., and Dill, M. 1985. Alterations in strength and maximal oxygen uptake consequent to Nautilus circuit weight training. *Research Quarterly for Exercise and Sport* 56 (4): 345–351.

Miller, W., Sherman, W., and Ivy, J. 1984. Effect of strength training on glucose tolerance and post glucose insulin response. *Medicine and Science in Sports and Exercise* 16 (6): 539–543.

Moreland, JD, Goldsmith, CH, Huijbregts MP, et al (2003). Progressive resistance strengthening exercises after stroke: a single randomized controlled trial. *Arch Phys Med Rehabil* 84 (10): 1433-1440.

National Center for Health Statistics (2009).Arthritis. 21 April.2009. www.cdc.gov/nchs/fastats/arthrits.htm.

National Institute of Arthritis, Musculoskeletal and Skin Diseases (2005). www.niams.nih.gov/Health_Info/Fibromyalgia/fibromyalgia_ff.asp

National Osteoporosis Foundation. 23 Nov.2009. Fast Facts. www.nof.org/osteoporosis/diseasefacts.htm.

National Stroke Association (2008). 9707 E. Easter Lane. Centennial, CO. 80112

Nelson, M., Fiatarone, M., Morganti, C., Trice, I., Greenberg, R., and Evans, W. 1994. Effects of high-intensity strength training on multiple risk factors for osteoporotic fractures. *Journal of the American Medical Association* 272 (24): 1909–1914.

Notelovitz, M., Martin, D., Tesar, R., Khan, F., Probart, C., Fields, C., and McKenzie, L. 1991. Estrogen therapy and variable resistance weight training increase bone mineral in surgically menopausal women. *Journal of Bone Mineral Research* 6: 583–590.

Paffenbarger, R., and Olsen, E. 1996. *Life fit: An effective exercise program for optimal health and a longer life*. Champaign, IL: Human Kinetics.

Pierson, LM, Herbert, WG, Norton, H, Kiebzak, GM, Griffth, P, Fedor, JM, Ramp, WK and JW Cook (2001). Effects of combined aerobic and resistance training versus aerobic training alone in cardiac patients. J Cardiopulmonary Rehabilitation 21 (2): 101-110.

Pratley, R., Nicklas, B., Rubin, M., Miller, J., Smith, A., Smith, M., Hurley, B., and Goldberg, A. 1994. Strength training increases resting metabolic rate and norepinephrine levels in healthy 50 to 65 year-old men. *Journal of Applied Physiology* 76:133–137.

Quirk, A., Newman, R., and Newman, K. 1985. An evaluation of interferential therapy, shortwave diathermy and exercise in the treatment of osteo-arthritis of the knee. *Physiotherapy* 71:55–57.

Rhodes, E.C., Martin, A.D., Taunton, J.E., Donnelly, M., Warren, J. and J. Elliot (2000). Effects of one year of resistance training on the relationship between muscular strength and bone density in elderly women. *Br J Sports Med* 34(1): 18-22.

Rimmer, J. (1997). Programming: Exercise guidelines for special medical populations. *IDEA Today* 15(5):26-34.

Risch, S., Nowell, N., Pollock, M., Risch, E., Langer, H., Fulton, M., Graves, J., and Leggett, S. 1993. Lumbar strengthening in chronic low back pain patients. *Spine* 18:232–238

Rooks, C., Silverman, C., and C. Kantrowitz (2002). The effects of progressive strength training and aerobic exercise on muscle strength and cardiovascular fitness in women with fibromyalgia: A pilot study. *Arthritis Care and Research* 47 (1) p 22-28.

Ryan, A., Treuth, M., Rubin, M., Miller, J., Nicklas, B., Landis, D., Pratley, R., Libanati, C., Grundberg, C., and Hurley, B. 1994. Effects of strength training on bone mineral density: Hormonal and bone turnover relationships. *Journal of Applied Physiology* 77:1678–1684.

Sequin, R., and Nelson, M. 2003. The benefits of strength training for older adults. *American Journal of Preventive Medicine* 25:141–149.

Sigal, J, Kenny, GP, Boule, NG, Wells, GA, Rud'homme, D, Fortier, M, Reid, RD, Tulloch, H, Coyle, D, Phillips, P, Jenngs, A and J. Jaffey. (2007) Effects of aerobic training, resistance training, or both on glycemic control in type 2 diabetics: a randomized trial. *Annuals of Internal Medicine* 147: 357-369.

Singh, NA, Clements, KM and MA Singh (2001), The efficacy of exercise as a long-term antidepressant in elderly subjects: a randomized, controlled trial. *J Gerontolo A Biol Sci Med Sci* 56 (8) 497-504.

Singh, N., Clements, K., and Fiatarone, M. 1997. A randomized controlled trial of progressive resistance training in depressed elders. *Journal of Gerontology* 52A (1): M27–M35.

Smutok, M., Reece, C., Kokkinos, P., Farmer, C., Dawson, P., Shulman, R., DeVane-Bell, J., Patterson, J., Charabogos, C., Goldley, A., and Hurley, B. 1993. Aerobic vs. strength training for risk factor intervention in middle-aged men at high risk for coronary heart disease. *Metabolism* 42:177–184.

Snow-Harter, C., Bouxsein, M., Lewis, B., Carter, D., and Marcus, R. 1992. Effects of resistance and endurance exercise on bone mineral status of young women: A randomized exercise intervention trial. *Journal of Bone Mineral Research* 7:761–769.

Stewart, K., Mason, M., and Kelemen, M. 1988. Three-year participation in circuit weight training improves muscular strength and self-efficacy in cardiac patients. *Journal of Cardio-pulmonary Rehabilitation* 8:292–296.

Stone, M., Blessing, D., Byrd, R., Tew, J., and Boatwright, D. 1982. Physiological effects of a short term resistive training program on middle-aged untrained men. *National Strength and Conditioning Association Journal* 4:16–20.

Tambalis, K, Panagiotakos, DB, Kavouras, SA, and LS Sidossis (2008). Responses of blood lipids to aerobic, resistance, and combined aerobic with resistance exercise training: a systematic review of current evidence. *Angiology* October 30 Epub (ahead of print) http://ang.sagepub.com.

Taunton, J., Martin, A., Rhodes, E., Wolski, L., Donnelly, M., and Elliot, J. 1997. Exercise for older women: Choosing the right prescription. *British Journal of Sports Medicine* 31:5–10.

Tokmakidis, SP, Zois, CE, Volaklis, K, and AM Touvra. (2004) The effects of a combined strength and aerobic exercise program on glucose and insulin action in women with type 2 duabetes. *European Journal of Physiology.* 92:437-442.

Tucker, L., and Sylvester, L. 1996. Strength training and hypercholesterolemia: An epidemiologic study of 8499 employed men. *American Journal of Health Promotion* 11:35–41.

Tufts University. 1992. An IQ test for losers. *Tufts University Diet and Nutrition Letter* 10 (March): 6–7.

Tufts University. 1994. Never too late to build up your muscle. *Tufts University Diet and Nutrition Letter* 12 (September): 6–7.

Ulrich, I., Reid, C., and Yeater, R. 1987. Increased HDL-cholesterol levels with a weight training program. *Southern Medical Journal* 80:328–331.

Weiss, A, Suzuki, T, Bean L and Fielding, R. (2000) High intensity strength training improves strength and functional performance after stroke. *Am J Phys Med Rehabilitation.* Jul-Aug;79(4):369-76.

Vander, L., Franklin, B., Wrisley, D., and Rubenfire, M. 1986. Acute cardiovascular responses to Nautilus exercise in cardiac patients: Implications for exercise training. *Annals of Sports Medicine* 2:165–169.

Westcott, W., and Howes, B. 1983. Blood pressure response during weight training exercise. *National Strength andConditioning Association Journal* 5:67–71.

Westcott, W. 1986. Strength training and blood pressure. *American Fitness Quarterly* 5:38–39.

Westcott, W. 1995. Keeping fit. *Nautilus* 4 (2): 5–7.

Westcott, W., and Guy, J. 1996. A physical evolution: Sedentary adults see marked improvements in as little as two days a week. *IDEA Today* 14 (9): 58–65.

Westcott, W., Richards, M., Reinl, G., and Califano, D. 2000. Strength training elderly nursing home patients. *Mature Fitness.* American Senior Fitness Association. www.seniorfitness.net.

Westcott, W. 2004a. Strength training for low back health. *Fitness Management* 20 (11): 26–28.

Westcott, W. 2004b. Strength training and blood pressure: A series of studies. *Fitness Management* 20 (3): 26–28.

Westcott, W. 2005. Weight loss approaches for older adults. *ICAA Functional U* 3 (4): 1–5.

Westcott, W. 2009. ACSM strength training guidelines. *ACSM's Health & Fitness Journal* 13 (4): 14–22.

Wolfe, F., Smyth, H, Yumus, M. et al. 1990. The American College of Rheumatology 1990 criteria for the classification of fibromyalgia. *Arthritis Rheumatology* 33: 160-172.

CHAPTER 2

American College of Sports Medicine. 2010. *Guidelines for exercise testing and prescription,* 8th ed. Philadelphia: Lippincott, Williams and Wilkins.

American College of Sports Medicine. 2006. *Guidelines for exercise testing and prescription,* 7th ed. Philadelphia: Lippincott, Williams and Wilkins.

Baechle, T., and Earle, R. 2008. *Essentials of strength training and conditioning,* 3rd ed. Champaign, IL: Human Kinetics.

Baechle, T., and Earle, R. 2006. *Weight training: Steps to success,* 3rd ed. Champaign, IL: Human Kinetics.

Baechle, T., and Earle, R. 2005. *Fitness weight training,* 2d ed. Champaign, IL: Human Kinetics.

Behm, D., et al. 2002. The effect of 5, 10, and 20 repetition maximums on the recovery of voluntary and evoked contractile properties. *Journal of Strength and Conditioning Research* 16 (2): 209–218.

Bemben, D., et al. 2000. Musculoskeletal response to high and low intensity resistance training in early postmenopausal women. *Medicine and Science in Sports and Exercise* 32 (11): 1949–1957.

Braith, R., Graves, J., Pollock, M., Leggett, S., Carpenter, D., and Colvin, A. 1989. Comparison of two versus three days per week of variable resistance training during 10 and 18 week programs. *International Journal of Sports Medicine* 10: 450–454.

Campbell, W., Crim, M., Young, V., and Evans, W. 1994. Increased energy requirements and changes in body composition with resistance training in older adults. *American Journal of Clinical Nutrition* 60:167–175.

Chestnut, I., and Docherty, D. 1999. The effects of 4 and 10 repetition maximum weight training protocols on neuromuscular adaptations in untrained men. *Journal of Strength and Conditioning Research* 13:353–359.

DeMichele, P., Pollock, M., Graves, J., Foster, D., Carpenter, D., Garzarella, L., Brechue, W., and Fulton, M. 1997. Isometric torso rotation strength: Effect of training frequency on its development. *Archives of Physical Medicine and Rehabilitation* 78:64–69.

Faigenbaum, A., Zaichkowsky, J., Westcott, W., Micheli, L., and Fehlandt, A. 1993. The effects of a twice-a-week strength training program on children. *Pediatric Exercise Science* 5:339–346.

Faigenbaum, A., Westcott, W., Micheli, L., Outerbridge, A., Long, C., LaRosa-Loud, R., and Zaichkowsky, L. 1996. The effects of strength training and detraining on children. *Journal of Strength and Conditioning Research* 10 (2): 109–114.

Fiatarone, M., Marks, E., Ryan, N., Meredith, C., Lipsitz, A., and Evans, W. 1990. High-intensity strength training in nonagenarians. *Journal of the American Medical Association* 263 (22): 3029–3034.

Fleck, S., and Kraemer, W. 1997. *Designing resistance training programs*, 2nd ed. Champaign, IL: Human Kinetics.

Frontera, W., Meredith, C., O'Reilly, K., Knuttgen, H., and Evans, W. 1988. Strength conditioning in older men: Skeletal muscle hypertrophy and improved function. *Journal of Applied Physiology* 64 (3): 1038–1044.

Harris, et al. 2004. The effect of resistance training intensity on strength gain response in the older adult. *Journal of Strength and Condition Research* 18 (4): 833–838.

Kelly, Stephen B., Brown, Lee E., Coburn, Jared W., Zinder, Stephen M., Gardner, Lisa M., and Nguyen, Diamond. 2007. The effect of single versus multiple sets on strength. *Journal of Strength Training and Conditioning Research* 21 (4): 1003–1006.

Kerr, D., et al. 1996. Exercise effects on bone mass in postmenopausal women are site-specific and load-dependent. *Journal of Bone and Mineral Research* (11) 2: 218–225.

Koffler, K., Menkes, A., Redmond, A., Whitehead, W., Pratley, R., and Hurley, B. 1992. Strength training accelerates gastrointestinal transit in middle-aged and older men. *Medicine and Science in Sports and Exercise* 24: 415–419.

Kraemer, W., Purvis, T., and Westcott, W. 1996. Everything you wanted to know about strength training. *IDEA Personal Trainer* 7 (6): 20–22.

McLester, J., Bishop, P., Smith, J., Wyers, L., Dale, B., Kozusko, J., Richardson, M., Nevett, M., and Lomax, R. 2003. A series of studies—a practical protocol for testing muscular endurance recovery. *Journal of Strength and Conditioning Research* 17 (2): 259–273.

Menkes, A., Mazel, S., Redmond, R., Koffler, K., Libanati, C., Gundberg, C., Zizic, T., Hagberg, J., Pratley, R., and Hurley, B. 1993. Strength training increases regional bone mineral density and bone remodeling in middle-aged and older men. *Journal of Applied Physiology* 74:2478–2484.

Miles, M., Li, Y., Rinard, J., Clarkson, P., and Williamson, J. 1997. Eccentric exercise augments the cardiovascular response to static exercise. *Medicine and Science in Sports and Exercise* 29:457–466.

Miranda, H., Fleck, S., Simão, R., Barreto, A., Dantas, E., and Novaes, J. 2007. Effect of two different rest period lengths on the number of repetitions performed during resistance training. *Journal of Strength and Conditioning Research* 21 (4): 1032–1036.

Nelson, M., Fiatarone, M., Morganti, C., Trice, I., Greenberg, R., and Evans, W. 1994. Effects of high-intensity strength training on multiple risk factors for osteoporotic fractures. *Journal of the American Medical Association* 272 (24): 1909–1914.

Pratley, R., Nicklas, B., Rubin, M., Miller, J., Smith, A., Smith, M., Hurley, B., and Goldberg, A. 1994. Strength training increases resting metabolic rate and norepinephrine levels in healthy 50 to 65 year-old men. *Journal of Applied Physiology* 76:133–137.

Shimano, T. Kraemer, W, Spiering, B, Volek, J, Hatfield, D, Silvestre, R., Vingren, J, Fragala, M, Maresch, C, Fleck, S, Newron, R, Spreuwenberg, L., Hakkinen, K. 2006. Relationship between number of repetitions and selected percentages of one repetition maximum in free weight exercises in trained and untrained men. *J Strength Cond Res.* 20 (4): 819-23.

Stadler, L., Stubbs, N., and Vukovich, M. 1997. A comparison of a 2-day and 3-day per week resistance training program on strength gains in older adults (abstract). *Medicine and Science in Sports and Exercise* 29:S254.

Starkey, D., Pollock, M., Ishida, Y., Welsch, M., Brechue, W., Graves, J., and Feigenbaum, M. 1996. Effects of resistance training volume on strength and muscle thickness. *Medicine and Science in Sports and Exercise* 28 (10): 1311–1320.

Taaffe, D., et al. 1996. Comparative effects of high and low intensity resistance training on thigh muscle strength, fiber area, and tissue composition in elderly women. *Clinical Physiology* 16 (4): 381–392.

Vincent, K., and Braith, R. 2002. Resistance exercise and bone turnover in elderly men and women. *Medicine and Science in Sports and Exercise* 34 (2): 17–23.

Westcott, W., Greenberger, K., and Milius, D. 1989. Strength training research: Sets and repetitions. *Scholastic Coach* 58:98–100.

Westcott, W. 1995a. *Strength fitness: Physiological principles and training techniques*, 4th ed. Dubuque, IA: Brown and Benchmark.

Westcott, W. 1995b. Transformation: How to take them from sedentary to active. *IDEA Today* 13 (7): 46–54. .

Westcott, W., and Guy, J. 1996. A physical evolution: Sedentary adults see marked improvements in as little as two days a week. *IDEA Today* 14 (9): 58–65.

Westcott, W. 2009. Strength training for frail older adults. *Journal on Active Aging*. 8(4): 52-59.

Westcott, W. 2002. A new look at repetition ranges. *Fitness Management FMY* 18 (7): 36–37.

Westcott, W., Winett, R., Annesi, J., Wojcik, J., Anderson, E., and Madden, P. 2009. Prescribing physical activity: Applying the ACSM protocols for exercise type, intensity, and duration across 3 training frequencies. *The Physician and Sportsmedicine* 37 (2): 51–58.

Westcott, W., Martin, W., LaRosa Loud, R., and Stoddard, S. 2008. Protein supplementation and body composition changes. *Fitness Management*, 24(5): 50-53.

CHAPTER 3

American College of Sports Medicine. 2006. *Guidelines for Exercise Testing and Prescription* (7th Edition). Philadelphia: Lippincott, Williams and Wilkins.

American College of Sports Medicine. 2010. *Guidelines for Exercise Testing and Prescription* (8th Edition). Philadelphia: Lippincott, Williams and Wilkins.

Arthritis Foundation. 2007. www.arthritis.org/learn-about-arthritis.php.

Baechle, T., and Earle, R., eds. 2008. *Essentials of strength training and conditioning*, 2nd ed. Champaign, IL: Human Kinetics.

Baechle, T., and Earle, R. 2006. *Weight training: Steps to success*. Champaign, IL: Human Kinetics.

Baechle, T., and Earle, R. 2005. *Fitness weight training*. Champaign, IL: Human Kinetics.

Caserotti, P., Aagaard, P., Buttrup, J., and Puggaard, I. 2008. Explosive heavy-resistance training in old and very old adults: Changes in rapid muscle force, strength and power. *Scandinavian Journal Medicine and Science in Sports* 18:773–782.

Earle, R., T. Baechle, eds. 2004. *Essentials of personal training*. Champaign, IL: Human Kinetics.

Fiatarone, M., Marks, E., Ryan, N., Meredith, C., Lipsitz, A., and Evans, W. 1990. High-intensity strength training in nonagenarians. *Journal of the American Medical Association* 263 (22): 3029–3034.

Frontera, W., Meredith, C., O'Reilly, K., Knuttgen, H., and Evans, W. 1988. Strength conditioning in older men: Skeletal muscle hypertrophy and improved function. *Journal of Applied Physiology* 64 (3): 1038–1044.

Graves, J., Pollock, M., Jones, A., Colvin, A., and Leggett, S. 1989. Specificity of limited range of motion variable resistance training. *Medicine and Science in Sports and Exercise* 21 (1): 84–89.

Jones, A., Pollock, M., Graves, J., Fulton, M., Jones, W., MacMillan, M., Baldwin, D., and Cirulli, J. 1988. *Safe, specific testing and rehabilitative exercise for the muscles of the lumbar spine*. Santa Barbara, CA: Sequoia Communications.

Koffler, K., Menkes, A., Redmond, A., Whitehead, W., Pratley, R., and Hurley, B. 1992. Strength training accelerates gastrointestinal transit in middle-aged and older men. *Medicine and Science in Sports and Exercise* 24:415–419.

Menkes, A., Mazel, S., Redmond, R., Koffler, K., Libanati, C., Gundberg, C., Zizic, T., Hagberg, J., Pratley, R., and Hurley, B. 1993. Strength training increases regional bone mineral density and bone remodeling in middle-aged and older men. *Journal of Applied Physiology* 74:2478–2484.

Nelson, M., Fiatarone, M., Morganti, C., Trice, I., Greenberg, R., and Evans, W. 1994. Effects of high-intensity strength training on multiple risk factors for osteoporotic fractures. *Journal of the American Medical Association* 272 (24): 1909–1914.

Pratley, R., Nicklas, B., Rubin, M., Miller, J., Smith, A., Smith, M., Hurley, B., and Goldberg, A. 1994. Strength training increases resting metabolic rate and norepinephrine levels in healthy 50 to 65 year-old men. *Journal of Applied Physiology* 76:133–137.

Risch, S., Nowell, M., Pollock, M., Risch, E., Langer, H., Fulton, M., Graves, J., and Leggett, S. 1993. Lumbar strengthening in chronic low back pain patients. *Spine* 18:232–238.

Westcott, W., and Baechle, T. 2007. *Strength training past 50*, 2nd ed. Champaign, IL: Human Kinetics.

Westcott, W., Winett, R., Annesi, J., Wojcik, J., Anderson, E., and Madden, P. 2009. Prescribing physical activity: Applying the ACSM protocols for exercise type, intensity, and duration across 3 training frequencies. *Physician and Sportsmedicine,37(2): 51-58.* .

Westcott, W. 2003. *Building strength and stamina,* 2nd ed. Champaign, IL: Human Kinetics.

Westcott, W., and Guy, J. 1996. A physical evolution: Sedentary adults see marked improvements in as little as two days a week. *IDEA Today* 14 (9): 58–65.

Westcott, W., Dolan, F., and Cavicchi, T. 1996. Golf and strength training are compatible activities. *Strength and Conditioning* 18 (4): 54–56.

Westcott, W. 1995. *Strength fitness: Physiological principles and training techniques*, 4th ed. Dubuque, IA: Brown and Benchmark.

CHAPTER 4

Westcott, W. 1994. Strength training for life: Weightloads: Go figure. *Nautilus Magazine* 3 (4): 5–7.

CHAPTER 5

Baechle, T.R., and Earle, R.E. 2008. *Essentials of strength training and conditioning*. Champaign, IL: Human Kinetics.

Baechle, T.R., and Earle, R.E. 2005. *Fitness weight training*. Champaign, IL: Human Kinetics.

Earle, R.E., and Baechle, T.R. 2004. *Essentials of personal training*. Champaign, IL: Human Kinetics.

Westcott, W.L. 2003. *Building strength and stamina*. Champaign, IL: Human Kinetics.

CHAPTER 7

American College of Sports Medicine. 2010. *ACSM Resource Manual for Guidelines for Exercise Testing and Prescription* (8th Edition). Philadelphia: Lippincott, Williams and Wilkins.

Annesi, J., and Westcott, W. 2007. Relations of physical self-concept and muscular strength with resistance exercise-induced feeling state scores in older women. *Perceptual and Motor Skills* 104:183–190.

Annesi, J., Westcott, W., La Rosa Loud, R., and Powers, L. 2004. Effects of association and dissociation formats on resistance exercise-induced emotion change and physical self-concept in older women. *Journal of Mental Health and Aging* 10 (2): 87–98.

Annesi, J., Westcott, W., and Gann, S. 2004. Preliminary evaluation of a 10-week resistance and cardiovascular exercise protocol on physiological and psychological measures for a sample of older women. *Perceptual and Motor Skills* 98:163–170.

Annesi, J., and Westcott, W. 2004. Relationship of feeling states after exercise and total mood disturbance over 10 weeks in formerly sedentary women. *Perceptual and Motor Skill* 99:107–115.

Baechle, T., and Earle, R. 2006. *Weight training: Steps to success*. Champaign, IL: Human Kinetics.

Dishman, R. 1988. *Exercise adherence*. Champaign, IL: Human Kinetics.

Girouard, C., and Hurley, B. 1995. Does strength training inhibit gains in range of motion from flexibility training in older adults? *Medicine and Science in Sports and Exercise* 27 (10): 1444–1449.

Rikli, R and C. Jones (2000). Senior Fitness Test Manual. Champaign, IL: Human Kinetics.

Varela, S, Ayan, C and J Cancela (2008). Batteries assessing health related fitness in elderly: a brief review. *Eur Rev Phys Act*. 5:97-105.

Varela, S, Ayan, C and J Cancela (2008). Batteries assessing health related fitness in elderly: a brief review. *Eur Rev Phys Act*. 5:97-105.

Westcott, W., Martin, W., La Rosa Loud, R., and Stoddard, S. 2008. Research update: Protein and body composition. *Fitness Management* 24 (5): 50–53.

Westcott, W. 1995. Strength training for life: Keeping fit. *Nautilus Magazine* 4 (2): 5–7.

Westcott, W. 2003. *Building strength and stamina*. Champaign, IL: Human Kinetics.

Westcott, W., Dolan, F., and Cavicchi, T. 1996. Golf and strength training are compatible activities. *Strength and Conditioning* 18 (4): 54–56.

Westcott, W. 1994. Strength training for life: Weightloads: Go figure. *Nautilus Magazine* 3 (4): 5–7.

Westcott, W. 1987. *Building strength at the YMCA*. Champaign, IL: Human Kinetics.

CHAPTER 8

American Association of Cardiovascular and Pulmonary Rehabilitation (AACVPR). 2004. *Guidelines for cardiac rehabilitation and secondary prevention program*, 4th ed. Philadelphia: Lippincott, Williams & Wilkins.

American College of Sports Medicine. 2006. *ACSM's health/fitness facilities and standards and guidelines*, 3rd ed. Champaign, IL. Human Kinetics.

American College of Sports Medicine. 2010. *ACSM's resource manual for guidelines for exercise testing and prescription*, 6th ed. Philadelphia: Lippincott, Williams & Wilkins.

American College of Sports Medicine. 2010. *ACSM's guidelines for exercise testing and prescription*, 8th ed. Philadelphia: Lippincott, Williams & Wilkins.

American Council on Exercise. 1999. *Clinical exercise specialist manual; ACE's source for training special populations*. San Diego: ACE.

American Diabetes Association. 2008. www.diabetes.org/diabetes-basics/.

American Diabetes Association. 2008. Ketoacidosis www.diabetes.org/type-1-diabetes/ketoacidosis.jsp.

American Heart Association (2007) Know the facts and get the stats. http://www.americanheart.org.

Baker, K., Nelson, M., Felson, D., Layne, J., Sarno, R., and Roubenoff, R. 2001. The efficacy of home based progressive strength training in older adults with knee osteoarthritis: A randomized controlled trial. *Journal of Rheumatology* 28:155–1665.

Bennell, K., Khan, K., and McCay, H. 2000. The role of physiotherapy in the prevention and treatment of osteoporosis. *Manual Therapy* 5 (4): 198–213.

Borg, G. 1998. *Borg's perceived exertion and pain scales*. Champaign, IL: Human Kinetics.

Campbell, W., Crim, M., Young, V., and Evans, W. 1994. Increased energy requirements and changes in body composition with resistance training in older adults. *American Journal of Clinical Nutrition* 60:167–175.

Clark, J. 1997. Programming for adults with age-related health challenges. *American Council on Exercise Certified News* 3 (5): 4–6.

Drought, J. 1995. Resistance exercise in cardiac rehabilitation. *Strength and Conditioning* 17 (2): 56–64.

Eriksson, J., Taimela, S., Eriksson, K., Parviainen, S., Peltonen, J., and Kujala, U. 1997. Resistance training in the treatment of non-insulin dependent diabetes mellitus. *International Journal of Sports Medicine* 18 (4): 242–246.

Evans, W., and Rosenberg, I. 1992. *Biomarkers*. New York: Simon and Schuster.

Eves, N.D., and Plotnikoff, R.C. 2006. Resistance training and type II diabetes: Considerations for implementation at the population level. *Diabetes Care* 29:1933–1941.

Faigenbaum, A., Skrinar, G., Cesare, W., Kraemer, W., and Thomas, H. 1990. Physiologic and symptomatic responses of cardiac patients to resistance exercise. *Archives of Physical Medicine and Rehabilitation* 70:395–398.

Faigenbaum, A., Zaichkowsky, L., Westcott, W., Lang, C., LaRosa-Loud, R., Micheli, L., and Outerbridge, A. 1997. Psychological effects of strength training on children. *Journal of Sport Behavior* 20 (2): 164–175.

Fiatarone, M.A., and Singh, M. 2002. Exercise comes of age: Rationale and recommendations for a geriatric exercise prescription. *Journal of Gerontology Series A: Biological Sciences and Medical Sciences* 57 (A): M262–28.

Fiatarone, M.A., O'Neill, E.F., Ryan, N.D., et al. 1994. Exercise training and nutritional supplementation for physical frailty in very elderly people. *New England Journal of Medicine* 330:1769–75.

Fiatarone, M., Marks, E., Ryan, N., Meredith, C., Lipsitz, L., and Evans, W. 1990. High-intensity strength training in nonagenarians. *Journal of the American Medical Association* 263 (22): 3029–3034.

Flood, L., and A. Constance (2002). Diabetes exercise safety. American Journal of Nursing Vol. 102, No. 6

Foltz-Gray, D. 1997. Bully the pain. *Arthritis Today* (July–August): 18–25.

Foreman, J. 1997. A big, bad, ugly disease. *Boston Globe* (August 4).

Frontera, W., Meredith, C., O'Reilly, K., Knuttgen, H., and Evans, W. 1988. Strength conditioning in older men: Skeletal muscle hypertrophy and improved function. *Journal of Applied Physiology* 64 (3): 1038–1044.

Ghilarducci, L., Holly, R., and Amsterdam, E. 1989. Effects of high resistance training in coronary heart disease. *American Journal of Cardiology* 64:866–870.

Hughes, V., Frontera, W., Dallal, G., Lutz, K., Fisher, E., and Evans, W. 1995. Muscle strength and body composition: Associations with bone density in older subjects. *Medicine and Science in Sports and Exercise* 7 (27): 967–974.

Jones, A., Pollock, M., Graves, J., Fulton, M., Jones, W., MacMillan, M., Baldwin, D., and Cirulli, J. 1988. *Safe, specific testing and rehabilitative exercise for muscles of the lumbar spine.* Santa Barbara, CA: Sequoia Communications.

Kalapotharakos, V., Michalopoulos, M., Tokmakidis, S., Godolias, G., and Gourgolis, V. 2005. Effects of heavy and moderate resistance training on functional performance in older adults. *Journal of Strength and Conditioning Research* 19 (3): 652–657.

Kelemen, M., Stewart, K., Gillilan, R., Ewart, C., Valenti, S., Manley, J., and Keleman, M. 1986. Circuit weight training in cardiac patients. *Journal of the American College of Cardiology* 7:38–42.

Kerr, D.T., Ackland, T. Masland, B., Morton, A., and Rice, R. 2001. Resistance training over 2 years increases bone mass in calcium replete postmenopausal women. *Journal of Bone and Mineral Research* 16:175–81.

Maddalozzo, G.F., and Snow, C.M. 2000. High intensity resistance training: Effects on bone in older men and women. *Calcified Tissue International* 66 (6): 399–404.

Menkes, A., Mazel, S., Redmond, R., Koffler, K., Libanati, C., Gunberg, C., Zizic, T., Hagberg, J., Pratley, R., and Hurley, B. 1993. Strength training increases regional bone mineral density and bone remodeling in middle-aged and older men. *Journal of Applied Physiology* 74:2478–2484.

National Health and Nutrition Examination Survey. 2004. National Institutes of Health (Publication No. 98-4083). www.nhlbi.nih.gov/.

National Heart, Lung, and Blood Institute. 2006. http://www.nhlbi.nih.gov.

National Institute of Arthritis and Musculoskeletal and Skin Diseases. 2005. www.niams.nih.gov/Health_Info/Fibromyalgia/fibromyalgia_ff.asp.

National Institute of Diabetes and Digestive and Kidney Diseases. 2004. www.nihseniorhealth.gov/diabetes/causes/0.3.html.

National Institute on Aging Information Center. 2008. www.nia.nih.gov.

National Institutes of Health (2007). Statistics related to overweight and obesity. Win.niddk.nih.gov/staitics table.

National Osteoporosis Foundation. 23 Nov.2009. Fast Facts. www.nof.org/osteoporosis/diseasefacts.htm.

National Stroke Association. 2008. Centennial, CO.

Nelson, M., Fiatarone, M., Morganti, C., Trice, I., Greenberg, R., and Evans, W. 1994. Effects of high-intensity strength training on multiple risk factors for osteoporotic fractures. *Journal of the American Medical Association* 272 (24): 1909–1914.

Nelson, M. 2002. *Strong women and men don't get arthritis.* New York: Penguin Putnam.

Noble, B.J., Borg, G.A.V., Jacobs, I., Ceci, R., and Kaiser, P. 1983. A category-ratio perceived exertion scale: Relationship to blood and muscle lactates and HR. *Medicine and Science in Sports and Exercise* 15:523–528.

Pierson, L.M., Herbert, W.G., Norton, H.J., et al. 2001. Effects of combined aerobic and resistance training versus aerobic training alone in cardiac rehabilitation. *European Journal of Cardiovascular Prevention and Rehabilitation* 21 (2): 101–110.

President's Council on Physical Fitness and *Sports Research Digest*. 1997. Physical activity and the prevention of type II (non-insulin dependent) diabetes. Series 2, no. 10.

Rhodes, E.C., Martin, A.D., Taunton, J.E., Donnelly, M., Warren, J., and Elliot, J. 2000. Effects of one year of resistance training on the relationship between muscular strength and bone density in elderly women. *British Journal of Sports Medicine* 34 (1): 18–22.

Rimmer, J. 1997. Programming: Exercise guidelines for special medical populations. *IDEA Today* 15 (5): 26–34.

Risch, S., Norvell, N., Pollock, M., Risch, E., Langer, H., Fulton, M., Graves, J., and Leggett, S. 1993. Lumbar strengthening in chronic low back pain patients. *Spine* 18:232–238.

Segal, K.R., Edano, A., Abalos, A., Albu, J., Blando, L., Tomas, M., and Pi-Sunyer, F. 1991. Effect of exercise training on insulin sensitivity and gucose metabolism in lean, obese and diabetic men. *Journal of Applied Physiology* 71:2402–2411.

Singh, N., Clements, K., and Fiatarone, M. 1997. A randomized controlled trial of progressive resistance training in depressed elders. *Journal of Gerontology* 52A (1): M27–M35.

Stewart, K.J. 2004. Exercise training: Can it improve cardiovascular health in patients with type II diabetes? *British Journal of Sports Medicine* 38:250–252.

Tufts University Diet and Nutrition Letter. 1994. Never too late to build up your muscle. Vol. 12 (September): 6–7.

Vander, L., Franklin, B., Wrisley, D., and Rubenfire, M. 1986. Acute cardiovascular response to circuit weight training in patients with cardiac disease. *Annals of Sports Medicine* 2:165–169.

Vega, C and C. Jimenez (2004) in Essentials of Personal Training, Earle, R. and T. Baechle editors. Champaign, IL: Human Kinetics, Inc

Weil, R. 1993. Mall walking can provide exercise, companionship, first chance at sales. *Diabetes in the News* 12 (1): 58–59.

Weiss, A., Suzuki, T., Bean, L., and Fielding, R. 2000. High intensity strength training improves strength and functional performance after stroke. *American Journal of Physical Medicine and Rehabilitation* 79 (4): 369–76.

Wenger, N.K., Froelicher, E.S., Smith, L.K., et al. 1995. *Cardiac rehabilitation as secondary prevention*. Clinical Practice Guideline No 17. Rockville, MD: U.S. Department of Health and Human Services, Public Health Service, Agency for Health Care Policy and Research and the National Heart, Lung and Blood Institute. AHCPR Publication No. 96-0672.

Westcott, W. 2009. ACSM strength training guidelines. *ACSM's Health & Fitness Journal* 13(4): 14-22.

Westcott, W. 1995. Keeping fit. *Nautilus* 4 (2): 5–7.

Westcott, W., and Guy, J. 1996. A physical evolution: Sedentary adults see marked improvements in as little as two days a week. *IDEA Today* 14 (9): 58–65.

Westcott, W., and O'Grady, S. 1998. Strength training and cardiac post-rehab. *IDEA Personal Trainer* 9 (2): 41–6.

Westcott, W., Dolan, F., and Cavicchi, T. 1996. Golf and strength training are compatible activities. *Journal of Strength and Conditioning* 18 (4): 54–56.

CHAPTER 9

Faigenbaum, A., Milliken, L., Moulton, L., and Westcott, W. 2005. Early muscular fitness adaptations in children in response to two different resistance training regimens. *Pediatric Exercise Science* 17: 237-248.

Westcott, W., Dolan, F., and Cavicchi, T. 1996. Golf and strength training are compatible activities. *Journal of Strength and Conditioning* 18 (4): 54–56.

Westcott, W. 1992. Fitness benefits of rock climbing. *American Fitness Quarterly*, 10(4): 28-31.

Westcott, W. 2009. ACSM strength training guidelines. *ACSM's Health & Fitness Journal* 13 (4): 14–22.

Westcott, W., Winett, R., Annesi, J., Wojcik, J., Anderson, E., and Madden, P. 2009. Prescribing physical activity: Applying the ACSM protocols for exercise type, intensity, and duration across 3 training frequencies. *The Physician and Sportsmedicine* 37 (2): 51–58.

CHAPTER 10

American Council on Exercise. 1996. *Personal trainer manual*, 2d ed. San Diego: American Council on Exercise.

American Dietetic Association: www.eatright.org.

American Heart Association. 1989. *Low-fat, low-cholesterol cookbook*. New York: Random House.

Anderson, L., Tufekovic, M., Zebis, K., et al. 2005. The effect of resistance training combined with timed ingestion of protein on muscle fiber size and muscle strength. *Metabolism* 54:151–156.

Ballor, D., and Poehlman, E. 1994. Exercise training enhances fat-free mass preservation during diet-induce weight loss: A meta analytic finding. *International Journal of Obesity* 18:35–40.

Campbell, W., Crim, M., Young, V., and Evans, W. 1994. Increased energy requirements and changes in body composition with resistance training in older adults. *American Journal of Clinical Nutrition* 60:167–175.

Campbell, W., Trappe, T., Wolfe, R., and Evans, W. 2001. The recommended dietary allowance for protein may not be adequate for older people to maintain skeletal muscle. *Journals of Gerontology Series A: Biological Sciences and Medical Sciences* 56:M373–M380.

Clark, N. 2009 *Sports nutrition guidebook*. Champaign, IL: Human Kinetics.

Cribb, P., and Hayes, A. 2006. Effects of supplement timing and resistance exercise on skeletal muscle hypertrophy. *Medicine and Science in Sports Medicine* 38 (11): 1918–1925.

Esmarck, B., Andersen, J., Olsen, S., Richter, E., Mizuno, M., and Kjaer, M. 2001. Timing of postexercise protein intake is important for muscle hypertrophy with resistance training in elderly humans. *Journal of Physiology* 535:301–311.

Fukagawa, N., and Young, V. 1987. Protein and amino acid metabolism and requirements in older persons. *Clinical Geriatric Medicine* 3 (2): 329–341.

Gersovitz, M., Motil, K., Munro, H., Scrimshaw, N., and Young, V. 1982. Human protein requirements: Assessment of the adequacy of the current recommended dietary allowance for dietary protein in elderly men and women. *American Journal of Clinical Nutrition* 35:6–14.

Haltom, R., Kraemer, R., Sloan, R., Hebert, E., Frank, K., and Tryniecki, J. 1999. Circuit weight training and its effects on excess postexercise oxygen consumption. *Medicine and Science in Sports and Exercise* 31 (11): 1613–1618.

Mann, T., Tomiyama, A., Westling, E., Lew, A., Samuels, B., and Chatman, J. 2007. Medicare's search for effective obesity treatment; diets are not the answer. *American Psychologist* 62 (3): 220–233.

Morais, J., Chevalier, S., and Gougeon, R. 2006. Protein turnover and requirements in the healthy and frail elderly. *Journal of Nutrition in Health and Aging* 10:272–283.

National Institutes of Health. 2004. National Health and Nutrition Examination Survey. www.nhlbi.nih.gov.

Ornish, D. 1993. *Eat more, weigh less: Dr. Dean Ornish's life choice program for losing weight safely while eating abundantly*. New York: Harper Collins.

Paffenbarger, R., and Olsen, E. 1996. *Lifefit: An effective exercise program for optimal health and a longer life*. Champaign, IL: Human Kinetics.

Pratley, R., Nicklas, B., Rubin, M., Miller, J., Smith, A., Smith, M., Hurley, B., and Goldberg, A. 1994. Strength training increases resting metabolic rate and norepinephrine levels in healthy 50- to 65-year-old men. *Journal of Applied Physiology* 76:133–137.

Rippe, J. 1992. *The exercise exchange program*. New York: Simon and Schuster.

Schardt, D. 2007. Saving muscle; how to stay strong and healthy as you age. *Nutrition Action Health Letter* 34 (3): 3–8.

Westcott, W., Martin, W., LaRosa Loud, R., and Stoddard, S. 2008. Protein supplementation and body composition changes. *Fitness Management* 24(5): 50-53.

Wilmore, J., Parr, R., Ward, P., Vodak, P., Barstow, T., Pipes, T., Grimditch, G., and Leslie, P. 1978. Energy cost of circuit weight training. *Medicine and Science in Sports* 10:75–78.

Index

Please note the following abbreviations that follow page numbers in the index:

Italicized *f* or *ff* indicates that there is a figure or figures on those pages, respectively.
Italicized *t* or *tt* indicates that there is a table or tables on those pages, respectively.

About the Authors

Thomas R. Baechle, EdD, CSCS,*D; NSCA-CPT,*D, competed in Olympic-style weightlifting and powerlifting and was an instructor of weight training and a strength and conditioning coach for 20 years. Currently he is a professor and chair of the exercise science department at Creighton University, where he directed phase III cardiac rehabilitation for 16 years. He is a cofounder and past president of the National Strength and Conditioning Association (NSCA) and for 20 years was the executive director of the NSCA Certification Commission.

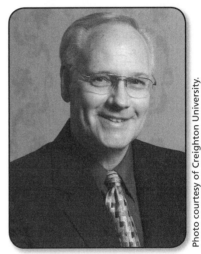

Thomas R. Baechle

Photo courtesy of Creighton University.

Baechle has been recognized as the force behind the creation of the Certified Strength and Conditioning Specialist and NSCA-Certified Personal Trainer examination programs. He has received awards for outstanding teaching and service from Creighton University, the NSCA's most coveted awards (Strength and Conditioning Professional of the Year and Lifetime Achievement) and other awards from international associations and organizations. Baechle also served on state and regional boards associated with the American Alliance for Health, Physical Education, Recreation and Dance, as president of the National Organization of Competency Assurance, and has served on various other regional, national, and international boards. Baechle has authored, coauthored, or edited 13 other books, the most popular of which is *Weight Training: Steps to Success*, that has been translated into ten languages and has sold almost 200,000 copies.

Wayne L. Westcott, PhD, CSCS, is fitness research director at Quincy College in Quincy, Massachusetts. As an athlete, coach, teacher, professor, researcher, author, and speaker, Westcott has more than 38 years of experience in strength training and is recognized as a leading authority on fitness.

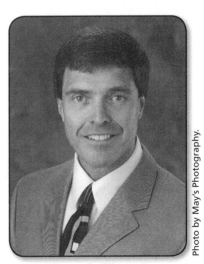

Wayne L. Westcott

Photo by May's Photography.

For over 25 years, Westcott has focused on strength training instruction and research for older adults (50 to 100 years). His landmark study at the John Knox

Village Nursing Home increased awareness of the benefits of strength training for seniors of varied health and fitness levels and led to the implementation of strength training centers within more than 500 nursing homes.

Westcott has served as a strength training consultant for numerous national organizations and programs, including Nautilus, the President's Council on Physical Fitness and Sports, the National School Fitness Foundation, the International Association of Fitness Professionals, the American Council on Exercise, the YMCA of the USA, and the National Youth Sports Safety Foundation. Through his work with these organizations, he has also received numerous awards, including the Hall of Fame Award from the International Fitness Professionals Association (IFPA), Fitness Industry Leader Award from the National Strength Professionals Association, the Massachusetts Governor's Council Lifetime Achievement Award, the IDEA Lifetime Achievement Award, the President's Council Healthy American Fitness Leader Award, and the Alumni Recognition Award from Pennsylvania State University.

Westcott has authored or coauthored 24 books on strength training, including *Building Strength & Stamina*, *Strength Training for Seniors*, and *Complete Conditioning for Golf*. In addition, he has served on the editorial boards of *The Physician and Sportsmedicine*, *ACSM's Health & Fitness Journal*, *On-Site Fitness*, *Prevention*, *Shape*, *Men's Health*, *Fitness*, *Club Industry*, *American Fitness Quarterly*, *Nautilus*, and *Fitness Management*. Westcott also serves on advisory boards for the International Council on Active Aging and the American Association for Health and Fitness. He is also an executive committee member for the New England chapter of the American College of Sports Medicine.

Westcott lives in Abington, Massachusetts, with his wife, Claudia. He enjoys staying physically active through running, cycling, and strength training.